What the Eye Reveals

What the Eye Reveals

by Denny Ray Johnson
with J. Erik Ness

First Published in 1995 by Rayid Publications
P.O. Box 17367 • Boulder • Colorado 80308 • USA

Library of Congress Catalog Card Number 94-068709
Johnson, Denny Ray.
What the Eye Reveals by Denny Ray Johnson with J. Erik Ness
Revised edition.
p. cm.
Includes: illustrations.
1. Rayid method (Personality assessment).
2. Iris (Eye) - Psychological aspects.
3. Personality assessment.
I. Ness, J. Erik
II. Title.
BF698.8.R28.J64 1994
138-dc20

ISBN 0-917197-04-6

Printed in Korea 1/95

Dedicated to:
The purpose of eternal increase
through the verb of light...
Love

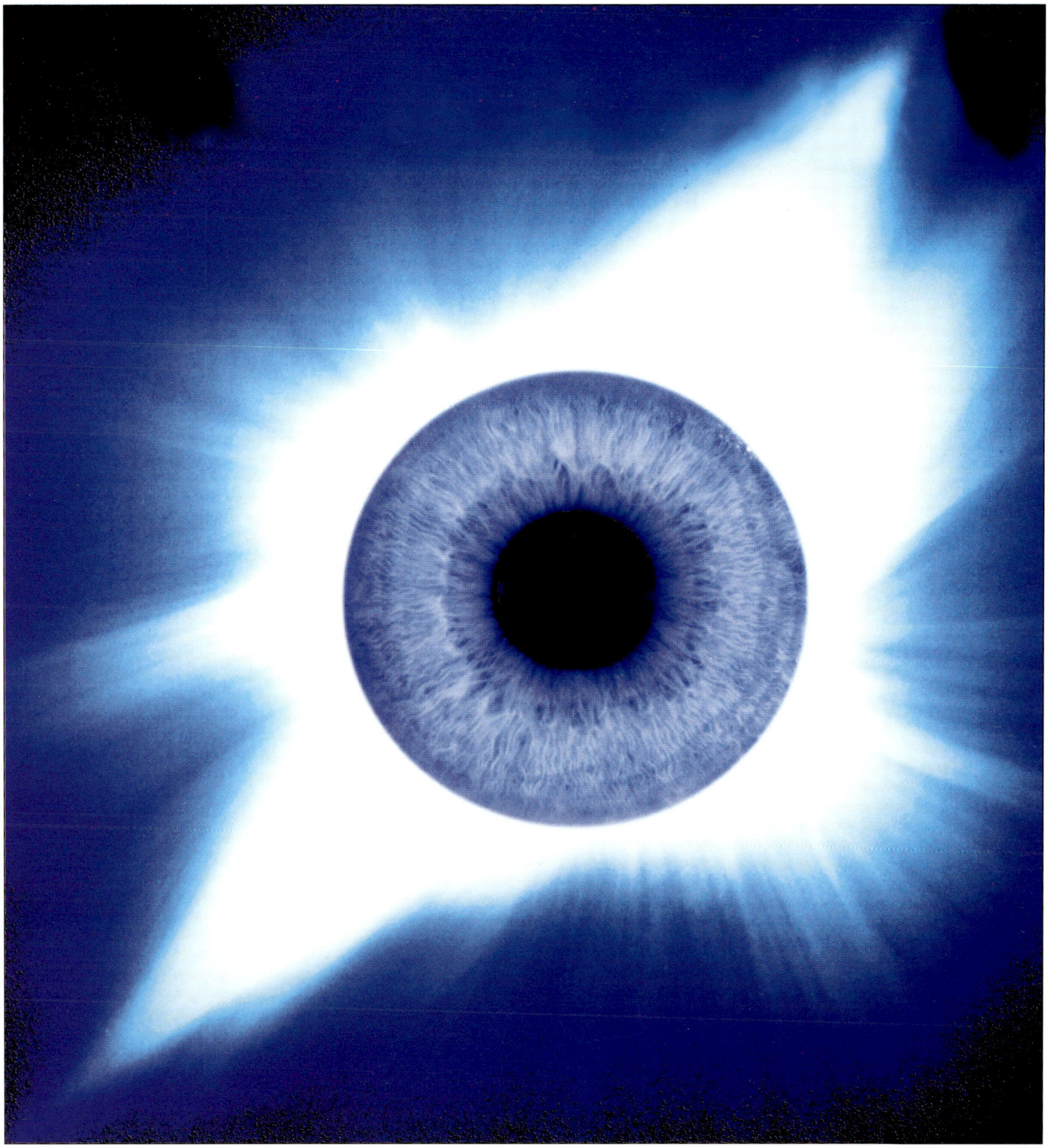

Rayid enables the harmonious integration of masculine and feminine energy. Like a full solar eclipse, in which the sun and the moon are perfectly aligned with the Earth, the Rayid Method of Iris Interpretation honors the presence of light flowing ~~through the~~ sacred union of a man and woman.

"SACRED UNION"
of a woman and a man.

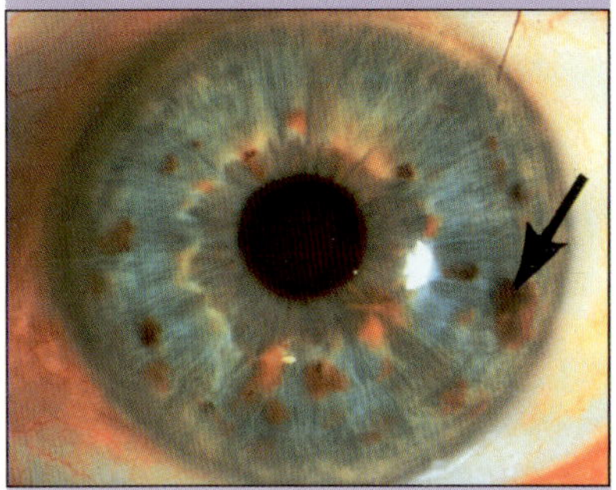

Jewel

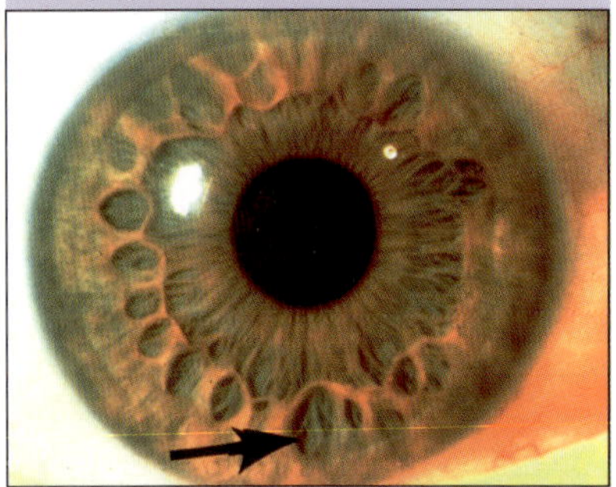

Flower

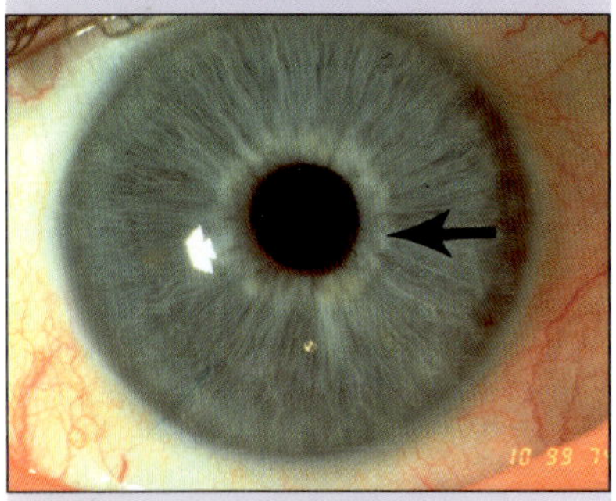

Introvert

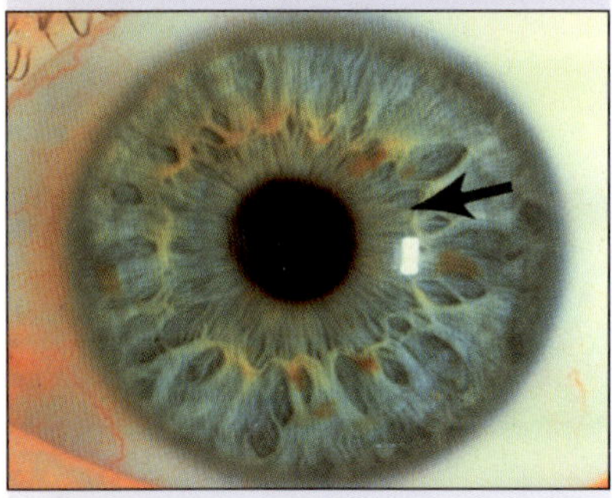

Extrovert

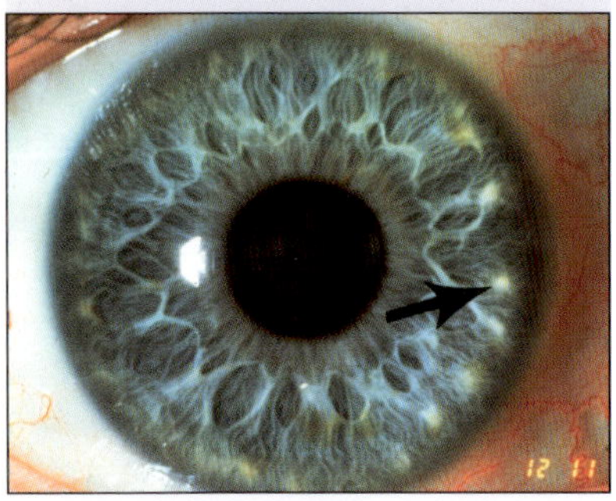

Ring of Harmony

Contents

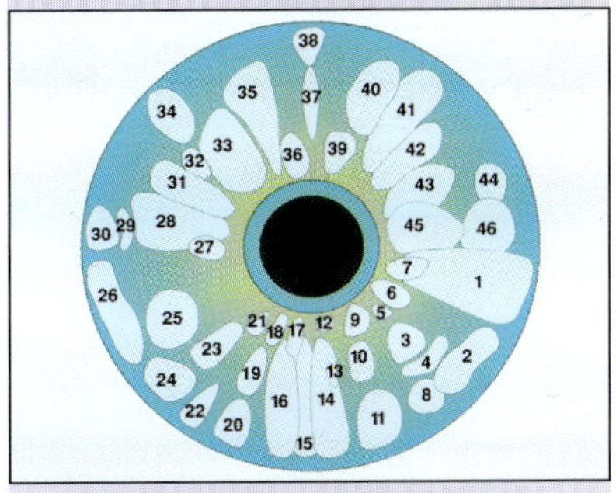

Iris positions (left eye)

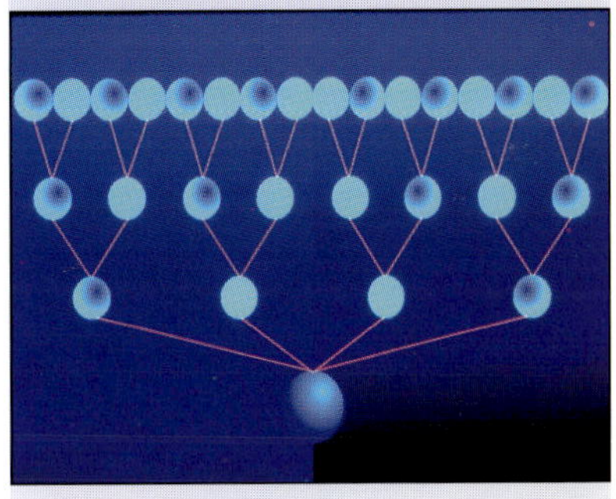

The family tree

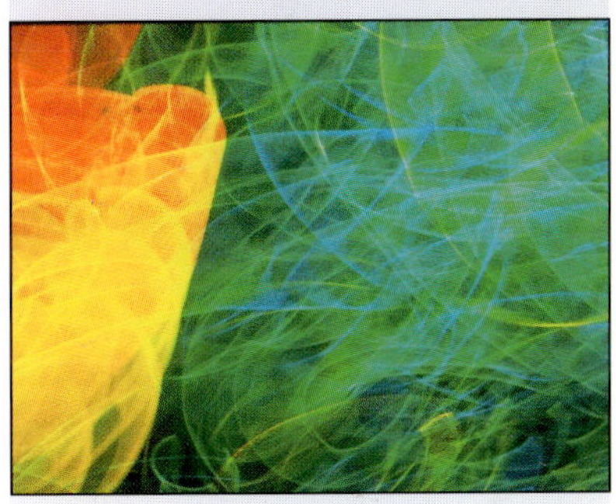

Masculine and feminine energies

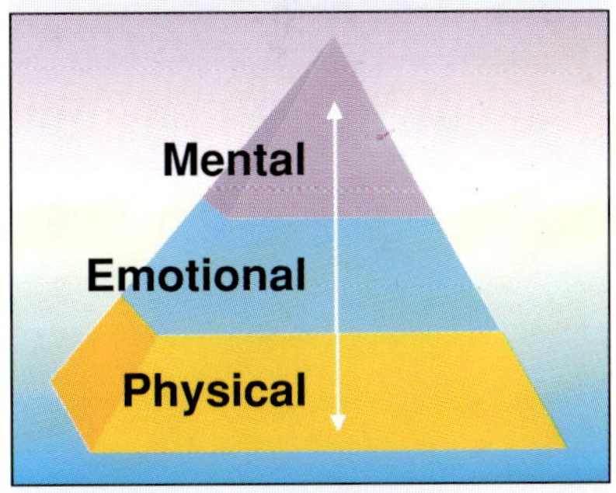

The healing pyramid

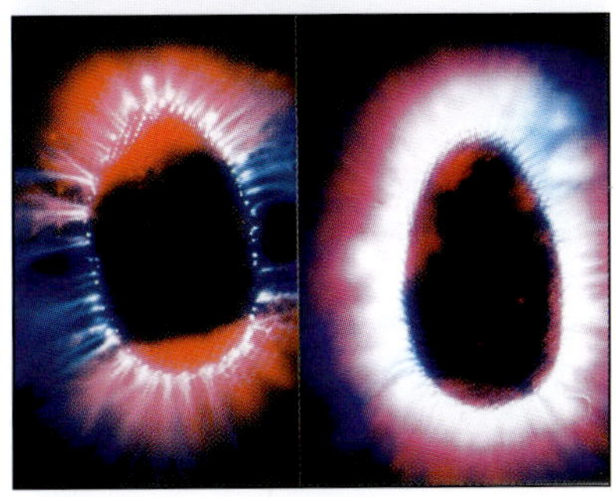

Before and after ritual

"If the doors of perception were cleansed, everything would appear to man as it is: infinite." - William Blake

Introduction

The iris of the eye is like a fingerprint. It is a long-term genetic pattern, a kind of blueprint of inheritance. If you look closely at the iris of the eye (the colored area encircling the pupil), you will notice small dark dots, streaks or rounded openings in the fibers. These characteristics provide the key to understanding your behavior and relationship patterns. The types of marking, their precise location and variations between your left and right eye each reveal different facets of your personality.

Much of personality has to do with the ways in which a person processes and responds to sensory information (auditory, visual, touch, etc.). We process information from the past and present through the internal, energetic systems of thought and emotion; our behavior, expressed through words, habitual postures and gestures, communicates information to the world around us. Different patterns in the iris of the eye are directly correlated with specific behavioral characteristics and ways of processing information.

The eyes have been called "the windows of the soul" and modern research is proving this old adage to be true. Forty percent of the cranial nerves going into or out of the brain are just for the eyes, which may be part of the reason why the Rayid Method of Iris Interpretation taps into the inner world so well.

Empirical studies have confirmed that patterns in the iris are genetically determined. By examining these patterns, we can see how the family tree influences character, relationship choices and health. For example, experience has shown that patterns in the left eye reflect traits acquired from the mother's side of the family. Traits in the right eye are from the father's side of the family. By comparing the irises, we can determine the influence of each parental relationship in shaping the personality of the individual. Rayid is therefore a model for understanding how the human character is transferred and modified from generation to generation.

There are, in essence, four primary iris structures, each of which is related to a specific personality profile (see photo below). A person's iris type is referred to as his constitutional structure. Each constitutional structure is a standing wave pattern in the physical vehicle of the body, just like the pattern light makes in a droplet of vibrating water. The photograph of the wave pattern, opposite, was made by shining light into a drop of water vibrating with sound. If you change the frequency of the sound, the pattern changes. People are like that. We each have a different frequency of vibration, a different pattern. And every pattern is beautiful. One type of iris structure is not better than another. Our responsibility is to clean up the murky water so that the pattern shines clear and bright, the way it was always meant to be seen.

Each of us is unique. Classifying human behavior into only a few fundamental personality types doesn't alter that. But most of us are not free. Our life experience is actually very predictable because our behavior today is regulated by patterns in the family tree. This may be hard for you to accept. The best way for you to know whether the

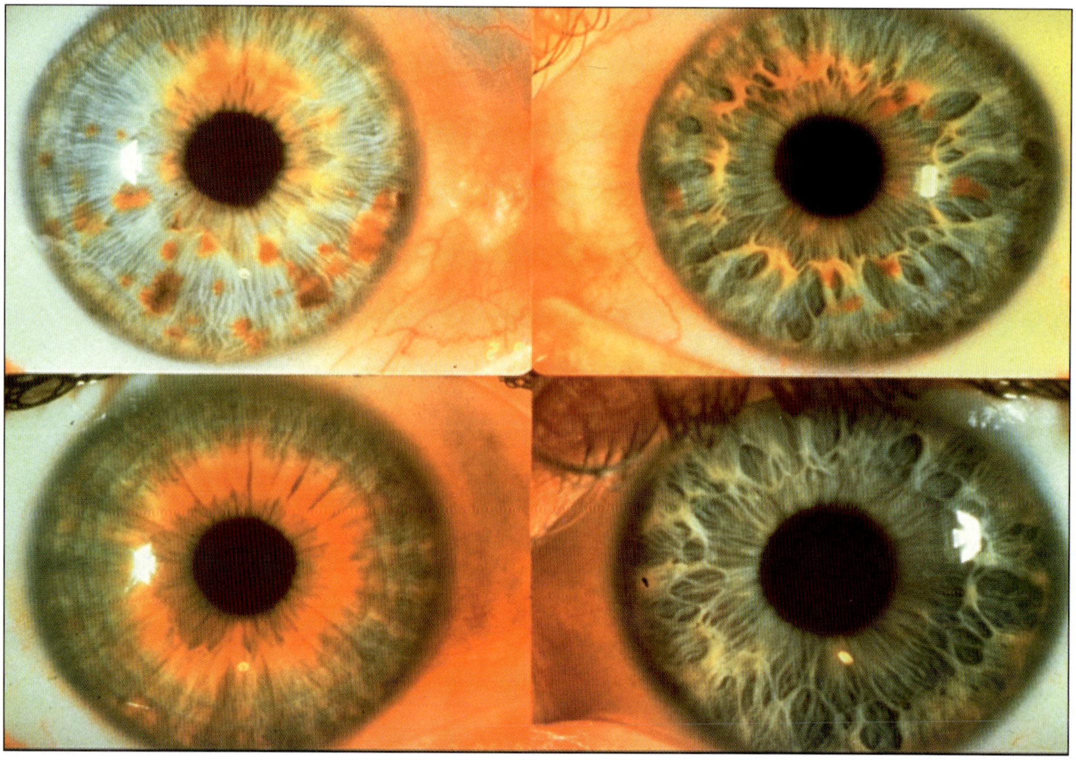

Four different types of iris. Clockwise from top left: Jewel, Shaker, Flower, Stream.

papercavalier

252 Java Street,
Suite 120
Brooklyn, NY 11222
United States

Biscuit Factory
Block J Unit 112A
100 Clements Road
London SE16 4DG
Great Britain

Hello. Here's your receipt:

Sales channel:	Amazon.co.uk
Order no:	205-8150178-3222760
Order date:	April 4, 2016
Bill to:	Agnieszka
Deliver to:	Agnieszka Kwiecien Flat 6, 2 Forest Road Kingswood BRISTOL BS15 8EG United Kingdom
This package contains:	What Your Eye Reveals [Paperback] [2002] Johnson, Denny R... Condition: Good Price: £23.47 Delivery: £2.80 VAT: 0 Total: £26.27 Paid in full

---

Find the best deals on new and used books online: http://www.part.ly

---

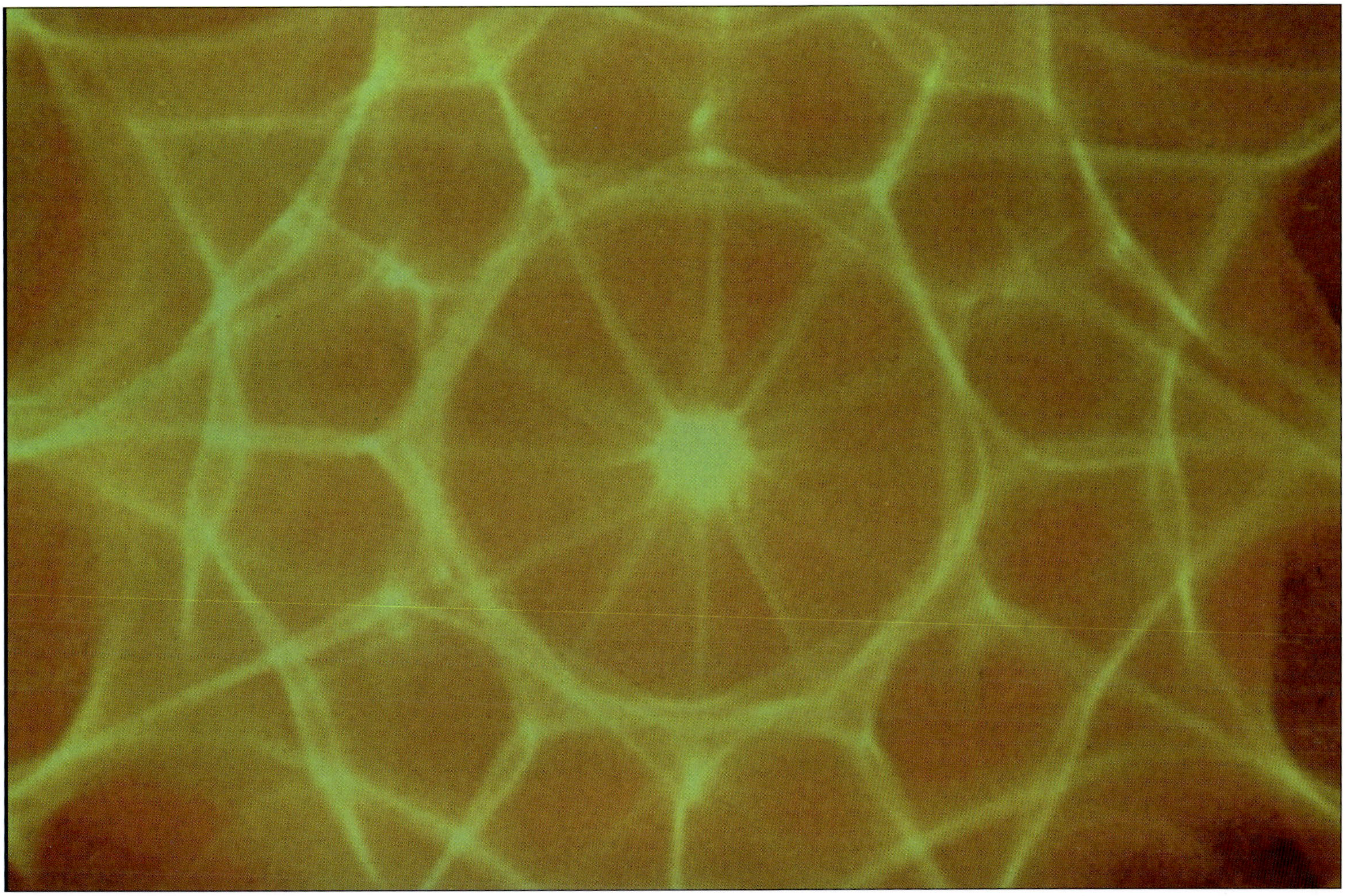

This standing wave pattern was photographed by shining a light through a droplet of water as it was being subjected to sound waves.

information in this book is correct is to test it. Do a few iris interpretations, then judge for yourself. Nothing in this book is meant to imply that people don't have the free will to change their transgenerational endowment. It's just that most of us don't exercise that will. Until we understand the extent to which our conscious expression is regulated by unconscious mechanisms, we can't choose to be free of that control.

The Rayid Method of Iris Interpretation, then, is not simply concerned with describing someone's personality; its primary purpose is to free the individual from any limitations associated with that personality. The structure of the iris is also a reflection of the individual's life potential, revealing character strengths and aspects of the personality that are undeveloped. Rayid uses the information contained in the iris of the eye to affirm and strengthen the innate character of the individual. Once he understands who he is and how he functions, which in itself can be a very freeing experience, a person can use Rayid therapies to help him to live life even more fully.

You are not the structure of your iris. It is important to realize this very early on. You are more. When we identify characteristics in the iris, we are identifying the mechanism of the personality. You are more than your personality. The goal of Rayid is to help you to harmonize with simple, natural laws that will allow your personality to perceive your true self, the presence within. Your personality, revealed in the structure of the iris, is in the process of changing, while your true self is constant and perfect. Rayid can help you to balance your physical, emotional and mental systems to become more sensitive to your true self. Some of the ways to do this are addressed in the chapter on therapies.

The Rayid Model of Iris Interpretation is unique. It is not based on any other system of personality evaluation. It does not have roots in iridology; it did not start in psychotherapy. It started in its own way. The theoretical insights have come from a continuing wave of inspiration that started in 1978, and have been thoroughly tested by conducting more than 20,000 case studies between 1978 and 1994.

Rayid is much more than a system of personality evaluation. It is a model of life. It is used by counselors, therapists and parents all over the world who seek a better understanding of others. And it is used by those who want to know themselves better, who long to be free.

The Essence of the Structures

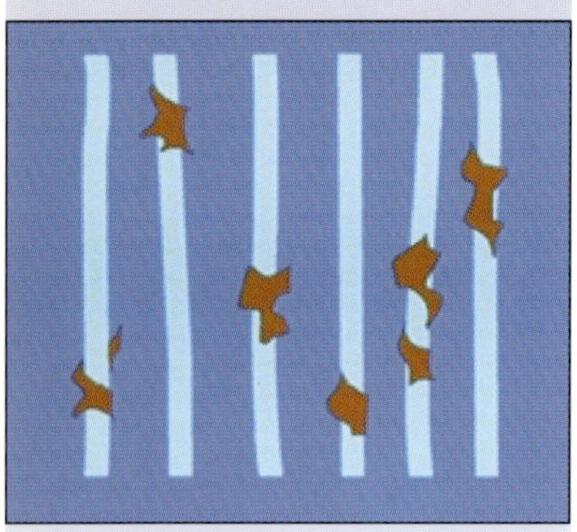

Jewel fibers

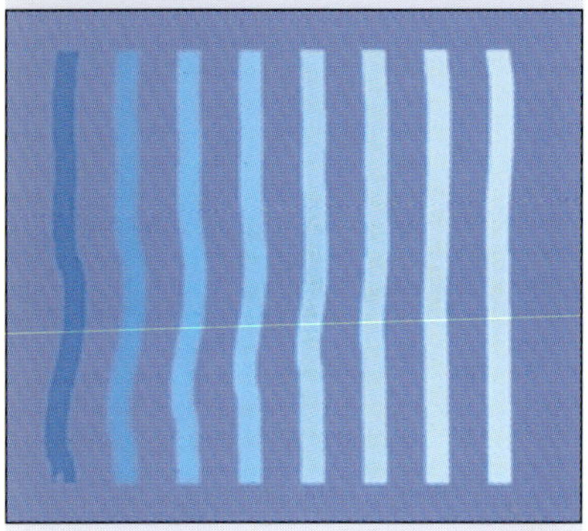

Stream fibers

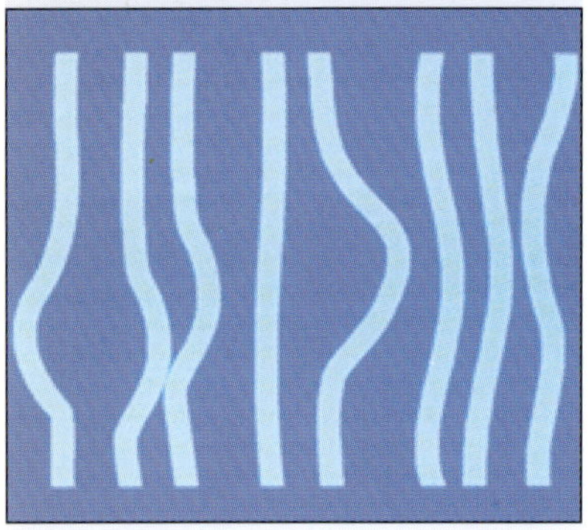

Flower fibers

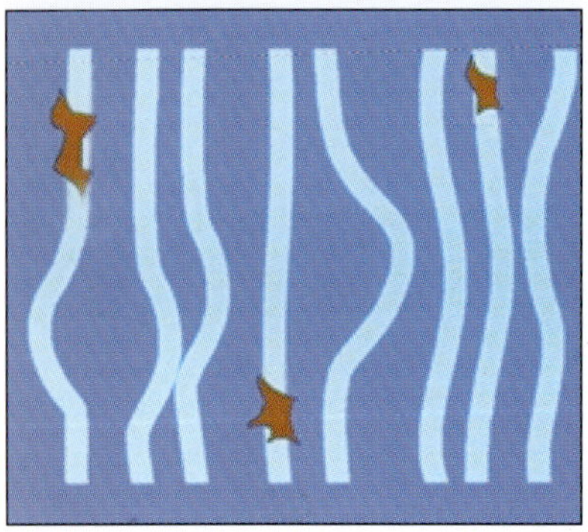

Shaker fibers

The diagrams above are representations of iris fibers, greatly magnified, showing the differing fiber structures in a Jewel, Stream, Flower and Shaker.

THE FOUR PRIMARY STRUCTURES

There are four primary iris structures referred to in the Rayid Method. These four constitutional types are the foundation stones of the mechanism of personality. Each represents a different aspect of personality: mental, emotional, physical and movement. They are defined as the mental (Jewel) type, the emotional (Flower) type, the kinesthetic (Stream) type and the extremist (Shaker) type. The first two create the framework for the other two.

If you understand the characteristics associated with the four basic structural types, you will have a good grounding for exploring some of the more advanced concepts, such as their relationship attractions, and for understanding how their characteristics are genetically passed on to future generations.

People with one of these four iris types will have a different way of being and different needs than the others. They will have a different mode of absorbing information (learning), a different mode of expression (output), and a lifetime of different social and physical experiences based on their natural tendency to be one polarized type. Because of that polarity, they attract someone with an opposite disposition as a mate, and draw experiences of the opposite pole in order to grow.

In the Rayid Method, the mental type and thc emotional type are opposites. The division between these two opposites is the foundation of duality; they are like opposite poles of a magnet. The Jewel is a constrictive, controlling type while the Flower is an expansive, emotional type. They are as far apart as the north and south poles, as different as the negatively charged electron and the positively charged proton. One constricts and binds, the other is expansive and radiant. The mental type is controlling, the emotional type is freeing. Almost paradoxically, these two types are attracted to each other.

When Jewels and Flowers interact, they create the energy of either the kinesthetic or the extremist type. If these north and south poles create a binding connection, they will manifest the stability, stillness and neutral energy of the Stream personality. The Stream personality represents the strength, the tenacity and the groundedness that is needed to nurture, support and hold. If the Jewel and Flower do not make a grounded connection with each other, they will manifest the unstable energy of the extremist type. In this case, instead of fusing, the Jewel and Flower energies perpetually chase each other, like the north and south end of a magnet spinning around trying to catch the other end. The personality of the Shaker is based on movement, and it is appropriate to think of it as a spinning magnet. That is the Shaker's primary mode of communication: movement, often expressed through gestures. Shakers represent the energy of attraction in constant motion.

Each one of these four types has its opposite. The Jewel has the Flower, the Stream has the Shaker. If you understand these four types and the relationships between them, you will understand the basic theory of the Rayid Model. A Jewel is like the force of gravity – a constant, binding force; the Flower represents expansion and freeing. The Stream represents physical, postural energy and stability; the Shaker represents gestures and movement. The motion of the Shaker is balanced by the stillness of the Stream. Analogies from nature can be helpful in understanding the different energies of the four structures.

The Jewel personality, like a rock, is created by a process of gradual change and compaction. The compacting process refines and compresses the material of the earth into its final, crystalline form. Like a large, solitary mountain, the Jewel is nearly impervious to seasonal changes. Rain and snow fall on the mountain, which it later releases as nourishment to the meadows and streams surrounding it. With an air of certainty, Jewels are typically strong, enduring and analytical; they are not as transient, emotional or quick to change as Flowers.

A flower is a seasonal and transient resident in a mountain meadow. Its bright explosion of color enhances the serene meadow for only a brief period of time. The emotional nature of the Flower personality is very similar in expression to the cycle of a meadow flower. In much the same way as the flower attracts the bee by its bouquet, radiance and beauty, so do feeling-oriented Flower types attract other people. With a sense of silent, breathless allowing, Flowers wordlessly accept the world around them.

Streams are the consolidating force in nature. They represent the water that moves through the earth, over and around the jewel, and up the flower. Entering all and a part of everything, this nourishing water brings life and support wherever it goes. Streams are nurturers, community-builders and nest-makers. They are the crib of creation.

Sustaining a sense of belonging, they touch and connect, inviting everyone to join in the experience of connectedness. They are the essence of embodiment.

Shakers are the power of nature in motion. Like the lightning that turns night into day and the thunderclap that jolts you awake, Shakers can effect a sudden and dramatic change in the consciousness of those around them. And like an earthquake, the Shaker sets all of the other structures in motion. There is sometimes a sense of holding back as the energy and pressure inside the Shaker builds, until it is released with the sudden drama of an avalanche racing down the mountainside, sculpting the rock into new shapes as it goes. Like a forest fire sweeping through the trees, Shakers don't stay in one place for long yet their influence is felt for a long time after they have passed. But the Shaker also represents the resurrection, the new life that springs forth from the ashes of the old forest, the renewal that always comes after any apparently destructive event.

These four basic personality types, in various combinations, create all the other personality types. In addition to their primary structural characteristics, Shakers and Streams also tend to have either Flower or Jewel characteristics (the secondary structure), something we will explore later in this chapter in the section on *Combination Structures*.

Every person, either consciously or unconsciously, is on a path that leads toward wholeness. People living in a relatively unconscious state tend to have a relatively shallow experience of reality – a world of black and white with few shades of gray. Such people tend to think in terms of there being only one truth, only one right way to do things and only one right way to be. Their personalities are often a reflection of this attitude: they (unconsciously) suppress many of their own subpersonalities and generally allow only one aspect of their inner reality to be present at a time. As people start to "wake up," they become less polarized and more accepting of diversity in the world and in themselves.

Ultimately, each of us will be able to gain access to all of the levels of consciousness represented by the Stream, Jewel, Flower and Shaker structures, and to move freely from one way of being to another. This is the wholeness that we seek.

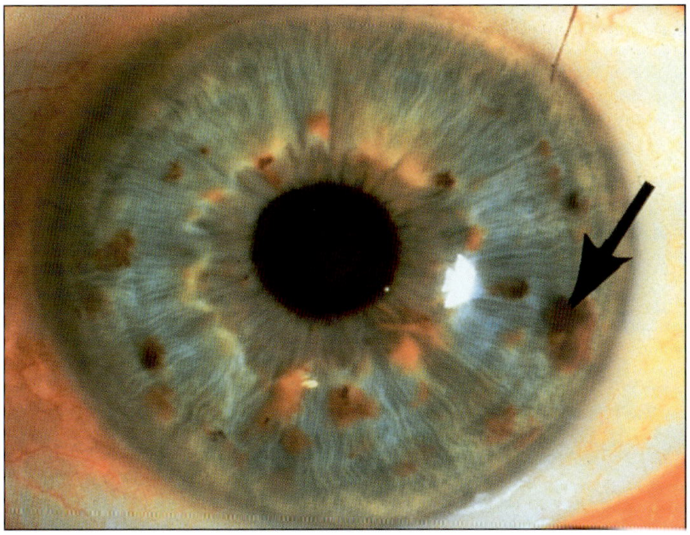

Jewel

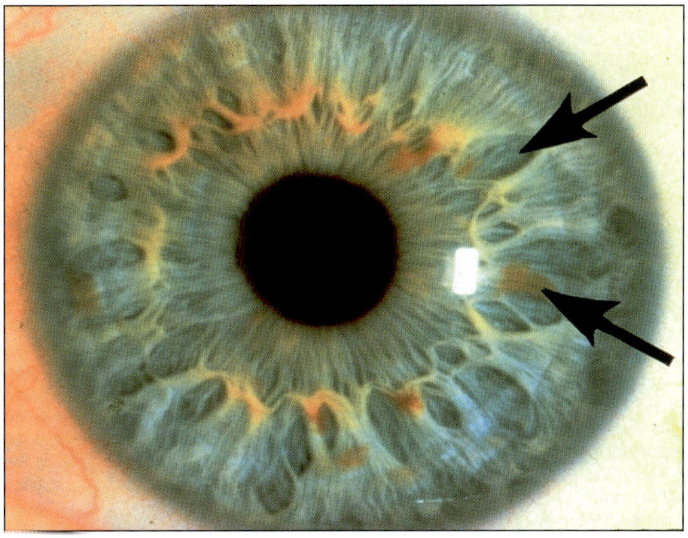

Shaker

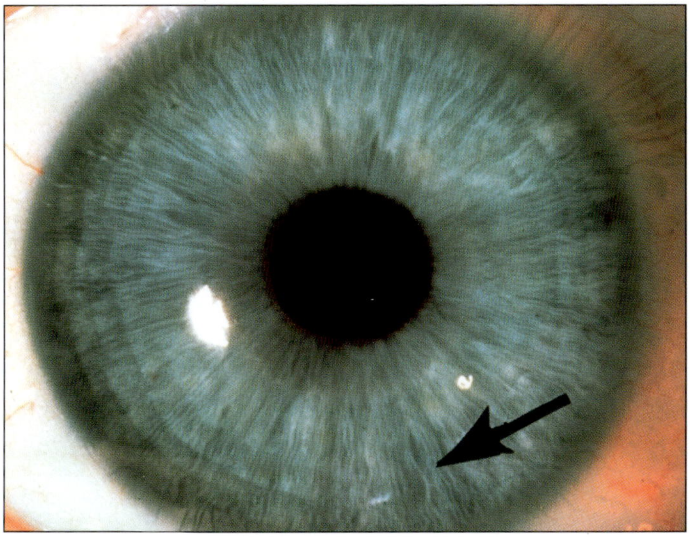

Stream

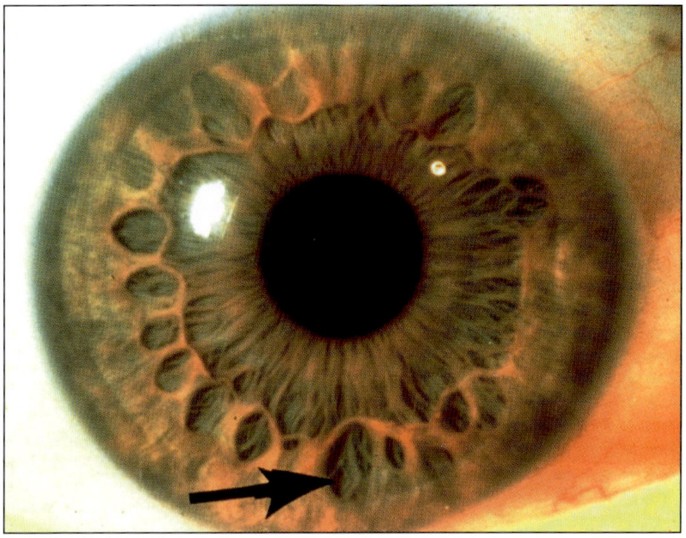

Flower

JEWEL

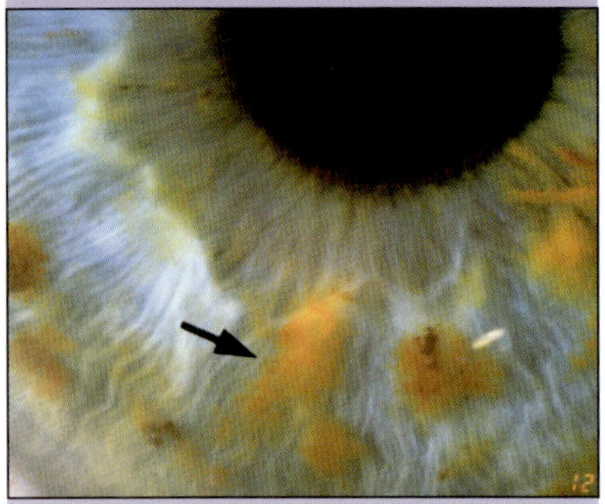

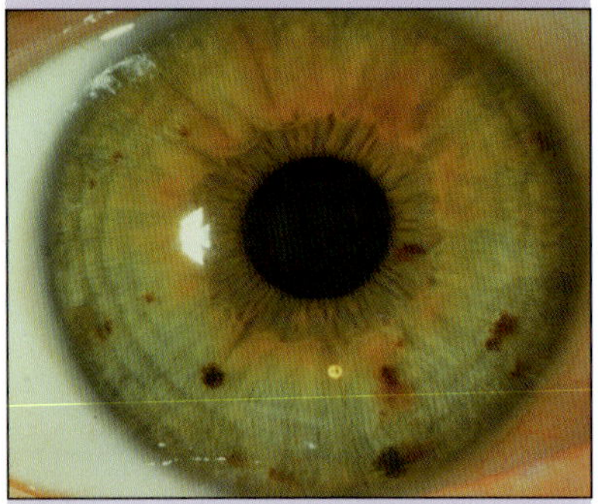

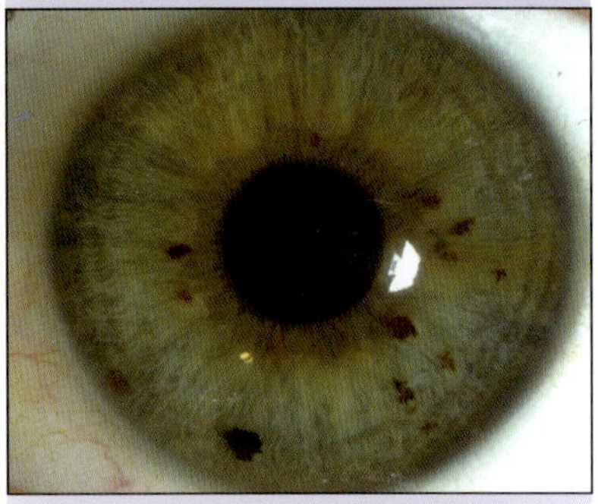

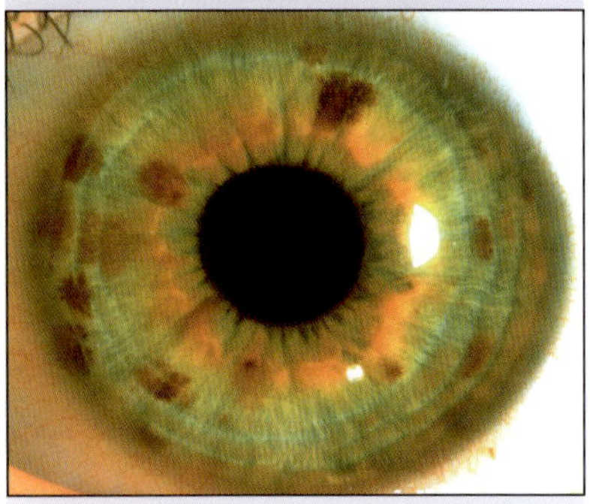

Four examples of Jewel irises (above).

Numerous, dot-like pigments in the iris indicate a thinking, intellectual person. These dots, which can be yellow or brown, large or small, are called jewels, and we refer to the mental type of person as a Jewel. Mental types direct their perceptions and feelings through internal thought and analysis. Every person thinks, and every person analyzes, but for Jewels these are recognizably their dominant personality characteristics.

When you see brown or gold flecks in an iris, it also indicates that the person has a tendency to take information in visually. This is the Jewel's primary mode of learning. Jewels like to watch, read and observe. They take information in through their eyes, process it, categorize it, name it, think of it and then explain it verbally. They are usually precise, verbal communicators. The Jewel temperament is perceptive and inquisitive, but introverted Jewels can be quite withdrawn. With a one-pointed, intense nature, the Jewel mind can enter the minute corners of human imagination, or spend hours examining the colors of a butterfly's wing. They love detail.

Jewels tend to control themselves, situations and other people. They like to tell people what to do. They generally show little emotion and use few, pointed gestures. Analysis and feeling are superficially mutually exclusive: Jewels are overtly very analytical and their feelings, which are actually as deep as anyone's, are hidden away rather than being on display. At times, their self-control and mental capabilities can give them the appearance of being aloof or self-righteous. Jewels seek freedom, and resent being controlled themselves. Some Jewels don't even like to wear seat-belts, because they don't like the feeling of constriction. They tend to find their freedom in abstract thinking, experiencing material reality as a prison. They abhor systems and organized structure for similar reasons (unless they themselves have created them), and have a tendency to uproot structures. They usually have a great need to be right, to interrupt and to have the final word, even to the point where they need to have the last word when saying goodbye.

Often intense, these deliberate, quietly driven people enjoy setting and attaining goals. Although they can sometimes be slow to accept new ideas, they often end up leading the way once they have thoroughly analyzed the possibilities. Their excellent speaking abilities endow them with traits of persuasion and inspiration. Future-oriented, with well-defined views, an attention to detail and a commanding presence, they excel as leaders, critics, teachers and scientists. Jewels are overtly quite interesting and active, and so find it superficially easier to relate to other people than Flowers.

When balanced, the mental types can contribute great clarity and wisdom to a social or work situation. When they are *very* balanced, they are clear without the need for analysis, and that is *knowing*. When they are out of balance, their thoughts start to become scattered, they become insatiably analytical and questioning, and their attention to detail can prove stifling to the realization of their highest potential.

Learning to flow with situations and to trust other people enables Jewels to better express their feelings and helps them to attain their long-term goals.

Needing release, or someone to listen, Jewels attract emotional types for long-term relationships. But although they may desperately want to have a relationship with someone who is emotional, the Flowers they attract are inevitably slower in expression; the Jewels end up either verbally or physically interrupting them all the time, creating tension in the partnership.

Jewels are usually closer to the mother in childhood, or to an older sister, and tend to have emotional issues or problems with the father or a brother.

The conscious fears of the Jewel are a fear of criticism and a fear of losing control. This stems partly from an uncomfortableness with their own vulnerability. They are attracted to intimacy but they also fear it. They are similarly attracted to the unknown but are afraid of actually experiencing it. Jewels tend to go looking for the experience of opening, but will stay closed to the experience while trying to have it.

There is some correlation between the ancient Chinese system of acupuncture and Rayid iris types. In Jewels, the governing meridian running up the back of the body is usually quite strong, while the female meridian, running up the front, is weak. So where do Jewels have most of their physical problems? In front, with such organs as the spleen, liver and pancreas. A denial of feeling in Jewels tends to create a soft, almost flaccid body, and an inner hardening with associated digestive problems. While *everyone* is either a Jewel or a Flower (see *Combination Structures*), only about 10% of people have a *pure* Jewel pattern.

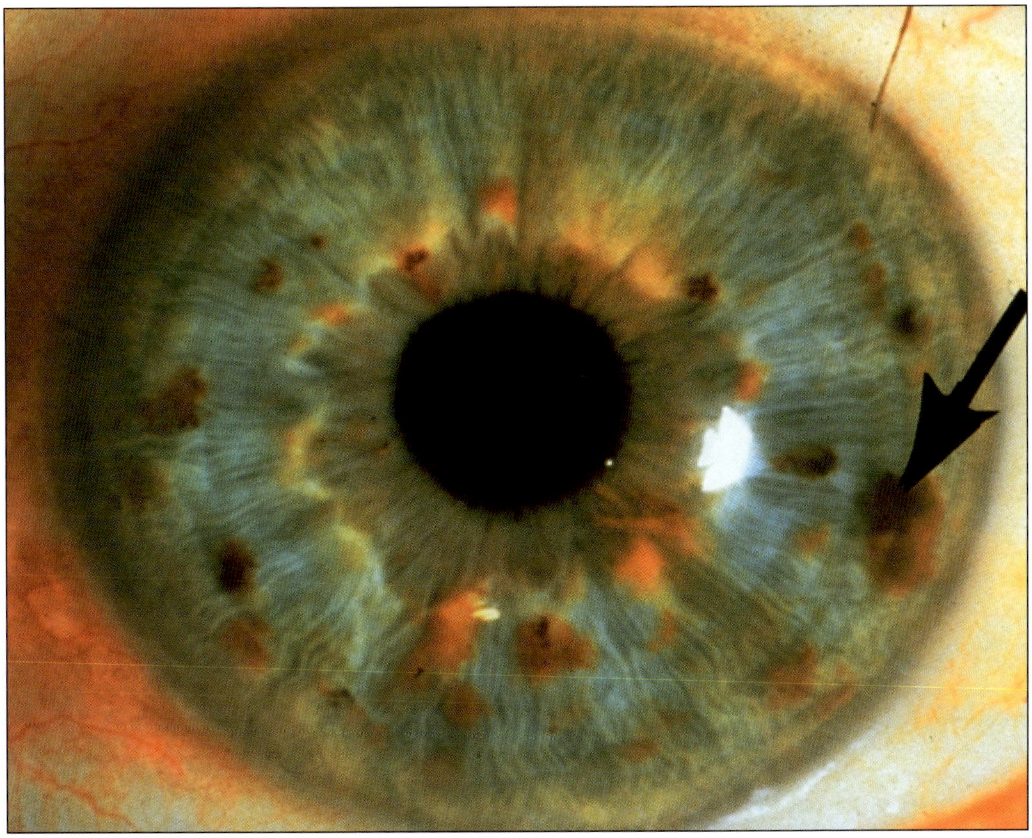

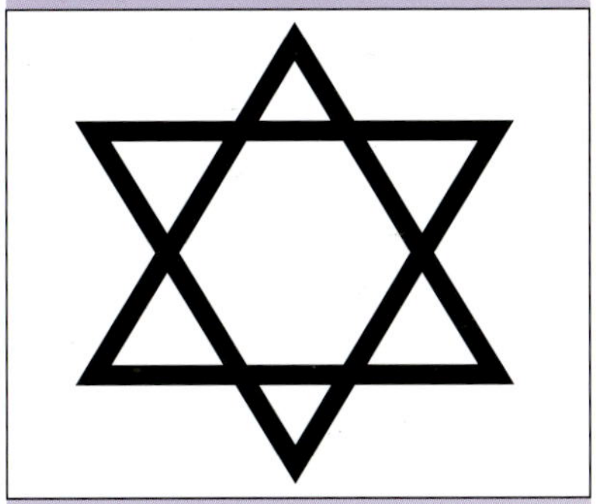

The angularity and precise focus of the Jewel is symbolically represented by a double triangle.

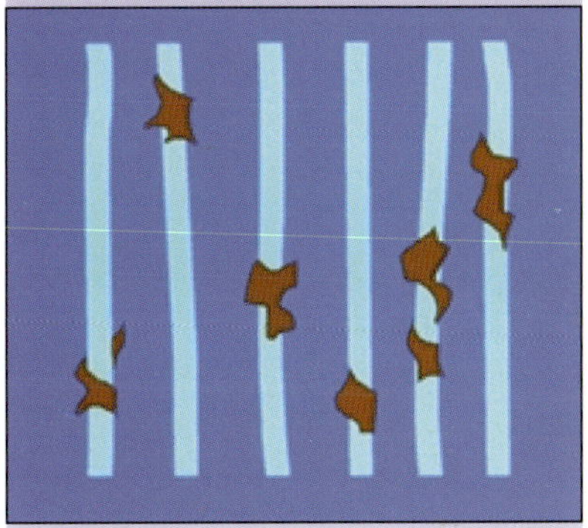

Jewel iris fibers

Summary of Jewel Characteristics

Iris traits:	Dot-like pigments
Personality:	Thinking, analytical, verbal, slow to change
Essence/Unique gift:	Clear, knowing
Gestures/Postures:	Controlled, pointed
Perspective:	I (1st person)
Gifts/Skills:	Leadership, attention to detail, clarity
Lessons:	Trust others, delegate, integrate, flow
Learning (subconscious):	Visual, and by association with emotions
Communication (conscious):	Verbal, using sounds and words
Family relationships:	Closer to mother/sister in childhood, problems with father/brother
Mate relationships:	Flowers
Activities/Disposition:	Star Trek fans, future-oriented
Energy pattern/Direction:	Build energy, direct it forward
Physical characteristics:	Sharp bone structure in face, cold hands
Interruptive pattern:	Verbal overanalysis, jittery hands/feet, abrupt body movements
Sleep:	Primarily on their left side, with partner on their right
Fears:	Letting go, criticism, intimacy, the unknown
Adaptation:	Emotional, spacey, forgetful
Stress imbalance:	Anxious, frustrated, avoiding, loss of confidence

Transformational Pathway

Positive expression:	Control, focus, analyze, plan
If blocked, they are:	Opionated, interruptive, avoiding
If they learn to:	Allow, flow, open
They experience:	Feeling, silence
Achieving a state of:	Knowing, truth

FLOWER

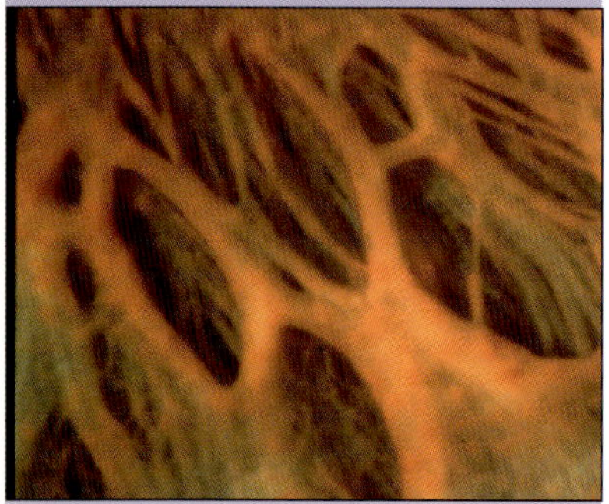

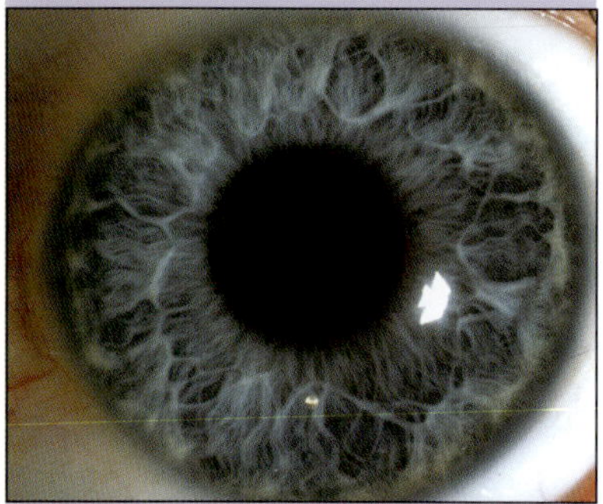

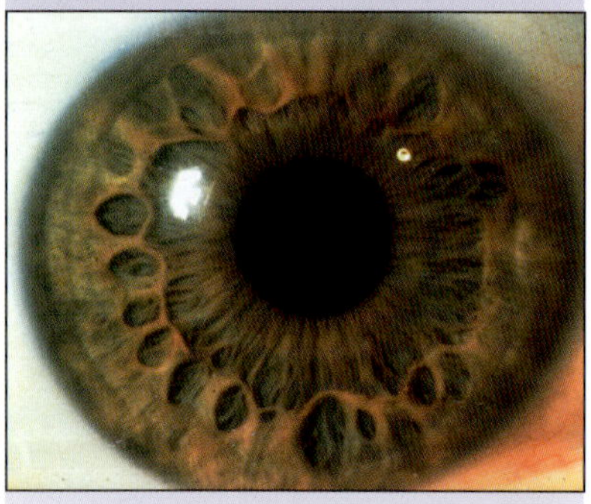

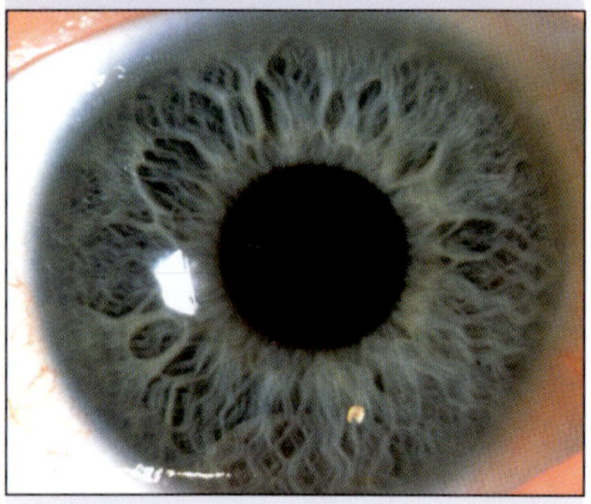

Four examples of Flower irises (above).

Distinctly curved or rounded openings in the fibers of the iris indicate an emotional type of person. These openings, which look as if the light-colored iris fibers actually have round holes within them, are called flowers, and we refer to the emotional type of person as a Flower. Feeling-oriented, they experience life through the sensitivities of the heart, with automatic emotional reactions to events.

Emotional types take life in auditorily, through sounds. They are fond of listening to music and learn most quickly when given specific auditory instructions. They communicate with imagery, emotions and gestures, and are generally animated and expressive, although introverted Flowers can be very soft and slow in social situations. When extroverted, these showy, demonstrative people use their bodies as active displays of their emotions. They can be sexy and flirtatious at a moment's notice, and then just as quickly can change their minds and move on to something else. Change is the hallmark of Flower personalities.

Flexible, spontaneous and changeable, they flow easily with social situations. Flowers are just as strong as Jewels, but express their strength in less direct ways. Exuding passion, fire and grace, Flowers generate excitement in others simply by their presence. They enjoy being on display, or even on stage, with the whole world as their audience. Overflowing with creative ideas, Flowers excel as artists, entertainers, musicians, inventors and engineers. Quick to embrace new concepts, they add vitality to any project, but may fail to see it through to completion. Living for the moment, their interest and enthusiasm often doesn't last their passion for experiencing life and tendency to overcommit can exhaust their energies.

Flowers like to be organized, but have difficulty sticking with any system for long. They tend to try out a new system for a while, believing it will improve their lives, then lose interest and go on to something else.

The great gift of the Flower is silent peace, expansiveness and a feeling of agelessness. When in balance, they are like a cool, quiet mountain lake. But when that mountain lake gets disturbed, it becomes reactive and muddy. When something goes wrong, Flowers easily become angry, blaming anyone but themselves for their misfortune. If they do blame themselves, however, they get depressed. Flowers are often in their minds, though unaware of it; when they get back into their bodies, they can experience ecstasy. When expressing their inner nature, they are poised and open, and contribute quiet calm to any social situation.

Flowers need to learn to trust themselves and their own abilities, and to accept responsibility for events. In order to fulfill their desires and find success, Flowers must learn to focus their energies.

Needing control, emotional types are attracted to mental types for long-term relationships. This particular combination of opposite temperaments produces relationships that are sometimes spectacular to watch.

Flowers usually prefer to be closer to the father in childhood, or to an older brother, and often have emotional issues or problems with the mother or a sister. However, their fathers are often not there for them. With most Flowers, there is a characteristic pattern of mother separation, a feeling of abandonment and anger. Superficially, Flowers seem to have no one, while Jewels have everyone. Pushed away from mother, with a father who was never *really* available, and with a more covert personality, the typical Flower can have a more difficult time relating.

The conscious fear of the Flower is a fear of being controlled. This may manifest as a fear of drowning, of suffocation or dying of thirst. Flowers never feel complete, and usually have a profound sense of aloneness. They feel as if they have been cut off from the source and experience this as a form of grief.

In Flowers, the meridian running up the back of the body tends to be weak, while the meridian running up the front is strong. They therefore tend to have problems with the back, neck, heart, gallbladder and kidneys, and enjoy having the neck, back and sometimes shoulders rubbed. Flowers also tend to burn themselves out and need periods of rest to overcome their self-induced states of exhaustion and depression. When they do take the time to be still, a kaleidoscope of inner passions fills their minds and they once again bubble forth with a newly discovered wave of enthusiasm. A denial of feeling in Flowers can create a physical hardening of the body, with associated tension, headaches and migraines.

About 10% of people have a pure Flower pattern. You will find 85% of all flowers in the mother eye (the left eye). The greater the number of flowers and the more rounded they are, the more spontaneous and emotional the individual's behavior is.

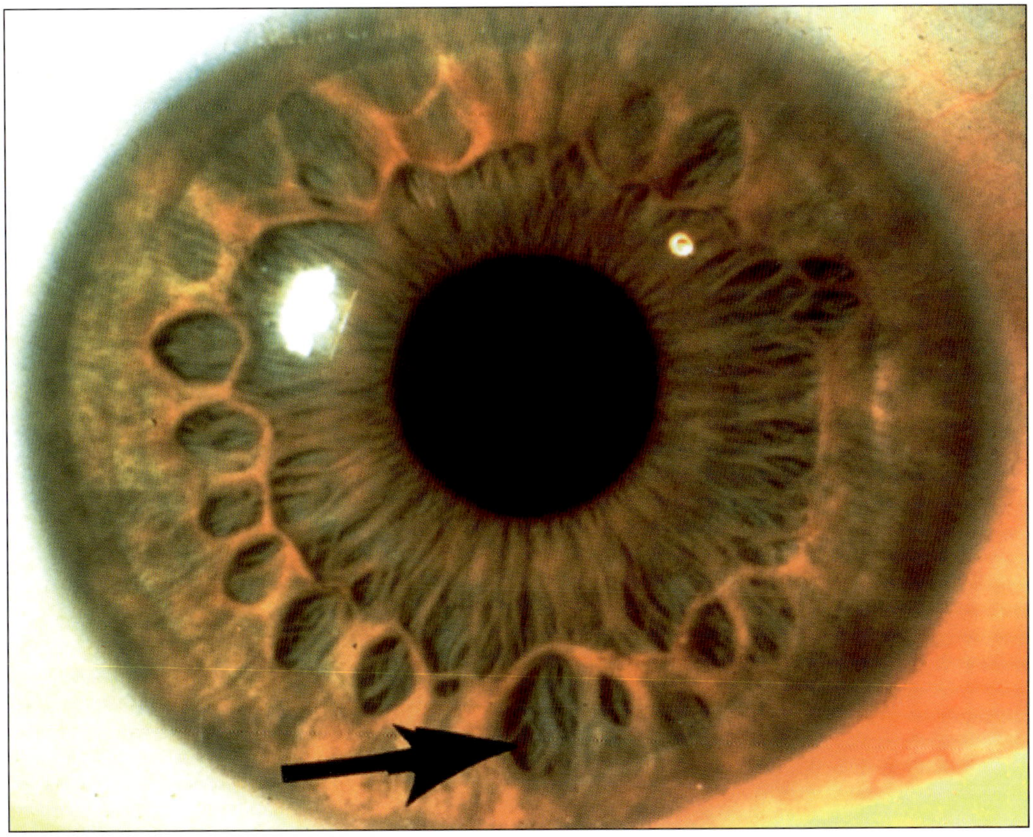

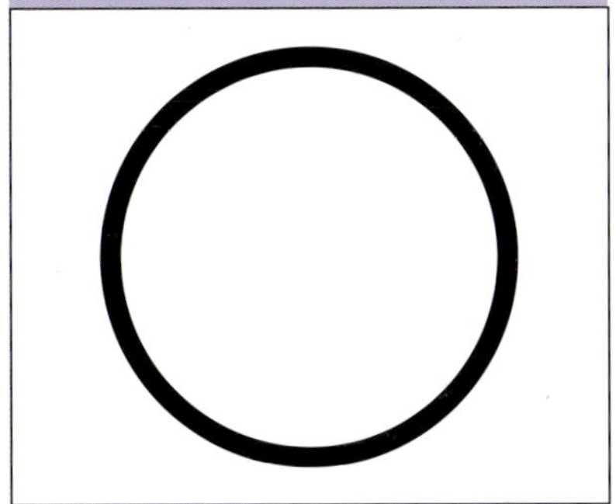

The openness and receptivity of the Flower is symbolically represented by a circle.

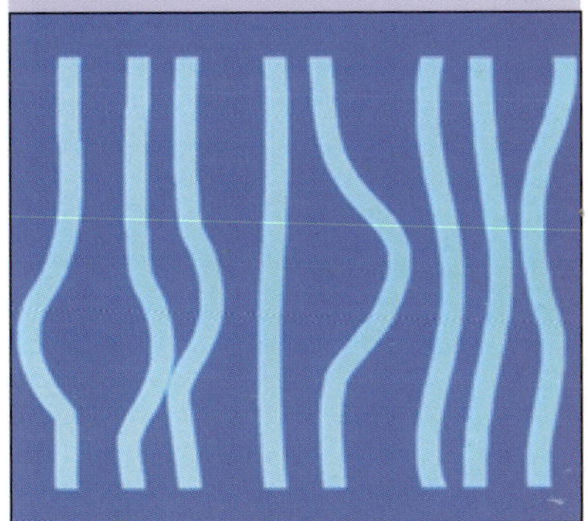

Flower iris fibers

Summary of Flower Characteristics

Iris traits:	Curved or rounded openings
Personality:	Emotional, feeling, expressive, changeable
Essence/Unique gift:	Spatial, peaceful
Gestures/Postures:	Spontaneous, animated
Perspective:	You (2nd person)
Gifts/Skills:	Joy, vision, sociability
Lessons:	Trust themselves, self-control, poise, focus and direct
Learning (subconscious):	Auditory
Communication (conscious):	Visual, using images and gestures
Family relationships:	Closer to father/brother, problems with mother/sister
Mate relationships:	Jewel
Activities/Disposition:	Music-lovers, romantic
Energy pattern/Direction:	Release energy, around
Physical characteristics:	Rounder face, hot or even sweaty hands
Interruptive pattern:	Develop a blank stare, interrupt by dispersal of energy
Sleep:	Primarily on their right side, with partner on their left
Fears:	Abandonment/separation, being controlled, suffocation
Adaptation:	Detailed, controlling
Stress imbalance:	Angry, depressed, blaming

Transformational Pathway

Positive expression:	Open, soothing, quiet
If blocked, they are:	Angry, depressed, blaming
If they learn to:	Accept, clarify, be self-responsible
They experience:	Certainty, joy
Achieving a state of:	Peace, warmth

SHAKER

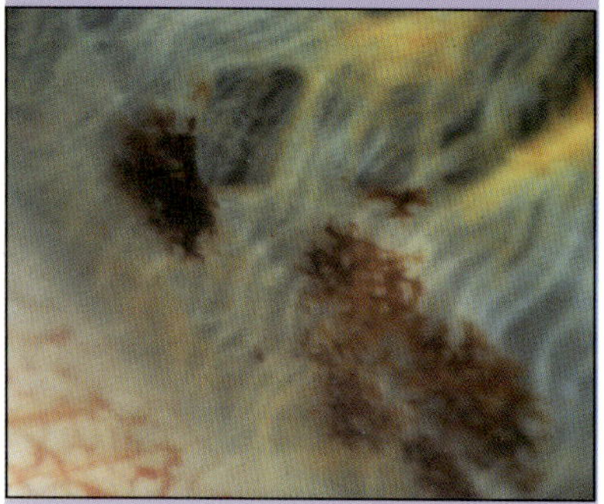

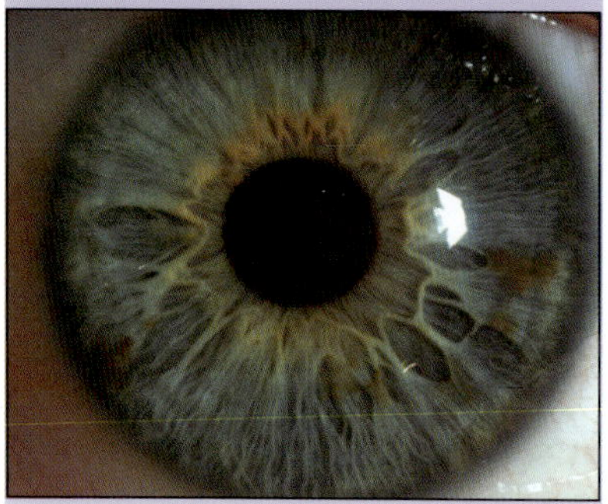

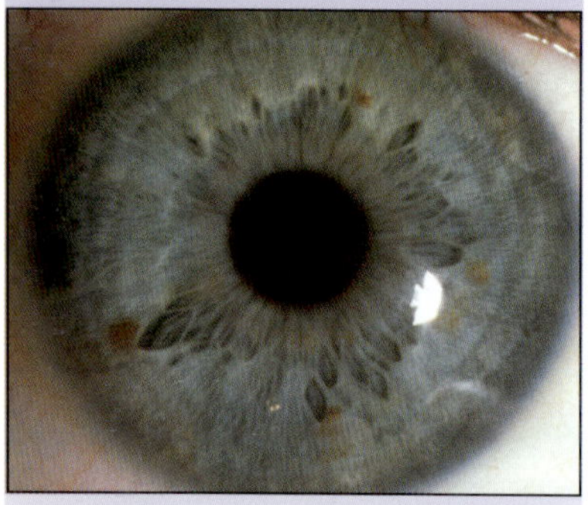

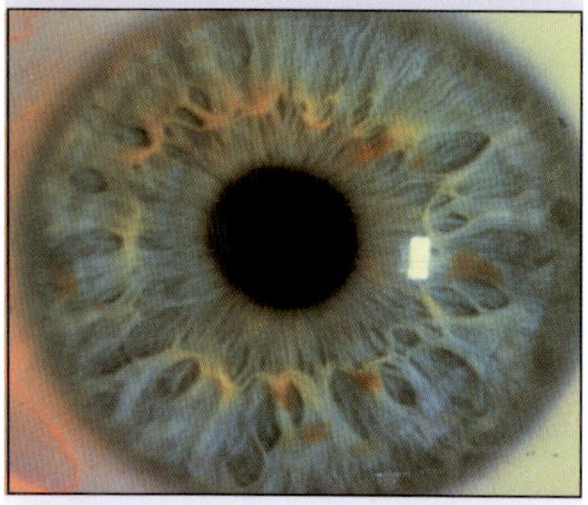

Four examples of Shaker irises (above).

Eyes that have both dot-like pigments *and* rounded openings indicate an extremist (Shaker) type of personality. Embodying the forces of attraction and repulsion, representing everything that moves, Shakers are highly motivated, dynamic and expressive. These radical, action-oriented people frequently venture beyond the limits of conventional thought and norms. They possess a bulldog-like tenacity that drives them to press on against all odds. Pioneering types, typically at the forefront of change and innovation, Shakers challenge life with abandon and zeal. Acting as the conscience of society, they often stand alone, sometimes attracting ridicule from their peers. Pure Shaker structures make up about 15% of the population.

With elements of both the Jewel and the Flower in their makeup, Shakers unify mental and emotional personality characteristics. They make decisions faster than a Jewel and stay with that decision longer than a Flower. Shakers learn best physically, while in motion (through the movement of their bodies) or by being touched. They have a strong intuitive sense and can learn through it, too. They communicate primarily by movement and gesture. They usually have a strong affinity for nature and the outdoors, where the physical connection with their environment increases their intuitive intake.

Shakers are the embodiment of ecstasy, joy and thankfulness, bringing feelings of exhilaration and excitement to any project they are involved in. People are initially attracted to Shakers because of their energy and conviction but they can be difficult to relate to because they are always in motion and frequently changing their focus. Adventurous and frequently devoted to a cause, Shakers excel as inventors, motivators and explorers.

As children, Shakers often prove to be quite a handful for their parents. Their extreme natures can make them difficult to teach or direct. They dislike confinement and resent any form of systematic control. They prefer to be physically active, which is good because they need to develop their bodies. If they develop a sense of concern for their families and the community at large, and learn to channel their energy, Shakers have the potential to create new and lasting changes in society.

Shakers know where they're going – or, at least, they *think* they know where they're going – and they can be inspiring leaders and motivators, eliciting one's conscience about a cause or bringing a sense of purpose to a project. Results-oriented, they are also prone to impatience they don't understand anything less than total commitment and find partial or half-hearted commitment to a project irritating. Shakers are the people who say, "Enough of the planning, let's go! Let's get up and do it!"

Driven to achieve, yet sometimes ungrounded, Shakers can experience cycles of great success and failure that exhaust their physical strength. They push themselves to the limit, typically with a complete disregard for their own bodies. When they are ungrounded, they can bring the whole group down through their recklessness, so they need to learn to plan. Their task in society is to expand the limits of humanity's self-imposed barriers and to pierce the shield of traditional values. Shakers are the tip of the spear.

When they get too excited, Shakers easily become scattered, which is when their intense energy can turn back on itself. They can become self-destructive, with a tendency to addiction, and their enthusiasm and desire to change the world can become obsessive, to the point where they start using blame to motivate people. Shakers rarely take a neutral stance on any topic; they are prone to being unfair and can be downright rude to anyone who disagrees with them. When unbalanced, their leadership potential can become subverted to lesser ends and they can turn out to be tyrants and ruthless dictators instead of inspiring and charismatic leaders.

When they can allow themselves to be still, to feel the integrity of who they are, Shakers can bring the experience of wakefulness, joy and thankfulness to any group. Learning moderation and consistency enables the Shaker to manifest change with stability.

Needing equilibrium in their lives, Shakers are attracted to kinesthetic (Stream) types for long-term relationships. Idealistic about romance, Shakers nonetheless place their life goals; uppermost on their list of priorities and want their partners to be supportive of those goals; they seek mates who are prepared to follow them on their sometimes precarious paths through life. Their perfectionism and demanding nature can make them quite a challenge as long-term partners.

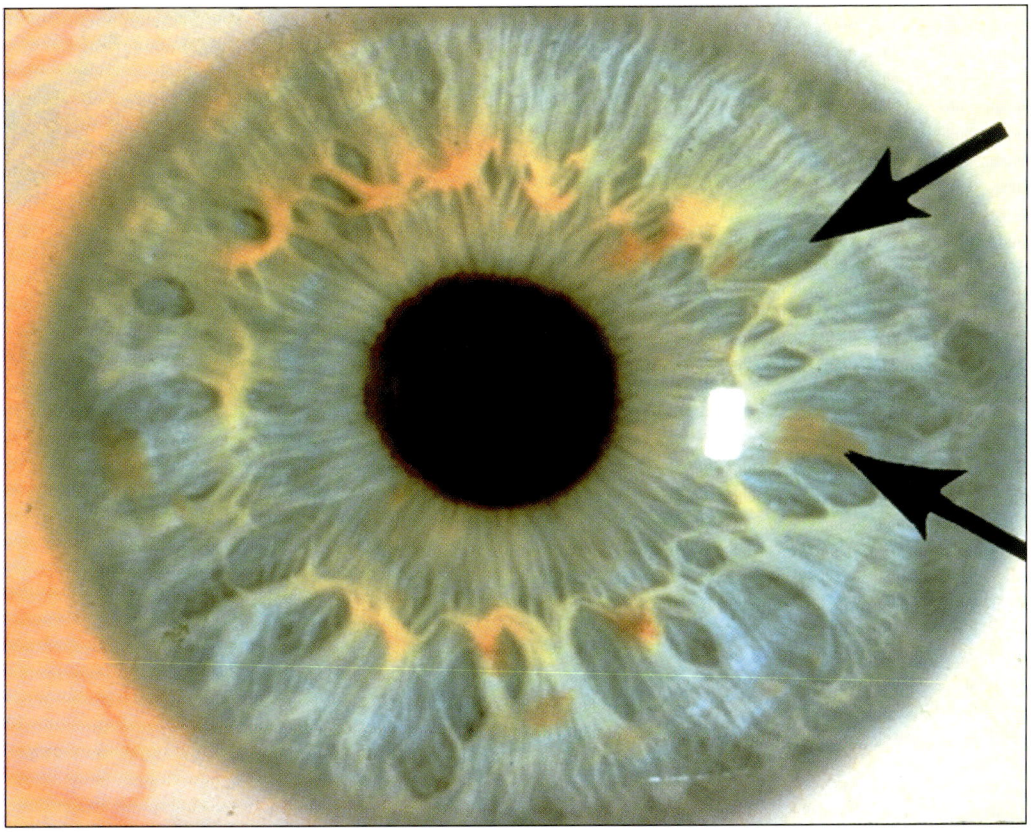

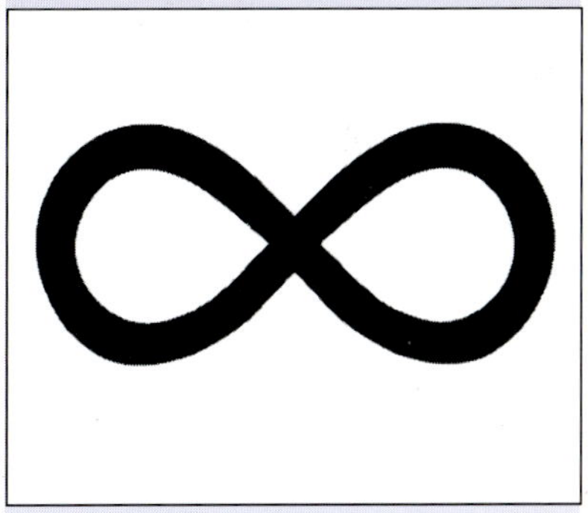

The motion and instability of the Shaker is represented by a spinning infinity symbol.

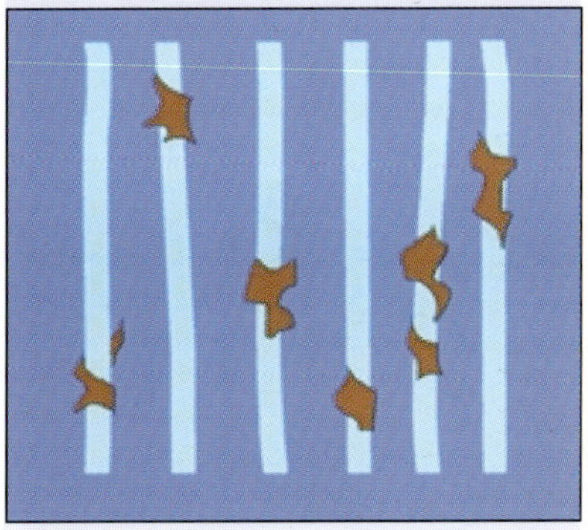

The Shaker structure includes both Jewel (above) and Flower (below) iris fibers.

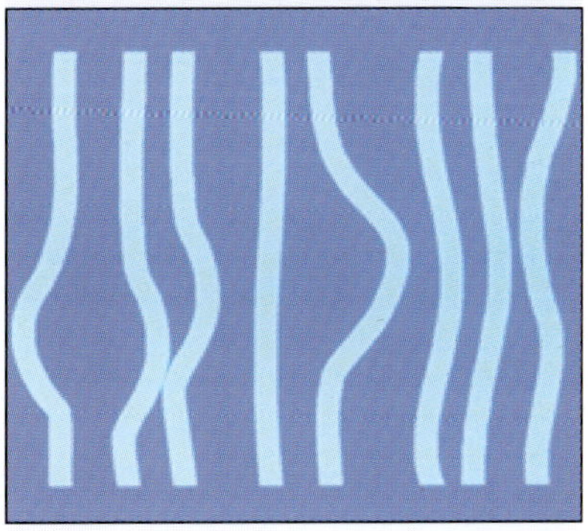

Summary of Shaker Characteristics

Iris traits:	Dot-like pigments and rounded openings
Personality:	Driven, progressive, in motion, unpredictable, extreme
Essence/Unique gift:	Vitality, joy
Gestures/Postures:	Dynamic
Perspective:	They (4th person)
Gifts/Skills:	Motivation, originality, zeal, achievement
Lessons:	Consistency, moderation, stability, trust the physical body
Learning (subconscious):	Through body experience/motion/intuitive feeling
Communication (conscious):	Alternating or unified (visual and verbal), and by gesture
Family relationships:	Depends on secondary structure
Mate relationships:	Stream
Activities/Disposition:	Travel and/or fighting for causes, enthusiastic, impatient
Energy pattern/Direction:	Moves energy, up and out
Sleep:	Depends on secondary structure
Fears:	Failure, being controlled, intimacy
Adaptation:	Inactive
Stress imbalance:	Autocratic

Transformational Pathway

Positive expression:	Drive, motivate
If blocked, they are:	Reckless, isolated
If they learn to:	Plan, join, connect
They experience:	Change, sense of purpose
Achieving a state of:	Conscience, aliveness

STREAM

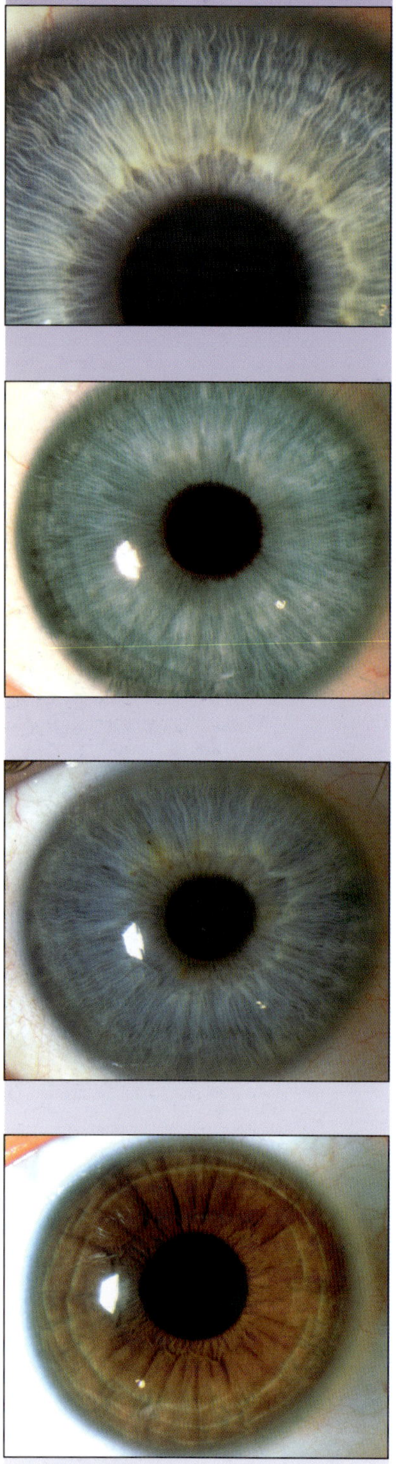

Four examples of Stream irises (above).

The fourth structural type in the Rayid Method is called the kinesthetic type, metaphorically referred to as a Stream. The iris of a Stream has a uniform fiber structure radiating out from the pupil, with only subtle variations or streaks of color. At first glance, Stream irises appear to have the fewest features of all iris structures, and it can take a little while before the Rayid student can easily discern all of the characteristics in a Stream eye.

Streams are the fabric that holds the world together. They are intuitive, grounded and amiable. Physical people, they perceive and integrate life through the sensory experience of their bodies. They subconsciously learn best when given the opportunity to experience their lessons, through movement or by doing. They also learn easily from teachers who alternate between verbal and visual instructions. They communicate by posture and by touch, or with delicately controlled gestures.

They are physically, mentally and intuitively sensitive. Automatically receptive to everything, their bodies act as receptacles for all that happens around them. Imagine Streams as having thousands of cat-like whiskers dangling in all directions. The slightest change or incident is immediately felt by them. Embodying the sensitivity of both the Jewel and the Flower natures, they are like walking radars, always being "touched" by things around them. Although they have a heightened sensitivity, they tend to control their subtle physical reactions to life through stillness. Their sensitivity is both a gift and a challenge.

With true empathy, they tend to nurture and balance others, mediating and balancing the extremes in society. Their subtle sensitivity gives them the capability to communicate with both Flowers and Jewels, increasing their mediating abilities. Slow to change, they like to do things in a group and to make decisions by committee. They are true visionary implementers, making things happen, getting the job done. Endowed with abundant physical energy and social skills, they are naturals in athletics, dance, health care, social work and public service.

Stream bodies become living pipelines of natural vitality as the energy of life pulses in and out of them. This makes them physically some of the most attractive people, and the uninhibited transfer of energy between people creates mental, physical and spiritual wellbeing in those around them. Streams provide the pathway for this essential nourishment to flow without them, the rest of humanity would wither and die.

These kinesthetic types provide a sense of belonging, a sense of nurturing, a sense of motherhood. Their presence evokes the feeling of being held or cuddled. When a Stream feels he belongs, everyone around him experiences a sense of relaxation. If Streams become fearful or reactive, their attentions can become overprotective, even stifling, instead of comfortably containing. When they become neurotic, they won't let go. Their sense of being connected with people can lead to confusion about their own self-worth or purpose in life and, when excessively sensitive, they can easily end up feeling hopelessly overwhelmed. When they are balanced in themselves, they bring a sense of integrity, stability and balance to any social situation.

By accepting the perfection in life and in themselves, Streams learn to touch others without taking on unnecessary burdens. Practicing perfect stillness heightens their kinesthetic sensitivity and allows the energy that is stored within them to be released. Channeling this energy into work allows Streams to realize their greatest potential.

Needing expansiveness, Streams are attracted to Shakers for long-term relationships. Their stabilizing influence helps to balance the radical nature of the Shaker.

Pure Stream structures account for about 15% of the population, and their eyes can initially be more of a challenge to interpret than other structures. If there are no distinct flowers or jewels in the eyes, the individual traits can be more difficult to pick out (see *Positions in the Iris*), and the overall iris structure can be more difficult to classify (see *Combination Structures* in this chapter). In Streams, positional characteristics are represented by any type of irregularity within the iris structure. Soft patches of color, dense concentrations of fiber or a markedly raised single fiber is indicative of Jewelness a noticeable *absence* of fiber in a particular area indicates Flowerness. A slight characteristic in a Stream iris can be as emotionally or physically significant as a very large characteristic in a Jewel or Flower iris, but the subtle variations in the fibers can be difficult to see without good lighting or photography. Dark eyes compound the difficulty.

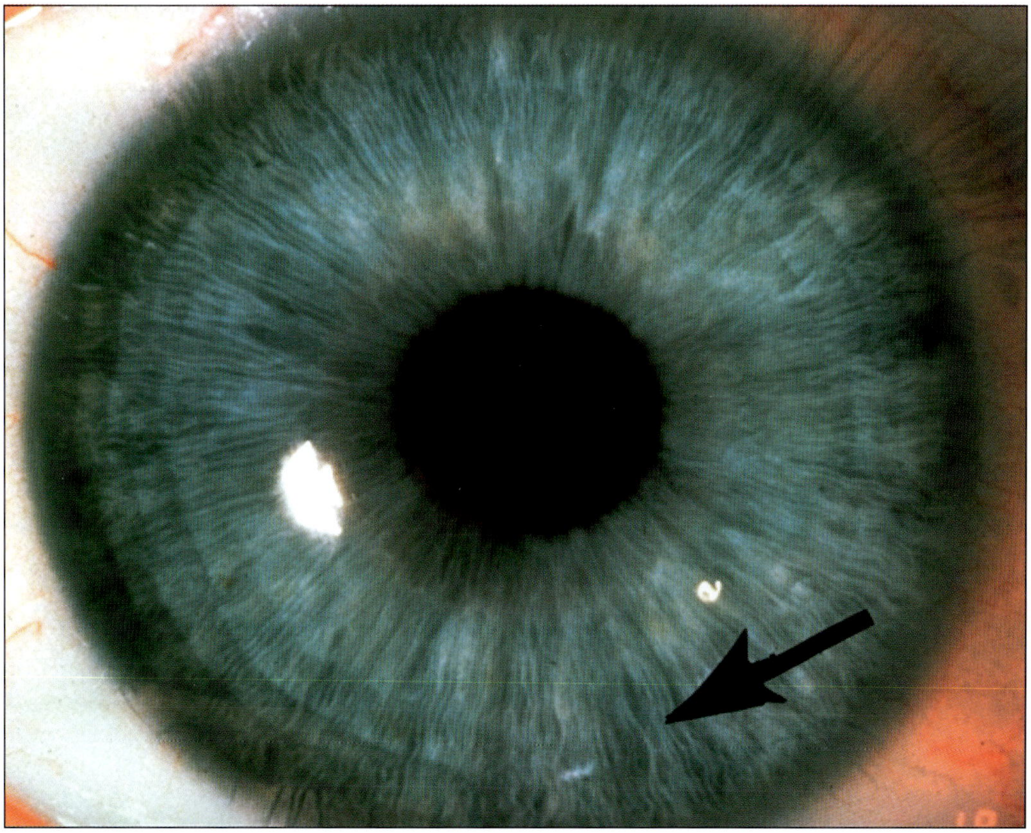

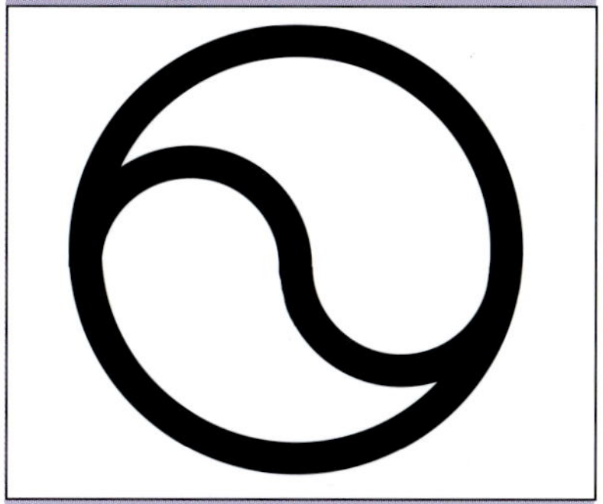

This symbol graphically represents the stability, strength and balance of the Stream.

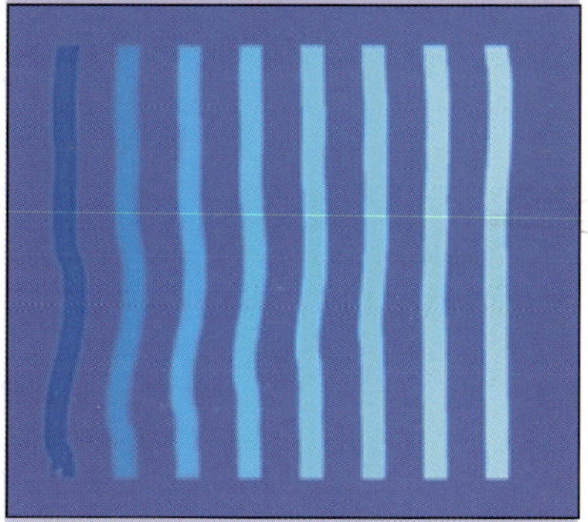

Stream iris fibers

Summary of Stream Characteristics

Iris traits:	Straight lines or streaks of color
Personality:	Amiable, intuitive, sensitive, grounded
Essence/Unique gift:	Stillness, connectedness, mediator
Gestures/Postures:	Subtle
Perspective:	We (3rd person)
Gifts/Skills:	Balance and stability, empathy, support, integration
Lessons:	Trust, release, find purpose
Learning (subconscious):	Experiential, by doing
Communication (conscious):	By touch and posture
Family relationships:	Depends on secondary structure
Mate relationships:	Shaker
Activities/Disposition:	Physically active, attentively concerned
Energy pattern/Direction:	Connecting and containing, directed downward (grounding)
Sleep:	Depends on secondary structure
Fears:	Change, initiation, mistakes, hurting others or being hurt
Adaptation:	Ungrounded
Stress imbalance:	Acquiescent, stymied, helpless

Transformational Pathway

Positive expression:	Support, serve, balance
If blocked, they are:	Blocked, indecisive
If they learn to:	Initiate, act, move, give
They experience:	Nurturing, unification
Achieving a state of:	Belonging, stillness

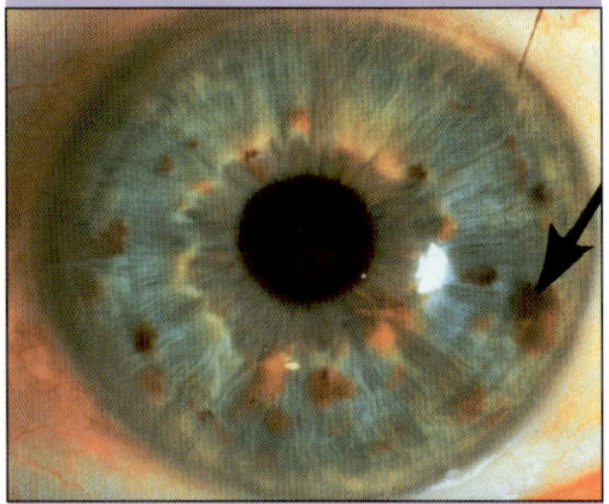

Jewel

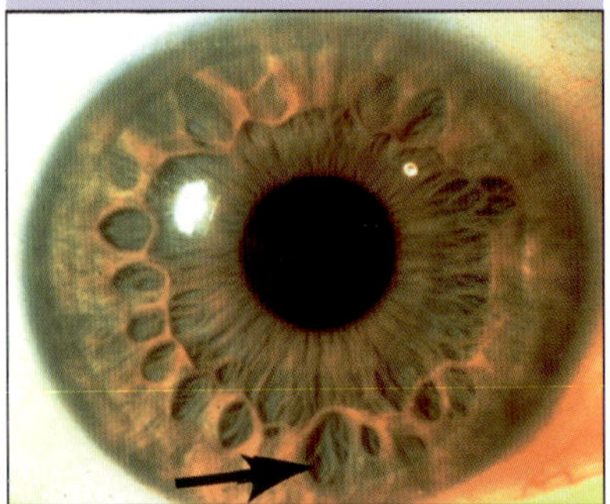

Flower

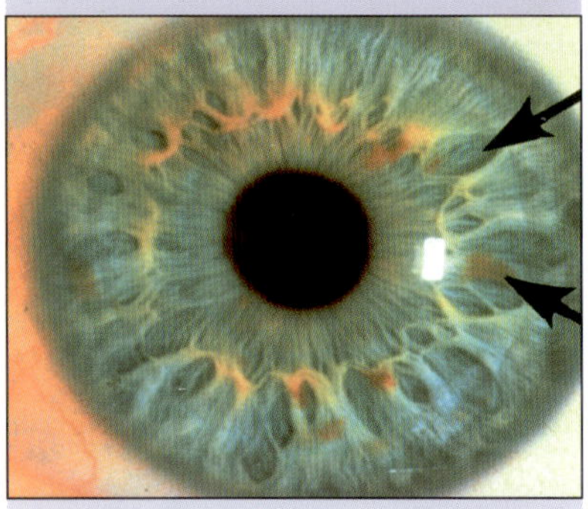

Shaker

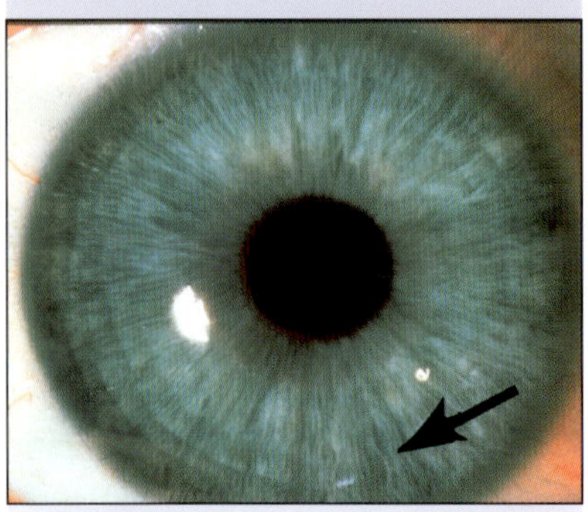

Stream

REVIEW OF THE PRIMARY STRUCTURES

As you study the Rayid Method, your ability to interpret fine details in the eyes will improve, giving you the means to be highly specific about individual behavior patterns. While this improves your accuracy in consultations, it is important not to lose sight of the primary structure of the iris and other overall patterns.

Each one of the iris structures represents a particular vibration, within which a particular individual may have a greater or lesser energy level or "amplitude" of vibration. Amplitude is the extent to which an individual expresses him particular pattern.

In the big picture, we are interested in raising and sustaining the overall vibration of the whole being (see *Beyond the Iris*). This increases the well-being of the person, and is much more important than tackling a symptomatic problem in the personality or body. If you raise an individual's amplitude, he will live more fully and express himself more fully, and is less likely to get ill.

There are just two vibrational frequencies that you really need to know: Jewels and Streams are constrictive, Flowers and Shakers are expansive. Understanding these two polarities is one of the keys to understanding to Rayid. The more fibers there are in the eye, the greater the tendency for the person to have Stream- or Jewel-type experiences. The lower the density of fibers, the more the person is likely to have Flower- or Shaker-like experiences. The more you can "see through" the eye, the more expansive the personality is.

Everyone has all four personality types within them. We all learn and communicate in all four of these modes, although we tend to use one more than others. The conscious personality, the dominant mode, is almost always the one represented by the constitutional structure of the iris. For example, if you have brown dots in your iris, your conscious personality is expressed primarily through analysis and words. The other three modes of learning and communicating are still there, but in the unconscious personality. One of the goals of the Rayid Method is to get all four of these inner personalities operating simultaneously in such a way that there is a harmonic rhythm between them, a synergistic fusion. Studying Rayid helps you to understand the mechanics of the system, so that you can objectively observe the interplay between the conscious and unconscious personalities. This helps you to bring all of them into the light where they can fuse and create a well-rounded, balanced personality living in the fullness of health.

A useful metaphor for this is to describe the structure of the eye as being representative of someone's vehicle, like a car. A car has four wheels, like four different iris structures. If the car is out of alignment, one of the wheels may well be tracking straighter than the other three. Similarly, most people have a tendency to operate from only one subpersonality, to drive primarily on one wheel at a time, without even knowing it. It becomes quite comfortable. Because they are driving mainly on one wheel and less on the other three, they wear out some parts of their personality, mind or body more than others.

Each personality type has different characteristic needs for nutritional healing programs, different forms of bodywork and other therapies, different types of affirmations, and different ways of gaining access to the unconscious. The ultimate goal, however, is always the same: to balance the physical vehicle, so that it can experience its true nature.

Each of the four constitutional types has an important contribution to make within one person (as a subpersonality) and within a social, family or community situation (as a member of the group). Each person has something special to offer, and each constitutional type within a person has something special to offer to the "vehicle," the personality, allowing it to experience something beyond the limitations of genetically predetermined behavior. Observing an awake Jewel and an awake Flower, it can be hard to tell them apart. It is possible to move beyond the personality.

COMBINATION STRUCTURES

In addition to the four primary iris structures and their associated personalities, there are a number of combination structures referred to in the Rayid Method. We have already discussed the way in which the energy of the Jewel and the Flower combine to make the Shaker and the Stream, each of which is attracted to its polar opposite. Other combinations are created in a similar way.

The strongest polarity, by far, is the one created by the tension between the Flower and the Jewel. Every person in the world has a tendency to fall onto one side of the balance scale or the other. They are going to be either some kind of an emotional type or some kind of a mental type, in varying degrees, even if their primary iris structure is that of a Shaker or a Stream. The resulting combinations are actually much more common than any of the four primary structures. Shakers and Streams usually have either Flower or Jewel characteristics as a *secondary structure* but the *predominant influence*.

Although there are other variations, the four most common combination structures are Shaker-Jewel, Shaker-Flower, Stream-Jewel and Stream-Flower. Each of these combination structures has its characteristic personality pattern and life history, just as do the primary structures. The most noticeable personality components will be those of the Jewel or the Flower, however. It is really worthwhile to develop a good understanding of the mental type and the emotional type, since virtually everyone is primarily one or the other.

With a little bit of practice, you will quickly learn to recognize whether a person is more like a Flower or more like a Jewel. With Shakers, remember that jewels are proportionately much more influential than flowers; with a few jewels in key positions (see *Positions in the Iris*), an otherwise Flower-like eye will be interpreted as a Shaker-Jewel. With Streams, you should interpret the eyes as being Flower-like if the network of iris fibers is loose or open, as Jewel-like if the fibers are dense, tightly-knit or have patches of color.

As with the descriptions of primary iris structures, the following personality profiles are archetypes. A person's actual behavior will be modified by hemispheric function, rings, individual trigger positions in the iris and the degree of introversion or extroversion.

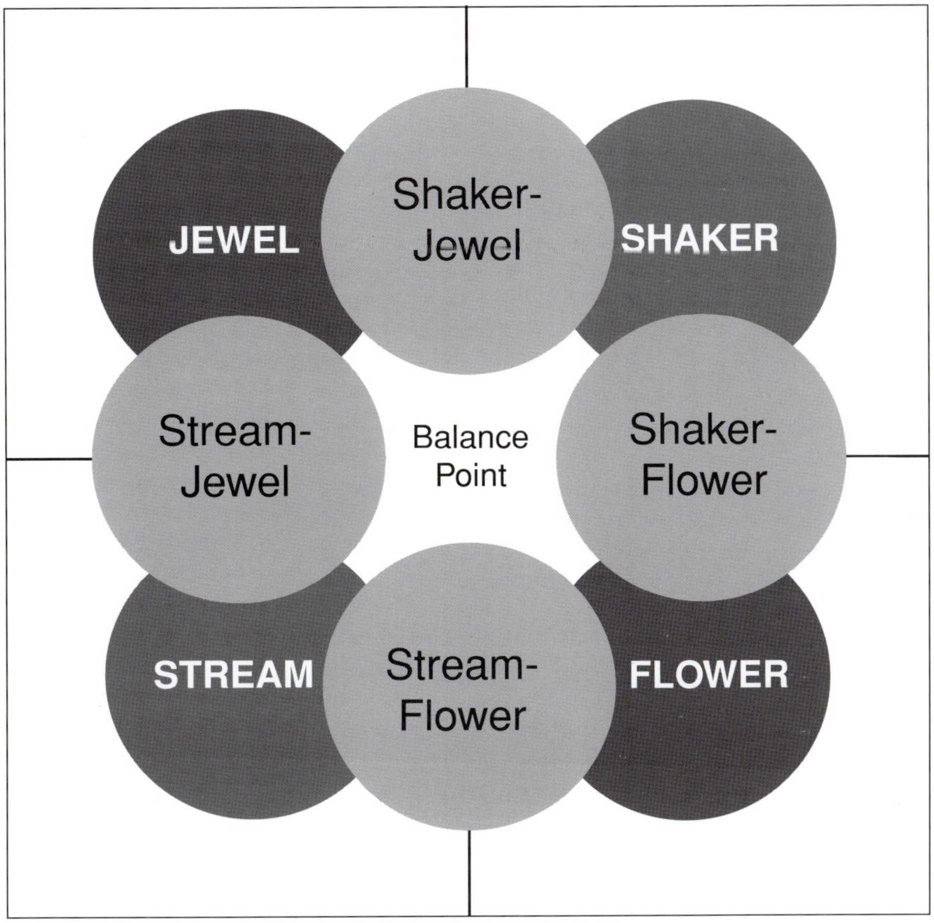

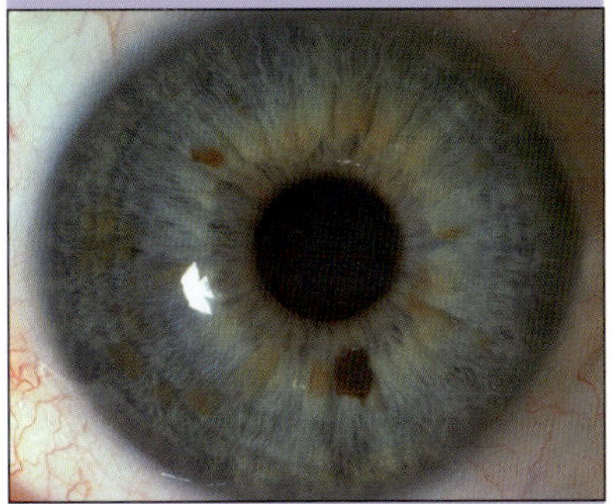

Stream–Jewel

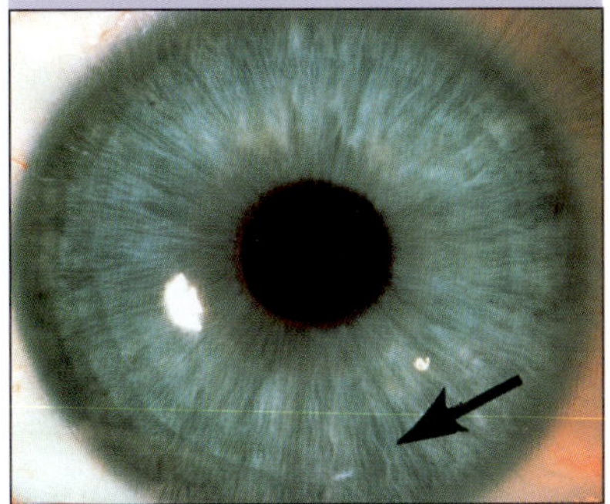

Stream–Flower

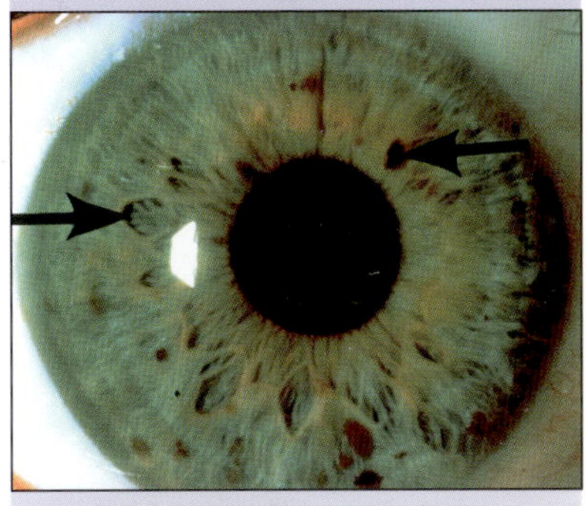

Shaker–Jewel

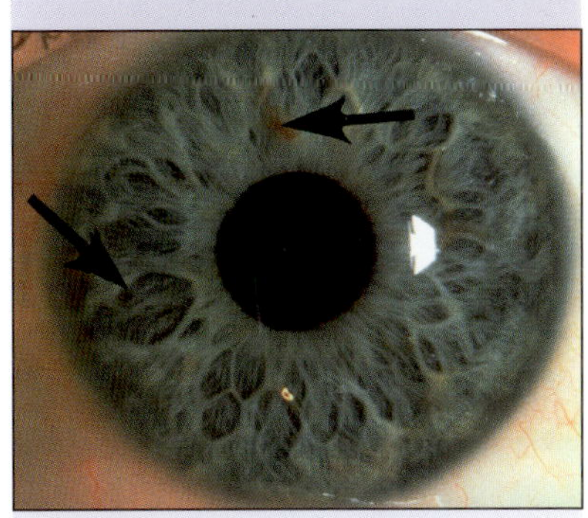

Shaker–Flower

The diagram (left) shows the relationship between the primary and secondary structures.

SHAKER-JEWEL

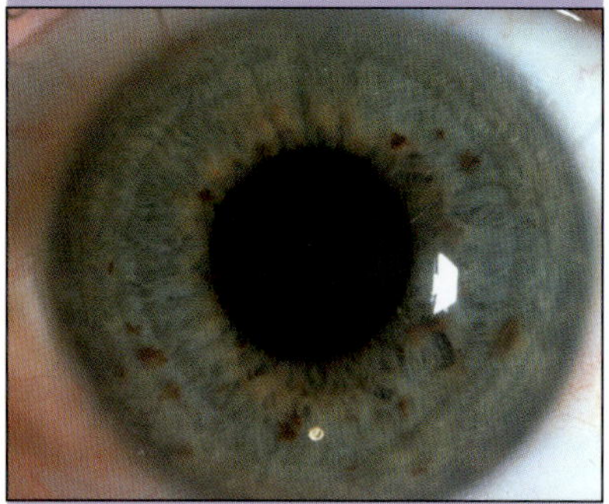

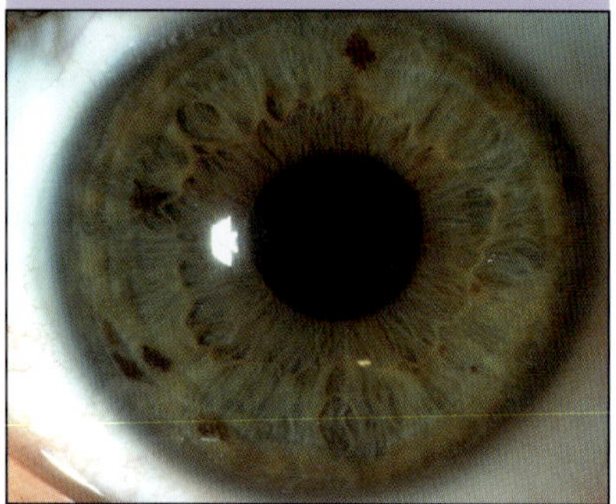

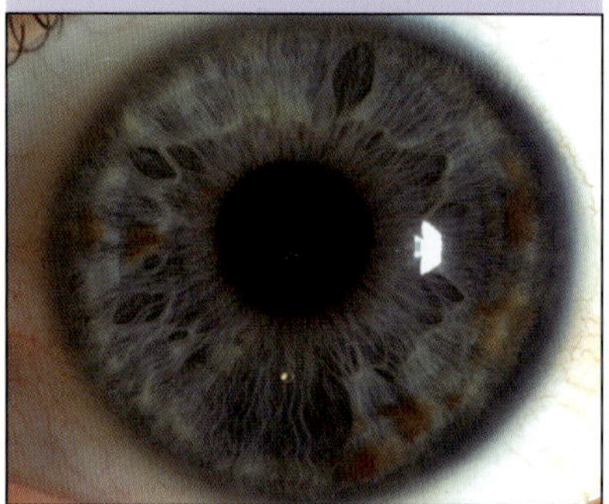

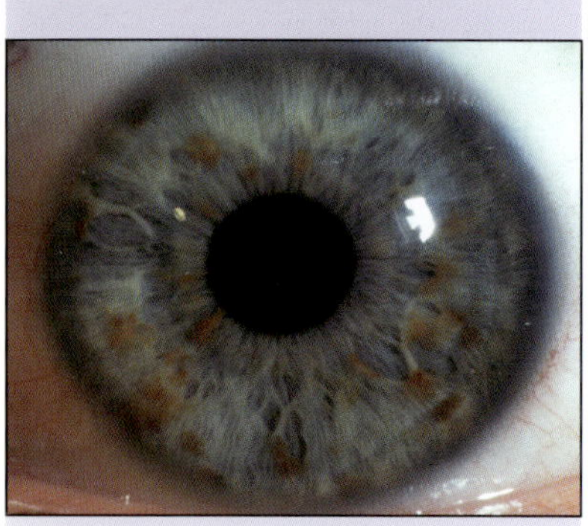

Four examples of Shaker-Jewel irises (above).

A Shaker with more dot-like pigments than flowers in the iris will behave, in many ways, like a Jewel. Like the outcast who breaks away from everything and seeks personal union with the infinite, Shaker-Jewels seldom walk the normal paths of life. Individualistic and self-reliant, these strong-willed people are often leaders of progressive thought or directed action.

Tenacious, dynamic and goal-oriented, Shaker-Jewels overcome obstacles with detailed analysis and strength of personal will. Synergistic communicators and excellent thinkers, they make superior scientists, philosophers and leaders. They are known for venturing far beyond the limits of conventional beliefs, creating pathways for the rest of society to follow. Far-sighted and prophetic, Shaker-Jewels are typically so future-oriented that they are often not appreciated in their own time.

Of all the structures, this one is the true revolutionary, the rock on the windshield, shattering the system. Rebelling against authority, abhorring established systems and structures, the Shaker-Jewel yearns for personal and global freedom. Former Soviet General Secretary Mikhail Gorbachev is a Shaker-Jewel. And, although we don't know what his iris structure was, former US President Lincoln, who fought for the emancipation of the slaves, had all the qualities associated with this structure. Shaker-Jewels are the iconoclasts and harbingers who are either ousted (like Gorbachev) or shot (like Lincoln) for their farsightedness, even though society later upholds their vision.

Shaker-Jewels aren't afraid of the unknown on the contrary, like the once-exalted explorer, Columbus, or like the crew of the USS Enterprise in the *Star Trek* television series, they boldly go in search of it. What they do fear, however, is loss of freedom, lack of fulfillment, dying with unfinished business. Imagine Daniel Boone, the American frontiersman, living out his life in an apartment complex and you have just pictured the Shaker-Jewel's worst nightmare. He is afraid of closeness, afraid of intimacy, afraid of being trapped. A classic *puer aeternus*, the Shaker-Jewel is attracted to the vigor of youth, the innocence of children and to endless change, making it difficult for him to choose from among the many options in life.

The Shaker-Jewel personality is given to extremes. Usually direct and abrupt, his shadow self is evasive and has a tendency to lie. While he usually fights for popular causes like saving the whales or saving the children, the Shaker-Jewel also loves conquest and war. Having such an extreme personality *can* allow him to see both sides of an issue, however.

Driven to understand and explain the world they live in, Shaker-Jewels have excuses, opinions and answers for everything. They are fascinated by words, concepts and philosophies. They have a tendency to be distant, lost in thought, and can become so wrapped up in their mental world that they forget to feed themselves. Like the mythical character Icarus, who got so excited by his new wings that he flew too close to the sun and perished, their minds have a tendency to outstrip the ability of their bodies to keep up. To realize their goals, they need to learn how to delegate responsibility while staying grounded, connected with life and surrendering to their inner guidance.

Usually right-brained, attracted to their mothers and with a feeling of early childhood abuse from their fathers, Shaker-Jewels often grow up nurturing women and other children. They develop their individuality early on they typically have issues with authority and hate being controlled. They usually reach their prime in their mid-40s. They are naturally solitary, even if they try to ignore this fact, and if they aren't comfortable with aloneness by the time they reach 45, they typically go into a panic or become reclusive.

Female-oriented, sensitive and caring, a Shaker-Jewel male moving from left to right will have no trouble finding a girlfriend. His tendency to be self-absorbed, distant and cool, however, can make it difficult for a woman to stay with him, and many Shaker-Jewels are loners. What Shaker-Jewels really crave in a relationship is to be understood, allowed to be who they are, to be emotionally and physically supported instead of forced to fit into a mold.

Eyes with just a few jewels and a lot of flowers will be interpreted differently depending on the exact location of the jewels. If they are in major trigger positions (see *Positions in the Iris*), the jewels can dominate the flower traits, and you should interpret the person as a Shaker-Jewel, even if the jewels are quite small. However, if the jewels are in less influential positions, and if the iris fibers are very open, then the Shaker is probably a Shaker-Flower, even if the few jewels in the eyes are quite large. There is no substitute for experience in making interpretations!

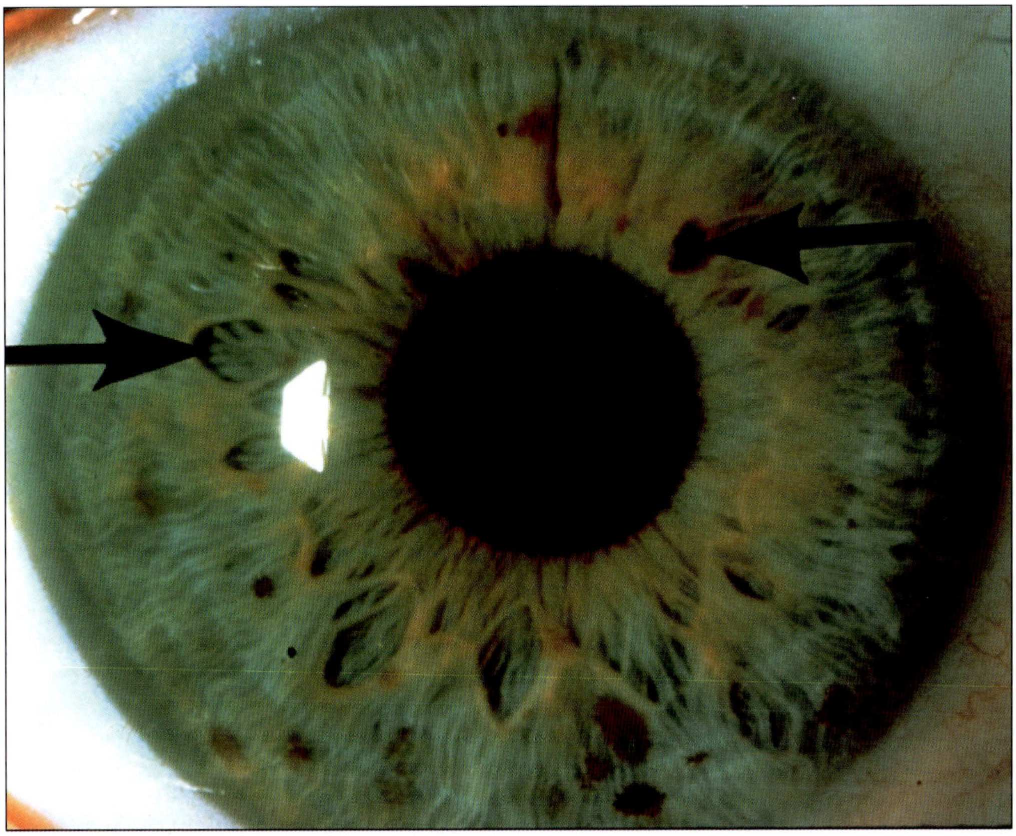

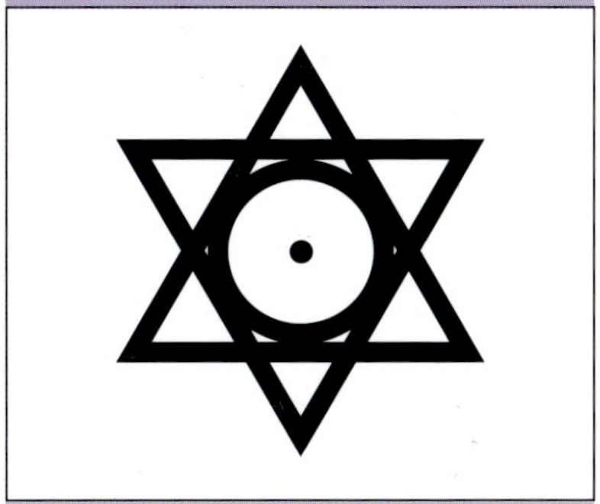

This symbol graphically represents the dynamism and precise focus of the Shaker-Jewel.

Summary of Shaker-Jewel Characteristics

Iris traits:	Dot-like pigments and curved/rounded openings (see text)
Personality:	Tenacious, individualistic, strong-willed, analytical, progressive
Essence/Unique gift:	Original insight
Gestures/Postures:	Dynamic and controlled
Perspective:	I, we (1st and 3rd person)
Gifts/Skills:	Clarity, attention to detail, prophetic leadership, motivated direction
Lessons:	Social empathy, allowing, simplicity, grounded flow
Learning (subconscious):	Through body experience and visually
Communication (conscious):	Synergistic and intense, both verbal and visual
Family relationships:	Closer to mother/sister in childhood, problems with father/brother
Mate relationships:	Stream-Flower
Activities/Disposition:	Individual sports, conceptual and seeking
Energy pattern/Direction:	Build and direct energy
Sleep:	Primarily on their left side, with partner on their right
Fears:	Criticism, being controlled, loss of freedom
Adaptation:	Melancholic, reclusive
Stress imbalance:	Reckless, ruthless, sarcastic, messiah complex

Transformational Pathway

Positive expression:	Seek and lead
If blocked, they are:	Interruptive and demanding
If they learn to:	Be compassionate
They experience:	Illumination
Achieving a state of:	Bliss

SHAKER-FLOWER

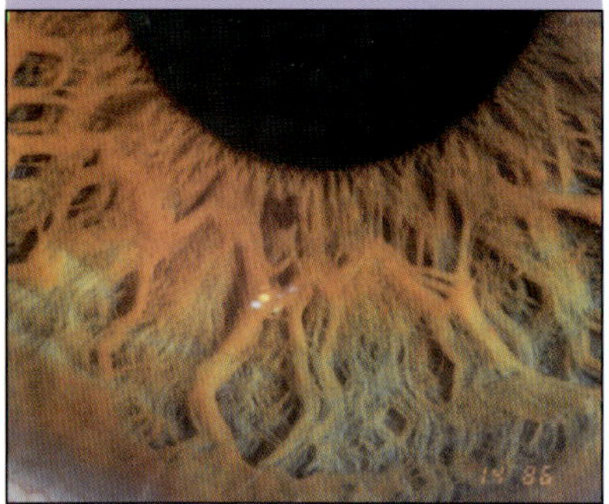

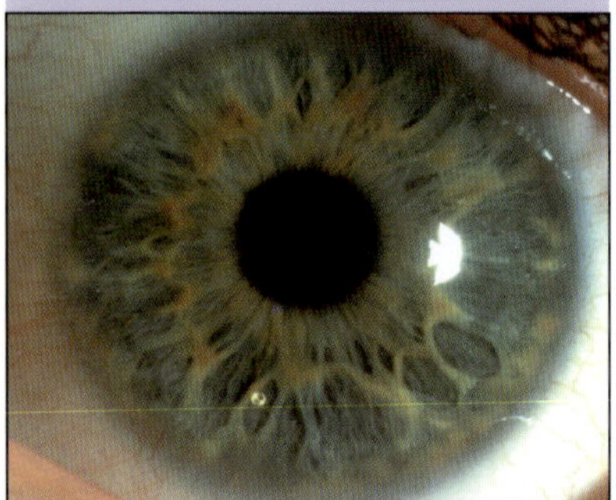

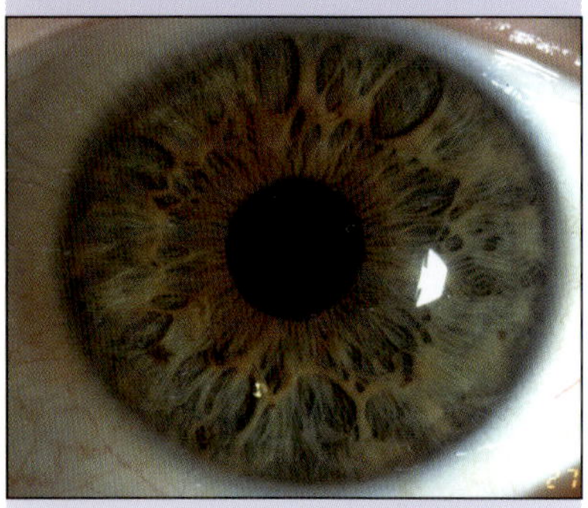

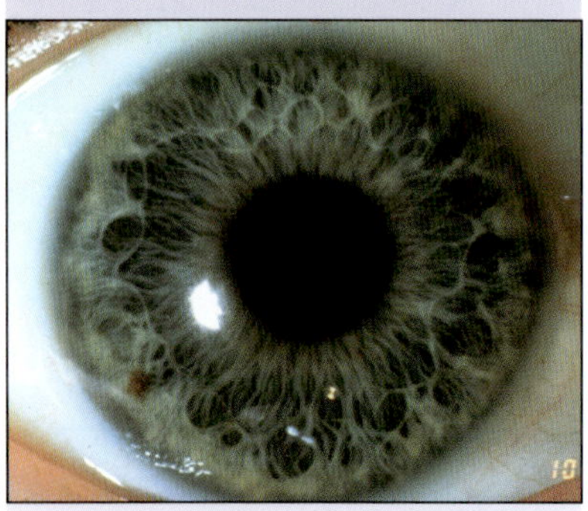

Four examples of Shaker-Flower irises (above).

If a Shaker iris has a predominance of rounded openings in the fibers, this will amplify the emotional tendencies, making the person behave more like a Flower.

With flashy imagination, radical insight and endless energy, Shaker-Flowers often lead the march of progress or conscience. Dynamic communicators, demonstrative and charismatic, they easily inspire groups with their visionary fervor. Easily distracted, they tend to do too many things at once and have a tendency to become depleted.

Shaker-Flowers yearn for recognition and generally like to be in the public eye. Consequently, they are attracted to the media, the arts, music, in fact any activity in which they are likely to be seen by others. They like systems, visual displays, social networks and the worlds of politics and economics. Comfortable in groups, they find it easy to engage in networking to their own advantage. They can immediately grasp the big picture in any situation but are less interested in the details. They make good social and political visionaries, interior designers and spontaneous flower arrangers. Give them the pieces of a system in disarray and they will reassemble it into a new whole that is better than the original.

As with all Shakers, the Shaker-Flower personality is given to extremes. In some cases physically and emotionally aggressive, even emotionally dictatorial, Shaker-Flowers can also be playful, happy, entertaining and light. They are the cheerleaders of life, encouraging others with their own dynamism. More traditional Shaker-Flowers are often attracted to the military as an outlet for their particular combination of aggression, enthusiasm and leadership qualities.

Shaker-Flowers are particularly prone to mood swings; they can be dynamically happy and expressive one moment, then equally depressive the next. They want to help the world but can be blaming, cynical and deeply disappointed in other people. They can be extremely generous or equally selfish and greedy. Sometimes this split shows itself in an automatic tendency to grab things for themselves, followed by a desire to give what they have acquired to the world, to be seen as a generous, almost Santa-Claus-like figure. A fear of poverty is often linked to this tendency toward acquisitiveness.

Intensely passionate, emotional people, Shaker-Flowers are equally capable of blocking the experience of feeling inside themselves. When this happens, their bodies harden and they tend to develop problems with the right shoulder, neck, knees, heart and kidney. This emotional block is usually the root cause of any tendency to be *continually* blaming, attacking, depressive or despondent. When balanced, Shaker-Flowers are unlikely to get stuck in depressive behavior.

To exist in the heart of passion and yet maintain poise is their ultimate challenge and also their grandest reward.

Usually from the father's side of the family, Shaker-Flowers often have an Anger pattern in the left eye that usually shows itself in difficult relationships with women and, in particular, the mother. Although they are too independent to be overtly clingy, Shaker-Flowers have a fear of abandonment, of being alone, that can make them quite manipulative in relationships. Other common fears include a fear of the unknown, of the dark, of suffocating or of drowning.

Both male and female Shaker-Flowers usually get along best with men; in the male, however, this is often particularly noticeable; in the workplace, his Anger pattern with women means that he has a tendency to treat them as if they are relatively insignificant. The Shaker-Flower female tends to be quite competitive at work, engaging in one-upmanship. In mate relationships, whether she expresses it or not, the Shaker-Flower female has a tendency to manipulate men to get what she wants, using subtle, feminine wiles. She typically becomes the matriarch of the family, although she may remain "second-in-command" behind the male head of the household. In both males and females, the quest for control of themselves and others can have its parallel in the development of fine motor skills and good physical coordination.

Shaker-Flowers usually reach their peak in their late 20s to mid-30s. If they aren't in a position of power/leadership by the time they reach their 40s, they may have a severe mid-life crisis that can take them into alcoholism and a tendency to reminisce about the "good old days." As they get older, Shaker-Flowers tend to develop high blood pressure, arthritis and swaybacks, and males have a higher-than-usual tendency to go bald.

Read the comments under the Shaker-Jewel description regarding the correct interpretation of Flower or Jewel tendencies in a Shaker iris.

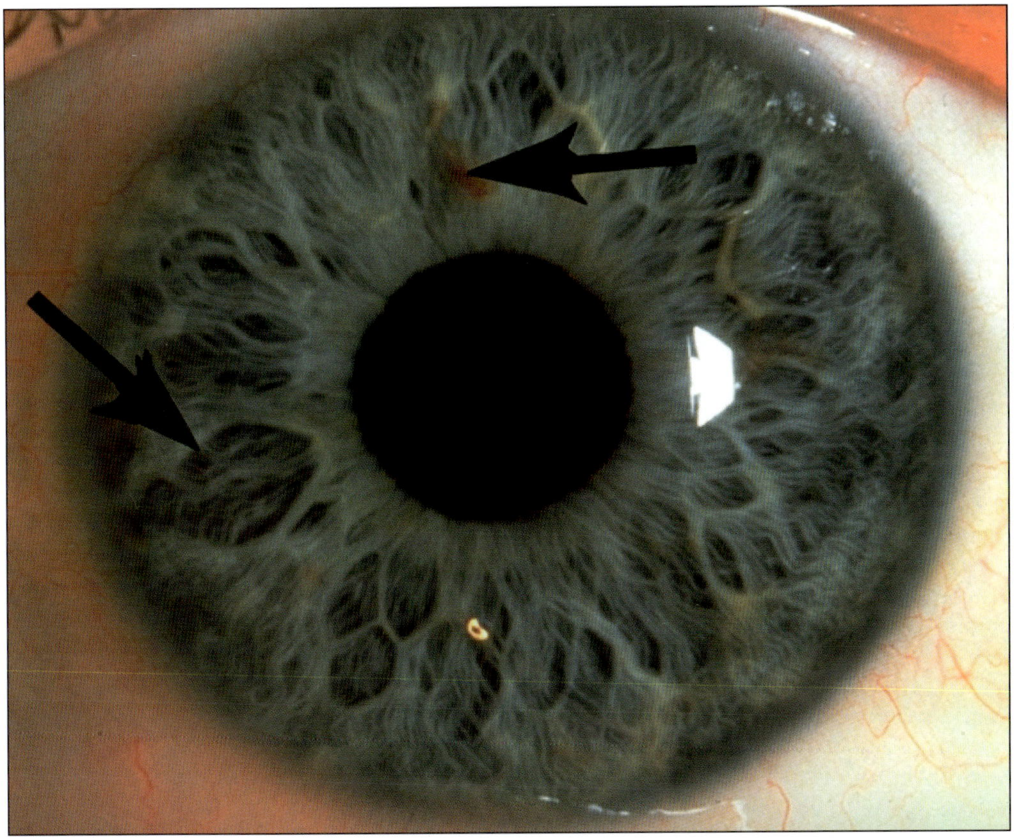

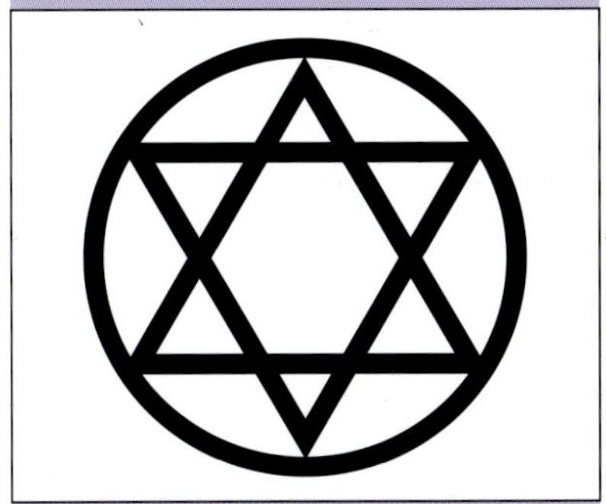

This symbol graphically represents the dynamism and openness of the Shaker-Flower.

Summary of Shaker-Flower Characteristics

Iris traits:	Curved/rounded openings and dot-like pigments (see text)
Personality:	Emotional, expressive, radical
Essence/Unique gift:	Visionary passion
Gestures/Postures:	Dynamic and animated
Perspective:	You, they (2nd and 4th person)
Gifts/Skills:	Inspiration, creativity, compassion, facilitating group dynamics
Lessons:	Physical control, use of power, focused attention
Learning (subconscious):	Through body experience and auditorily
Communication (conscious):	Synergistic and animated, both verbal and visual
Family relationships:	Closer to fathor/brother, problems with mother/sister
Mate relationships:	Stream-Jewel
Activities/Disposition:	Social entertaining, playful
Energy pattern/Direction:	Move and release energy
Sleep:	Primarily on their right side, with partner on their left
Fears:	Abandonment, separation, suffocation, unknown
Adaptation:	Detailed, methodical, compulsive
Stress imbalance:	Selfish, evasive, blaming

Transformational Pathway

Positive expression:	Exhilaration
If blocked, they are:	Cynical
If they learn to:	Be still, focus, show concern
They experience:	Unification, belonging
Achieving a state of:	Ecstasy

STREAM-JEWEL

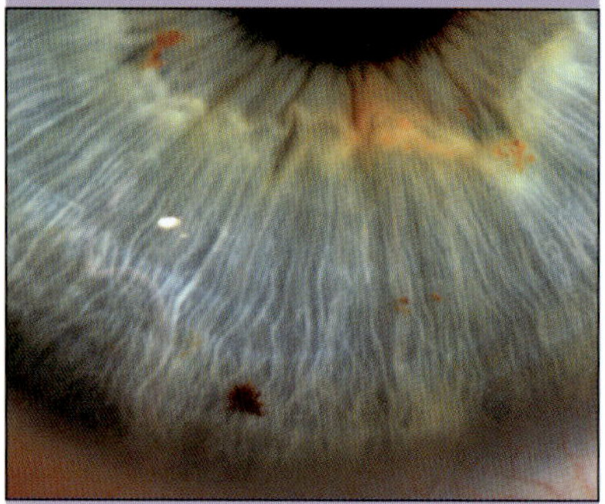

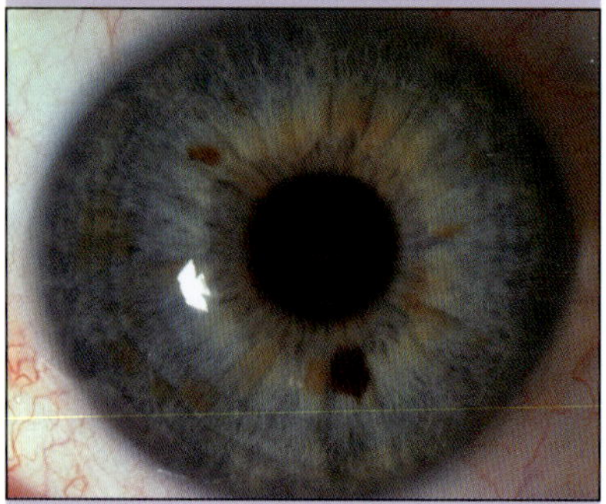

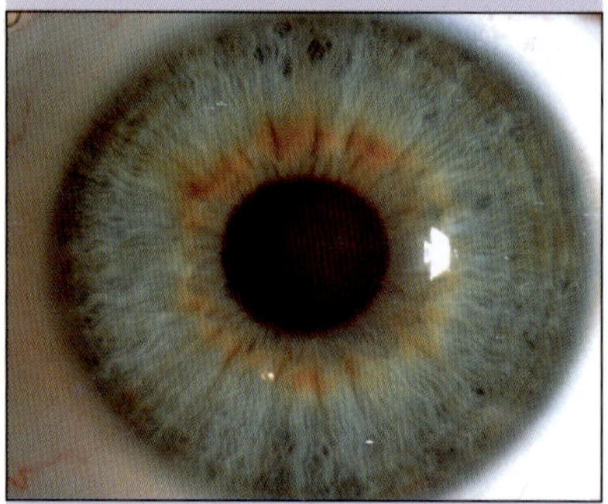

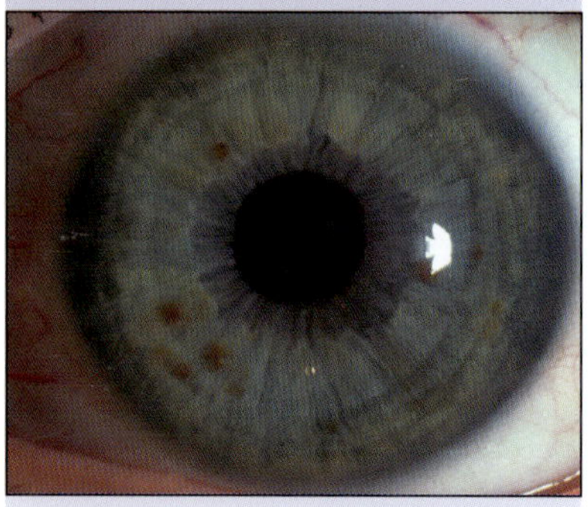

Four examples of Stream-Jewel irises (above).

The presence of small or very few dot-like pigments in a predominantly kinesthetic type of iris will accentuate that person's mental tendencies. Sensitive and alert, these clear thinkers lead the way to balance and stability.

Showing genuine concern for others, Stream-Jewels extend their presence to embrace all around them with a sense of security. Communicating with caring words and controlled body language, they offer a sense of support and gentleness that soothes the wounds of society. With the ability to unify thoughts, they extend their presence into a group, leading it to cohesiveness. Their insight and stability is useful in any social or work situation, and their natural skills with people make them supreme healers, teachers and managers.

Stream-Jewels have an ongoing need to comprehend and explain things, and have a habit of collecting information as supporting evidence. They are the kind of people who have subscriptions to three daily newspapers and hold onto interesting articles for 20 years. Natural gatherers and synthesizers, Stream-Jewels can become hoarders and system addicts. These "pack rats of consciousness" tend to collect reams of data about systems that they believe will improve their lives, whether that is a system of healing or teaching or simply another system for organizing all of their information! They then figure out which system works best by doing a systematic evaluation so as to fairly compare the alternatives. They like to have the cream of the crop; if information is meal, they don't just get to the nitty-gritty of things, they grind it up into a fine flour. These information junkies eventually try to synthesize all of the systems they have collected into a system of their own.

Like a huge glacier, Stream-Jewels are generally slow-changing and certain. They seldom take big risks and don't make decisions hastily. This structure is sometimes referred to as the bureaucratic, committee type. Their glacial slowness is also reflected in a tendency to have problems with blood circulation to the periphery, and they typically have cold hands and feet. In some cases, these circulation issues cause them to be dizzy and forgetful.

Consolidating and domestic, these nesters generally provide nurturing through touch and information. They are naturally mothering, the complete opposite of the domineering, matriarchal or patriarchal Shaker-Flowers. Walking libraries, Stream-Jewels make excellent teachers because of their fascination with knowledge and their love for the spontaneity of children. In traditional cultures, the wise woman of the village is often a Stream-Jewel, exuding a quality reminiscent of Mother Earth becoming curious about the mind. If they learn to loosen up, Stream-Jewels can do well in public relations and sales, serving their accounts well. Being interactive and social helps to animate them, making them more expressive and feelingful.

Stream-Jewels have a tendency to interrupt, and to be out of touch with their own feelings. Quietly restless, they can be chatterboxes when given free rein to express their opinions. Subject to worry, concern and being overburdened, Stream-Jewels need spontaneity in their lives.

Usually from the mother's side of the family, with a fear of criticism from father, Stream-Jewels often have an associated fear of making mistakes. This gives them a strong need to be right, and they have a tendency to see other people as inadequate. Attracted to Shaker-Flowers for long-term relationships, Stream-Jewels tend to be caring but closed with their partners. They typically consider themselves to be more intelligent than other people, and tend to take the lead in their partnerships. In women, this doubly constricted structure tends to give them masculine qualities, and they can have issues with their femininity. When imbalanced, they can become domineering, nagging mothers, the opposite of their natural expression. Stream-Jewels are usually particularly interested in spiritual or relationship rituals (see the *Therapies* chapter).

They need to learn to surrender, to let go of control. Learning to allow will ease the Stream-Jewel's frustration with carrying the mental burdens of others, leading to the experience of wholeness and embodied understanding. At their most balanced, Stream-Jewels are caring, nurturing and all-knowing while retaining simplicity and a quality of innocence.

The density of fiber in a Stream iris indicates the level of Jewelness, so a very dense Stream would be classified as a Stream-Jewel, even if there are no distinct dot-like pigments visible in the eye.

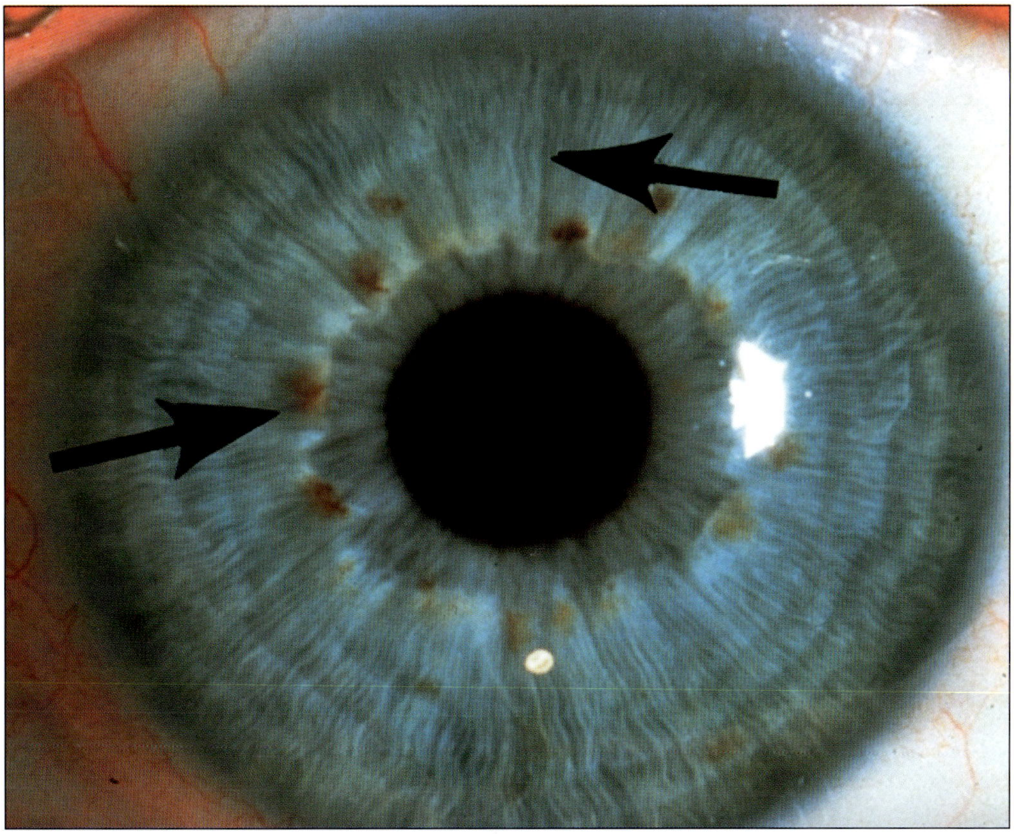

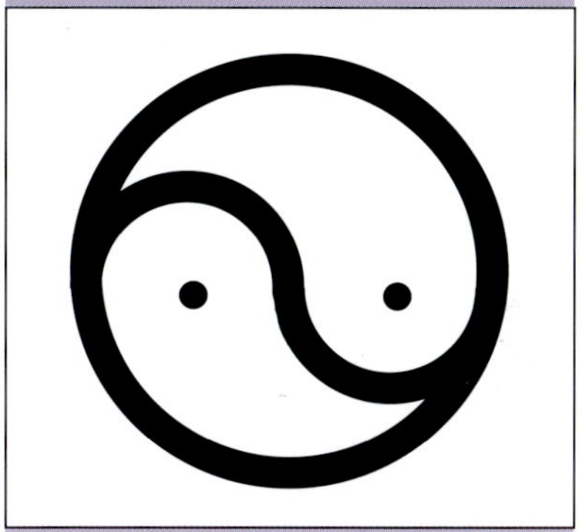

This symbol graphically represents the stability and alert sensitivity of the Stream-Jewel.

Summary of Stream-Jewel Characteristics

Iris traits:	Straight iris fibers; a few dot-like pigments may be visible
Personality:	Sensitive, alert, intuitive, analytical
Essence/Unique gift:	Physically and mentally nurturing
Gestures/Postures:	Controlled and subtle
Perspective:	I, we (1st and 3rd person)
Gifts/Skills:	Strength, healing
Lessons:	Receptivity, surrender, allowing
Learning (subconscious):	Visually and by doing
Communication (conscious):	Kinesthetic and auditory, using touch and words
Family relationships:	Closer to mother/sister in childhood, problems with father/brother
Mate relationships:	Shaker-Flower
Activities/Disposition:	Information addicts, caring
Energy pattern/Direction:	Build and channel energy
Sleep:	Primarily on their left side, with partner on their right
Fears:	Change, mistakes
Adaptation:	Spacey, ungrounded, irrational
Stress imbalance:	Demanding, impatient

Transformational Pathway

Positive expression:	Caring
If blocked, they are:	Impatient
If they learn to:	Allow
They experience:	Fulfillment
Achieving a state of:	Embodied understanding

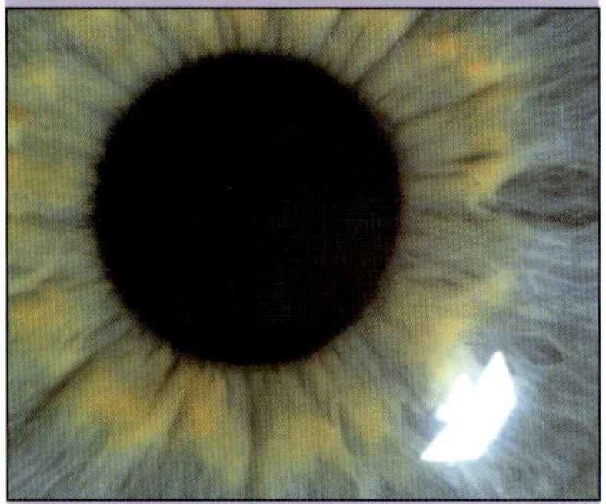

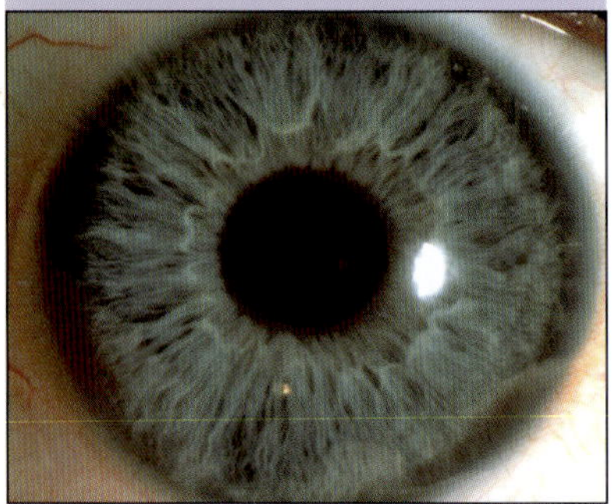

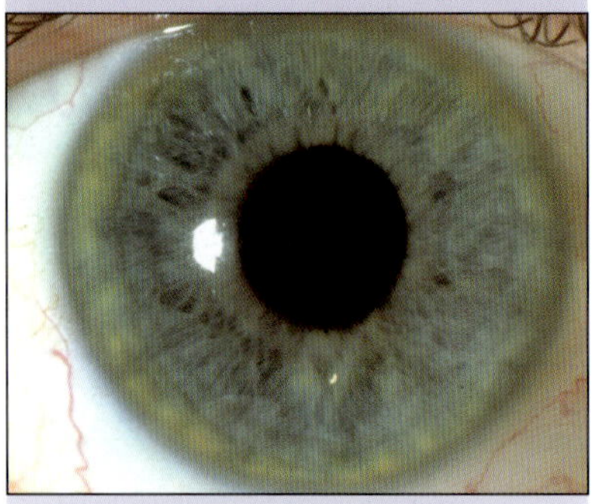

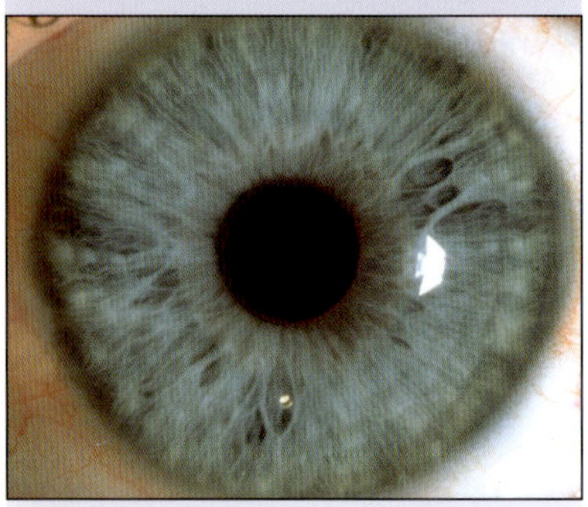

Four examples of Stream-Flower irises (above).

STREAM-FLOWER

A few curved openings or wavy fibers in a predominantly Stream iris will enhance that person's emotional traits. These physically vital individuals tend to be compassionate and responsive.

Combining emotional sensitivity with a natural, physical awareness, Stream-Flowers communicate with other people at a very deep level. Reaching out with tender-hearted calm, they can touch others deeply just with their presence. With quiet ease, they can circulate in a group of people, bringing comfort, stimulation or excitement where it is needed.

Their social connectedness and physical skills make Stream-Flowers exceptionally good performers, athletes and healers. Usually the picture of health and well-being, Stream-Flowers often have the most beautiful bodies. They are very kinesthetic, naturally symmetrical and shapely. Their physical beauty and physical awareness make them well suited to being dancers, gymnasts, models or beauticians. If they do have physical problems, the weak spots in a Stream-Flower tend to be the spine, neck, kidney and, in women, the ovary.

Female Stream-Flowers are the essence of tenderness. Kind, compassionate and warm, they have the quiet enthusiasm of an unblossomed flower. Motherly without being matriarchal, they have the sensuality of the soft, moist earth at twilight and the gentleness of a bunny rabbit, deer or golden retriever. When combined with their physicalness, these qualities make them excellent midwives, gardeners, water-color artists and caretakers of the earth. Exceptional chefs and with an eye for beauty, Stream-Flowers are capable of turning the chores of housework into an art form.

This dove-like being is attracted to the lone wolf, the Shaker-Jewel, for long-term relationships. Touched by flattery and words of appreciation, her inner sense of aloneness and need for security lead her to build a comfortable castle for her partner, hoping that its beauty and peace will encourage him to stay for more than just a while. Male Stream-Flowers, on the other hand, are more likely to take care of themselves, even giving up on women altogether.

These gentle souls have a great deal of strength, too. Usually slightly left-brained as an adaptation to their structure (see next chapter), this gives them some masculine, practical qualities. Materially oriented and goal-oriented, they are attracted to wealth, to the beauty and raw power of horses, and to the quality and elegance of beautifully bound books. They may act emotional, like a Flower, but they have much greater physical prowess.

Of all the iris structures, this is the one that is the most complete, the most stable and effective in life by itself. Stream-Flowers do very well alone but generally tend to follow more than they lead. They want to help people but are not driven and so are quite happy to follow in the wake of a Shaker-Jewel.

Stream-Flowers are not usually the people who originate the great ideas, but are the ones who sustain them in the long run. They are the real workers and achievers, the manifesters and implementers, illuminating the details of the grand plan and carrying it from concept into physical reality. Because of these qualities, this structure is sometimes referred to as the "delivery system of consciousness."

Stream-Flowers are sometimes so sensitive to the social and physical environment that they can lose the certainty of who they are, causing them to feel confused or hurt. Learning detachment will help allay the confusion or self-doubt that comes up when they are overly empathetic with others. Learning the poise and direction that comes from inner "knowing" brings them safely to the completion that they sense around them.

A Stream iris with no distinct dot-like pigments or rounded openings is interpreted as a Stream-Flower if the fibers are very open or wavy, and as a Stream-Jewel if the fibers are more dense and concentrated. In a Stream-Flower iris that has few flowers, or if the flowers are primarily very open, a *distinct* (closed) flower will have particular significance. It carries a lot of charge and may indicate particular volatility around the issue associated with that position, especially if it is in the emotional area of the iris.

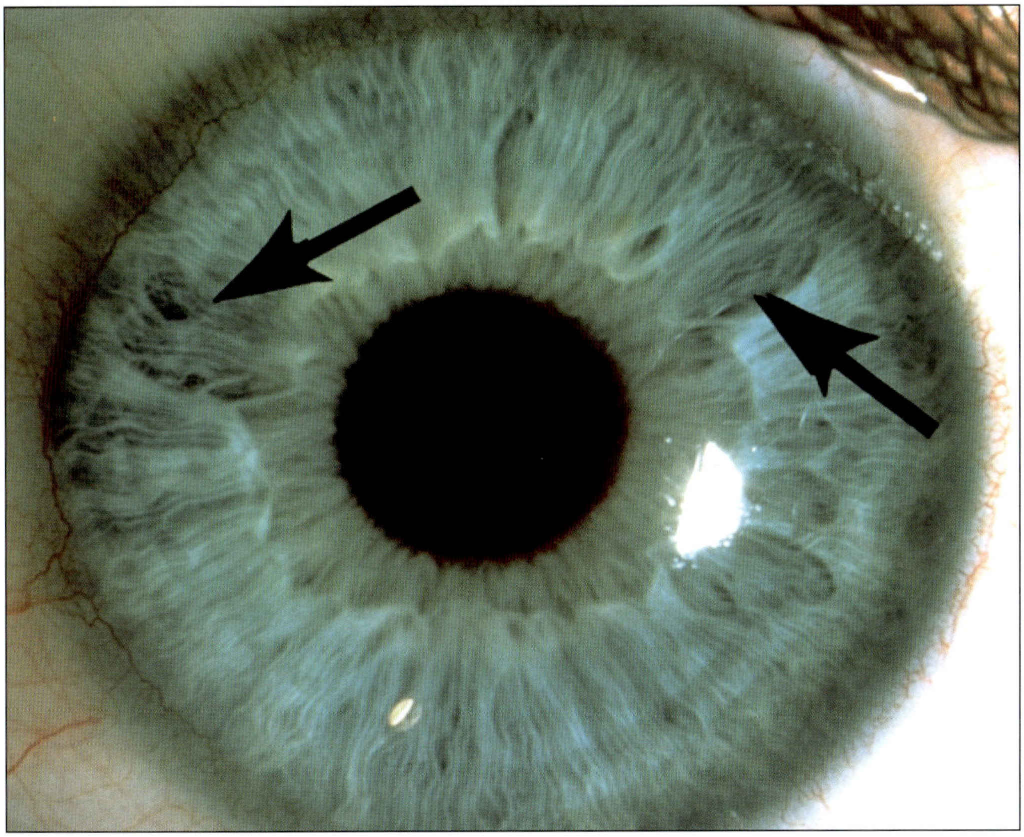

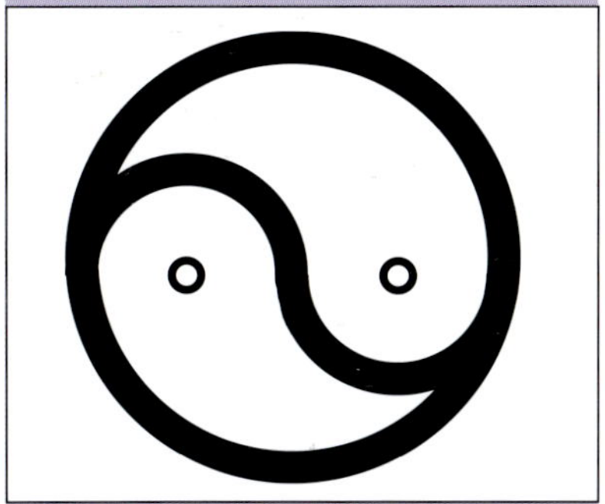

This symbol represents the stability and empathetic approachability of the Stream-Flower.

Summary of Stream-Flower Characteristics

Iris traits:	Straight lines or streaks of color and curved/rounded openings
Personality:	Sensitive, intuitive, emotional
Essence/Unique gift:	Physically creative
Gestures/Postures:	Animated and subtle
Perspective:	You, they (2nd and 3rd person)
Gifts/Skills:	Integration, mediation, healing
Lessons:	Truth, poise, direction
Learning (subconscious):	Auditorily and by doing
Communication (conscious):	Kinesthetic and visual, using images and gestures
Family relationships:	Closer to father/brother, problems with mother/sister
Mate relationships:	Shaker-Jewel
Activities/Disposition:	Physical, nurturing
Energy pattern/Direction:	Containment and flow
Sleep:	Primarily on their right side, with partner on their left
Fears:	Change, poverty, manipulation
Adaptation:	Impulsive, excessively rational, goal-fixated
Stress imbalance:	Neurotic, indecisive, confused

Transformational Pathway

Positive expression:	Compassion
If blocked, they are:	Depressive, angry
If they learn to:	Express choice and act
They experience:	Thankfulness
Achieving a state of:	Elation

Hemispheric Polarity and the Direction of Flow

THE PULSES OF LIFE: OUTWARD AND INWARD

In the Rayid Model, every structure has its opposite. The existence of these opposites creates the likelihood that any given structure will come to understand its lesson and its gift. For example, if you are a mental type, your lesson is to become consciously more like the emotional type, to awaken your ability to be open, *without* suppressing your strong analytical talents. There are many polarities in the Rayid Model, and each one of them has its opposite, its gift and its lesson.

One of the polarity systems, or pulses of life, is that of introversion and extroversion. Whatever your structural type, you are going to have a tendency to hold your personality close to yourself in an introverted (inner-directed) way, or to be more extroverted (outer-directed) in your expression. Introversion and extroversion add depth and substance to the way people handle the energy and vitality that moves through their bodies, with the direction of flow being either inward or outward. Extroverts generally express their sense of superiority over introverts, while introverts tend to be more quietly superior.

These polar opposites are attracted to each other in mate relationships to create harmony and balance. Without its opposite, the life experience of the introvert or the extrovert is lopsided, just as the natural rhythm of breathing in and out falters if either the inhalation or the exhalation is emphasized over the other.

While the constitutional structure of the iris seems to be created exclusively by long-term, genetic patterns that are very difficult to change, the characteristic of introversion or extroversion is only about 90% determined by inheritance. Environmental influences play a part, and fundamental changes in the direction of flow between extroversion and introversion *can* be observed in the eye. This is in sharp contrast to the primary iris structure, which can be added to but not reduced. No change in *fundamental* constitutional structure has been observed in anyone over the age of eight, by which time the primary iris structure is well-established. Flower traits and stream fiber patterns seem to be established prior to birth, while jewels start being added from about the age of two; we even have photographic evidence of individual jewel traits developing in late adulthood. See the *Iris Development* section for more information on this fascinating subject.

About 10% of people have switched at some point in their lives from an inherently introverted nature to extroverted behavior or vice-versa. It appears that the family environment has the effect of allowing or denying the expression of the genetic pattern which determines introversion and extroversion. It is easier to drive an extrovert in than to bring an introvert out, however; sufficient pain is all that is required to drive a person inward.

In any case, introversion and extroversion are more consciously accessible than the primary structures; it is easier to choose to be an extrovert than it is to choose to be a Flower. This could be likened to the process of breathing; although breathing is normally an autonomic activity, it is also possible to consciously regulate the in-breath and the out-breath.

Unlike hemispheric polarity (dealt with later in this chapter), which can radically modify the outer behavior of the individual, introversion and extroversion simply modify the *degree* of expression. What expression there is will still be consistent with the primary structural type.

Ultimately, Rayid aims to give people the ability to *fully* and consciously express the personality characteristics associated with both introversion and extroversion, so that they need not be limited to either mode of expression. To some extent, many people already oscillate back and forth between a personality expression that is slightly more extroverted and one that is slightly more introverted. Being able to fully occupy either mode is simply a matter of harnessing this pulse.

Considerable research is now being done on the subject of introversion and extroversion, and our understanding of this aspect of iris interpretation is currently in transition. It is beginning to become apparent that introversion is primarily determined by the mother's side of the family, while patterns of extroversion are somehow linked to the father's side of the family. It is possible that the tendency toward either introversion or extroversion may be determined by a specific great-great-grandmother. If this is the case, introversion/extroversion may act like a sextant that allows us to pinpoint the origin of the constitutional structure.

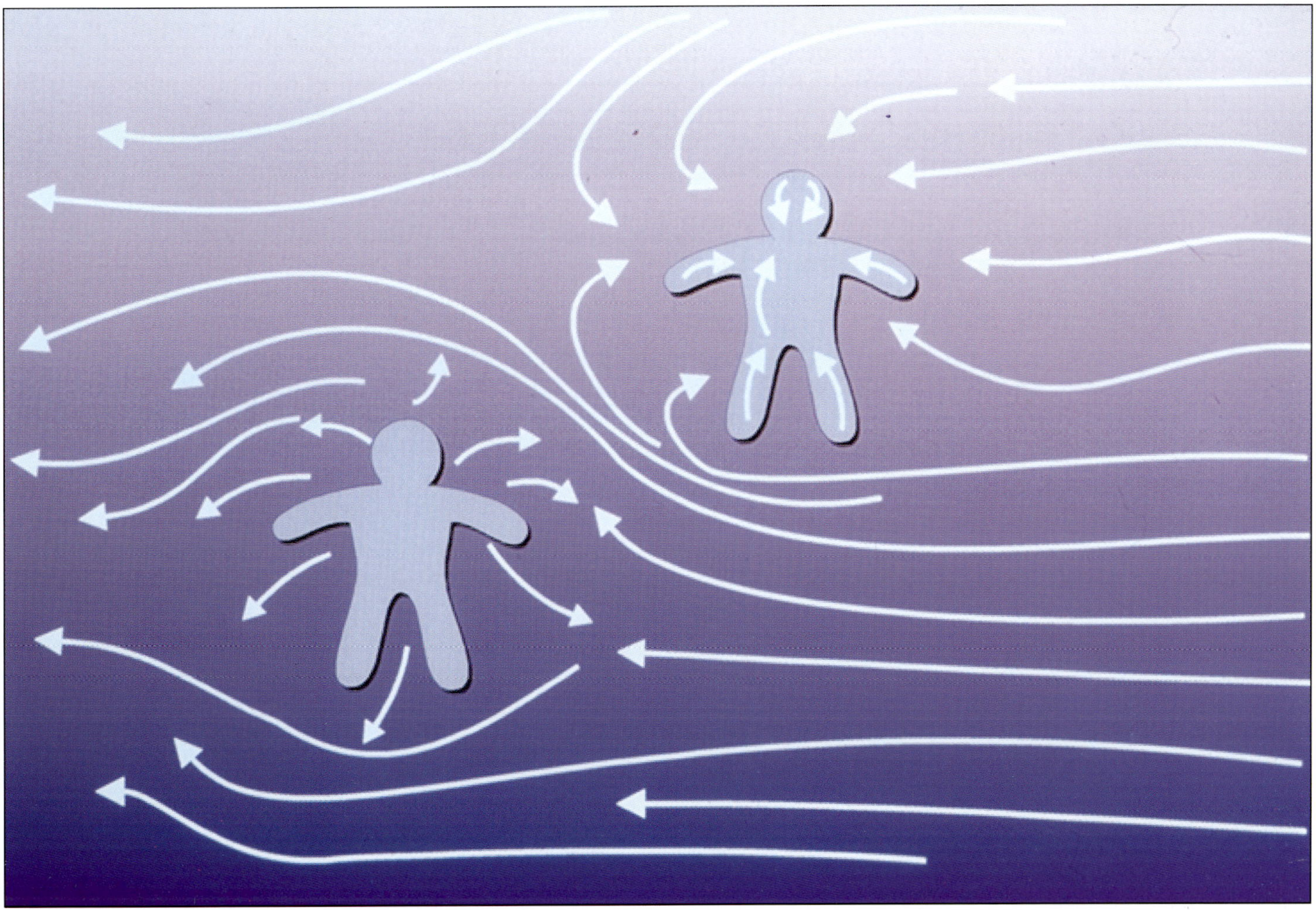

Extroverts deflect and release life energy

Introverts gather and store life energy

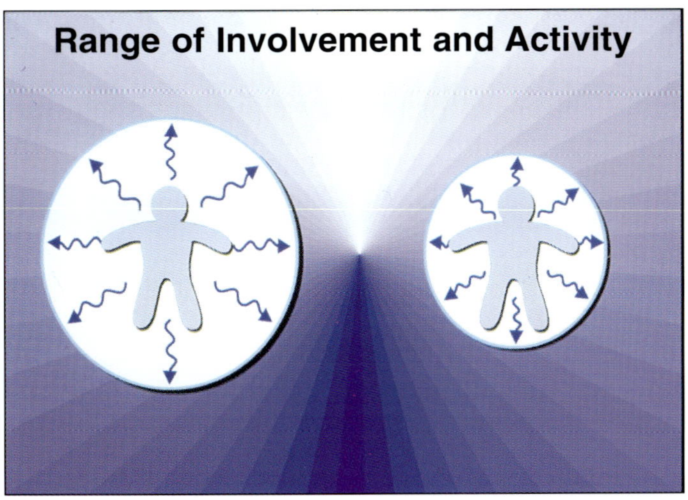

EXTROVERT
Greater range of social influence

INTROVERT
Lesser range of social influence

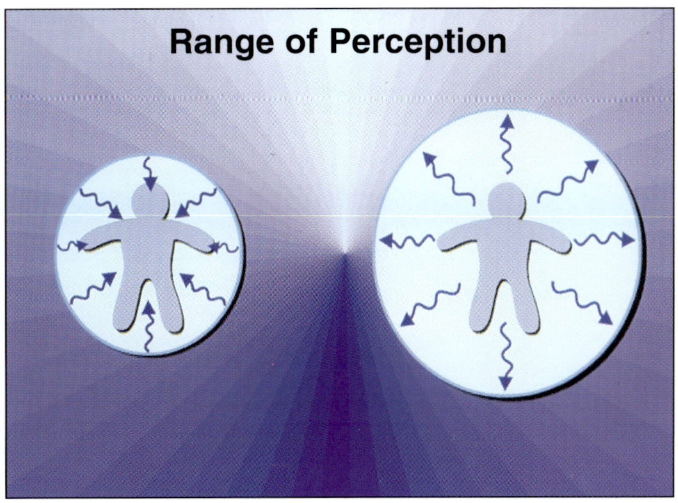

EXTROVERT
"Everyone is looking at me"

INTROVERT
"I am watching everyone"

INTROVERSION

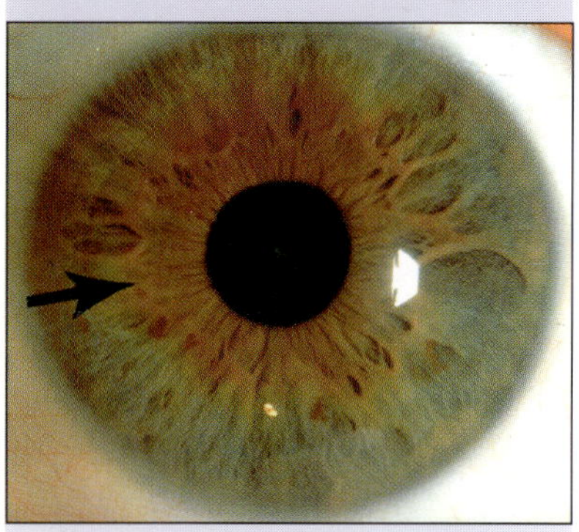

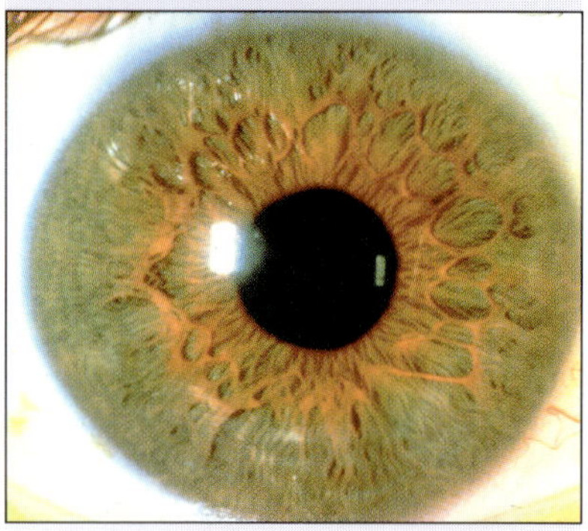

Two examples of extroverts gone in. All introverts have a concentrated band of color encircling the pupil but, in this case, there is also a noticeable Ring of Expression. Color on the inside of that ring indicates a movement inward.

A concentrated band of gold or brown color encircling the pupil signifies an introspective nature. These sensitive individuals tend to be reserved, observant and secretive. By internalizing their thoughts and emotions, they are developing wisdom and building vitality. While genuinely tolerant and understanding of others, they often hide their true feelings behind a facade of congeniality in order to avoid conflict. Without the feeling of release that comes from action and open, honest communication, they can become restless or stagnant.

Their gentle receptivity and willingness to listen makes introverts good counselors, teachers and friends. Introverts are also easier to teach because they are good at both listening and observation. By learning to be more communicative and expressive, inner-directed people can bring their inner fullness and beauty out into the world.

Introversion is the inward movement of emotional and physical vitality. This movement is a consequence of reward systems and attitudes based on inner gratification. Introversion internalizes the expression of any one of the constitutional structures. An introverted Flower, for example, will be less animated than an extroverted Flower; similarly, an introverted Jewel will talk less and use fewer gestures.

Introverts are often secure and happy people, and it is important not to misinterpret their quietness as a sign of insecurity or weakness. Their years of quiet listening and observation have given them a different type of strength. It is from this lifestyle that a deep inner knowing and security develops. Introverts are doing what wise men have been advising us all to do for thousands of years: "Go within." It is from this inward silence that they have developed independence, and they are not easily swayed by the falseness of outer stimulation. Introverts possess the seeds of creativity and the wisdom to use them correctly.

The inward flow of energy into the core of his being creates a channel that leads the introvert to the deeper levels of inspiration, inventiveness and imagination. Introverts are often future-oriented and conceptual. This inward flow also enhances the life force within the body. If this vitality remains unexpressed, however, it can become physically destructive to the body and mind.

Introverts are the "silent majority" in the world, since about 60% of people exhibit some tendency toward this pattern.

In Consultation

It is usually a good experience to interpret the eyes of an introvert. Introverts possess a soft receptivity that enables them to listen to the comments of others. They also seem to be more accepting and genuinely appreciate the half-hidden mysteries within themselves. Their inner calm allows the interpretation to penetrate to depths that are more difficult to reach with an expressive extrovert.

There is something unique about the reservoir of sensitivity within the introvert. Once this reservoir is stirred, many joys and pains can come bubbling to the surface. It is this process of bubbling and release that makes the experience of looking into an introvert's eyes so rewarding and enjoyable.

Depending on the underlying color of the iris, the band of color around the pupil that signifies introversion can make the eye appear green or hazel in color. In a brown eye, it makes the area next to the pupil appear even darker than the rest of the iris.

As the degree of introversion increases, the color intensity of the band also increases. It can range in color from a slight gold ring to a dark orange. If the band is burnt orange or dark brown, the individual will be prone to hyperactivity, incessant chattering and sugar addiction. This hyperactivity is the result of energy building up inside the person, which the body and mind needs to express.

In introverts, the Ring of Expression (see photos and description under *Extroversion*) is either absent or very close to the pupil. In general, the more introverted a person is, the closer the Ring of Expression is to the pupil. This ring also provides a clear indication of any shift between introversion and extroversion in the individual temperament. Such changes usually center around childhood experiences that involve anger, pain or great joy.

When the Ring of Expression is visible and there is a greater degree of coloration between the ring and the pupil, it generally indicates an extroverted temperament that is now moving inward or toward the left brain. A greater intensity of gold or orange *outside* the Ring of Expression usually means that the person had an introverted temperament but is now becoming more extroverted (or right-brained).

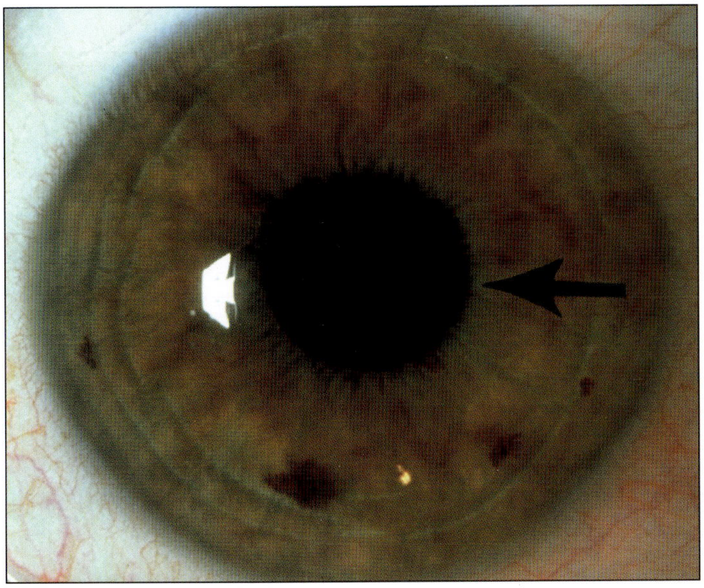

Jewel introvert

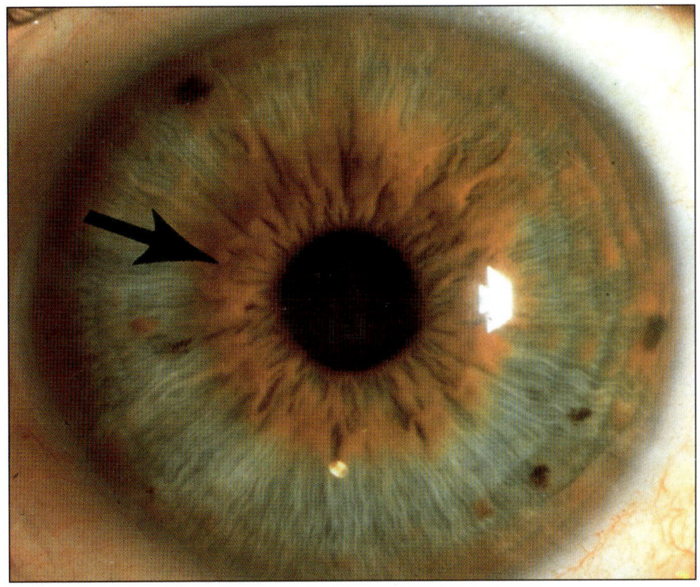

Shaker introvert

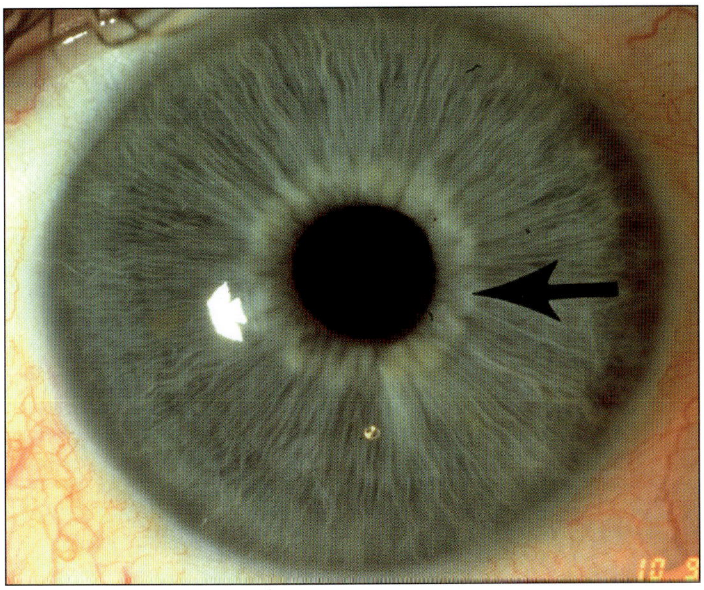

Stream introvert

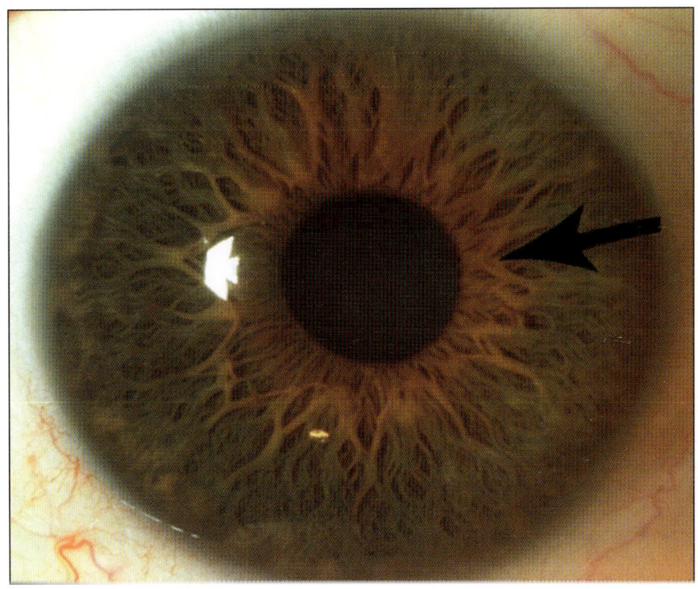

Flower introvert

Characteristics Associated with Introversion

Breathe:	Primarily through the nose, slowly
Energy pattern:	Build and store internal energy
Essence:	Sensitive, congenial, tolerant, insightful, conceptual
Communication style:	Quiet and observant
Gestures:	Less animated, more contained
Behavioral effects:	Decreases communication Increases sensitivity Increases wisdom
Professions:	Teaching, counseling, design
Gifts:	Stability, empathy, integration, appreciation
Lessons to be learned:	Self-expression, truthfulness, decisiveness

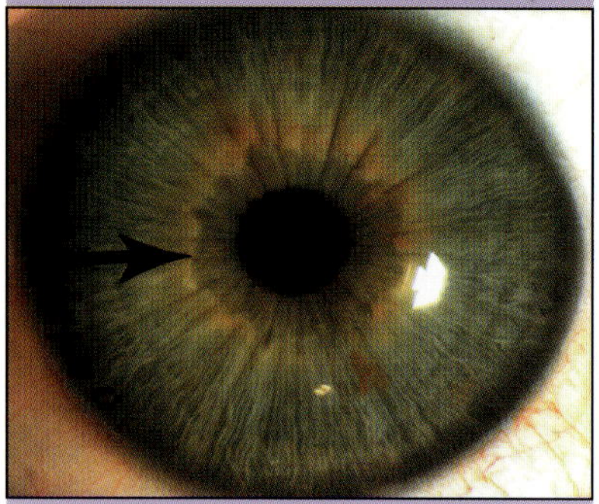

Two examples of introverts gone out. There is color on the outside of the Ring of Expression, indicating a movement outward. Similarly, any *clearing* on the inside of the Ring also indicates a movement outward, away from the pupil.

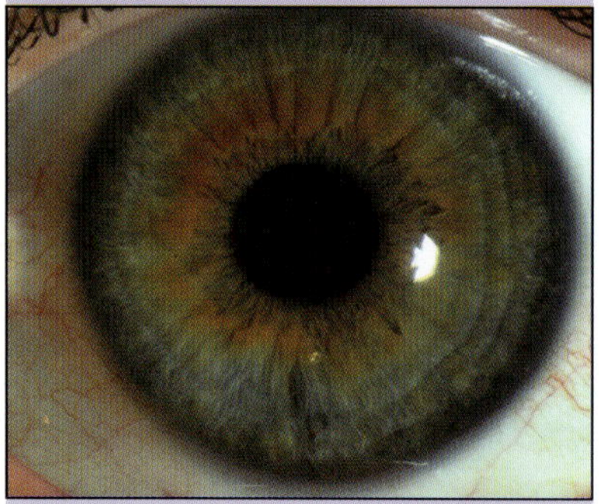

EXTROVERSION

Not only do extroverts have a noticeable absence of concentrated color immediately surrounding the pupil, they also have a distinct ridge or cord (the Ring of Expression) encircling the pupil, usually about a third of the way out toward the periphery of the iris, or more. This ring marks the junction between the region of the iris representing the mental body and that representing the emotional body. The mental region is closest to the pupil, on the *inside* of the Ring of Expression. Flowers are seldom found in the mental region, only jewels. Being a boundary between these two spheres of energy, it delineates the beginning of expression as a force moving outward.

Outgoing, expressive and honest, extroverts generally externalize their thoughts, words and emotions, thereby creating movement and change in their environment. They are achievement-oriented, active and productive. Tending to forego proper planning however, outer-directed people often overextend themselves, wasting their energy and causing fatigue. They also have a tendency to be impatient and compulsive, and are often honest to the point of being insensitive.

Socially active, they are usually good at management, public relations and marketing. By learning introspection and self-restraint, extroverts acquire sensitivity and grace; when this happens, they are capable of achieving extraordinary goals while remaining poised and balanced.

If it took six days to create heaven and earth, extroverts would want to finish the job in half that time. They provide the energy that keeps the wheels of society moving, and the means by which goals and dreams are accomplished. Many of the day-to-day functions of living would simply come to a halt without their impulsive qualities. They can draw out the highest potential of those around them and provide the atmosphere for others to communicate how they really feel. The energy born out of their natural enthusiasm makes them the cogs and wheels of many industries.

Extroverts have the rare quality of living completely in the "now." They prefer the gratification that comes from a total commitment to the present, rather than the whimsical dreaminess that can be characteristic of long-range planning. In their active need to communicate to the outside world, extroverts can be honest to a fault, without ever really sharing their deeper thoughts and feelings. This can lead to them living in a state of denial, using extroversion as a means of avoiding true intimacy.

They are socially active people and yet desire the intimacy of a deep one-to-one relationship. Mixed in with their urge for domestic security is their ever-present need for social recognition. They seem to want the best of all worlds, and are willing to totally expend themselves to achieve it.

Extroversion is the outward movement of emotional and physical vitality. This movement increases self-expression regardless of the primary structural type, while decreasing sensitivity. It is a consequence of reward systems and attitudes based on outer gratifications.

Even while they are resting, extroverts are constantly releasing vitality. This vitality is the fuel that keeps the world moving and binds together some of the reasons for human existence. This quality alone makes extroverts worthy of the recognition they so earnestly desire.

The extroverted temperament releases more energy than it takes in. People with an extroverted eye structure are usually optimistic and positively oriented in their relationships with others. They find comfort and well-being in socially interacting with groups of people.

As with most relationship patterns, the opposite qualities of the extrovert and introvert create a balance. It is the automatic pursuit of this balance that drives the extrovert to seek out the cool refreshment of a silent introvert. The natural attraction and interaction between them produces a transfer of energy between the extrovert and the introvert, ultimately bringing balance to both. The extrovert thrives on the storehouse of energy built up by the introvert, while the extrovert in turn provides a channel for the expression of the introvert's ideas and insights.

In Consultation

It is easy to interpret the iris structure of a true extrovert. Before you even start your interpretation, they usually begin explaining what it is that you're probably going to see. Their inherent urge for self-expression can have its rewarding and its irritating moments. If you succeed in keeping them quiet for a brief period, you can learn much about their style of self-expression from the shape of the Ring of Expression.

As the distance between the Ring of Expression and the pupil increases, you will also notice that the degree of extroversion increases proportionately. When the Ring is perfectly round, the overall behavior is "steady" and even-natured. If the Ring is irregularly shaped, then the individual will probably experience many highs and lows.

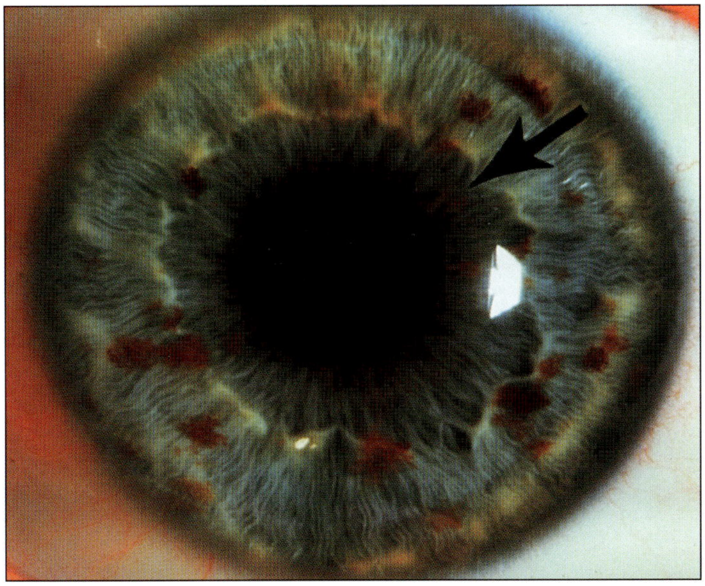

Jewel extrovert

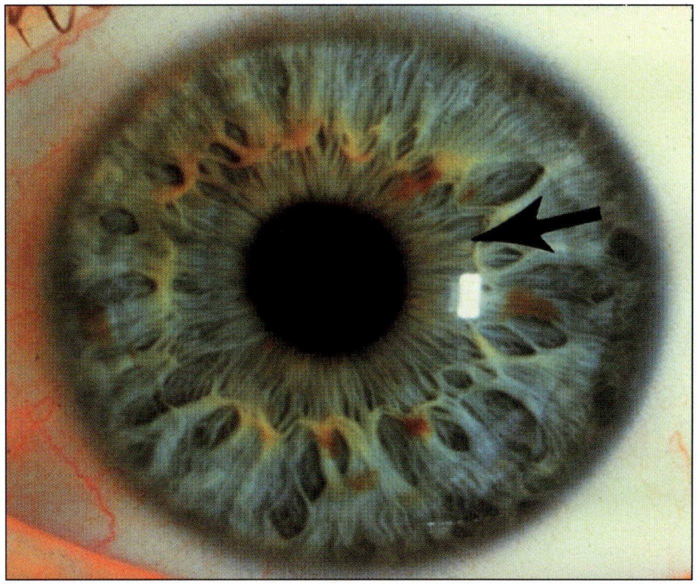

Shaker extrovert

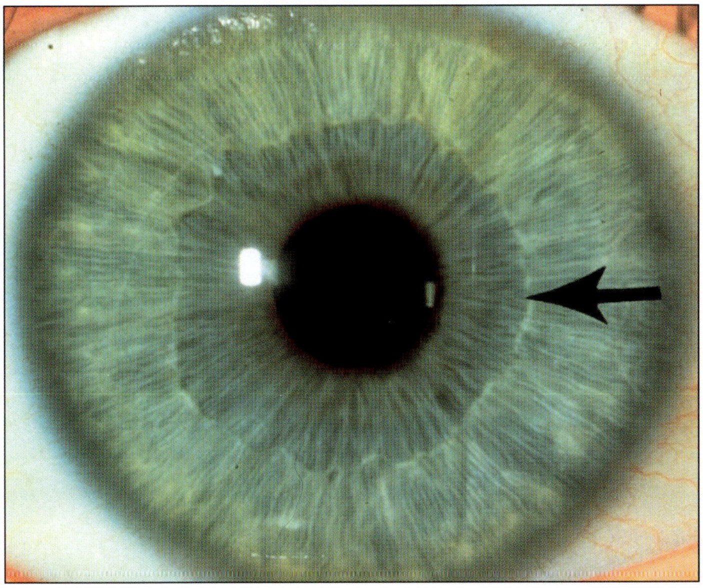

Stream extrovert

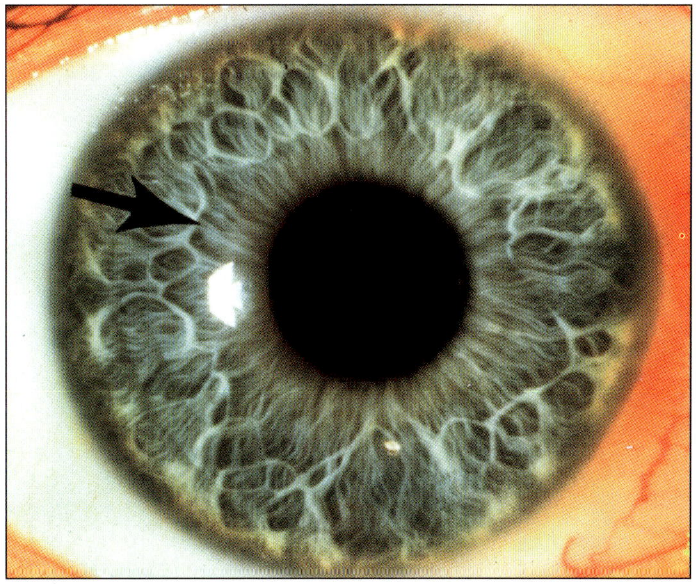

Flower extrovert

Characteristics Associated with Extroversion

Breathe:	Primarily through the mouth
Energy pattern:	Release energy, generate peripheral energy
Essence:	Forthright, social, practical
Communication style:	Expressive
Gestures:	Animated
Behavioral effects:	Increases communication
	Decreases sensitivity
	Increases honesty and directness
Professions:	Management, public relations, entertainment
Gifts:	Achievement, coordination, manifestation
Lessons to be learned:	Stillness, respectfulness, patience, inner giving

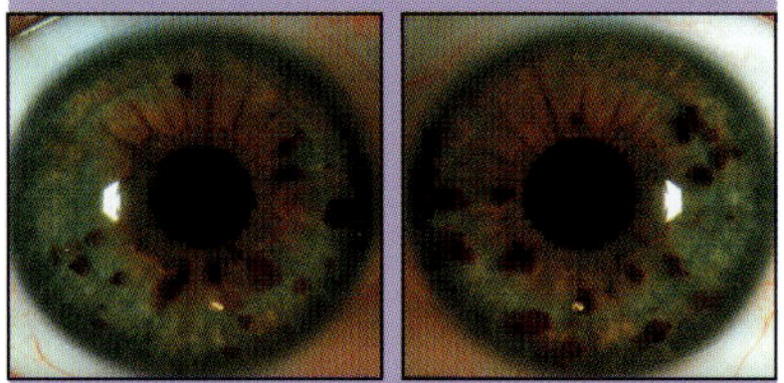

Right-brain dominance

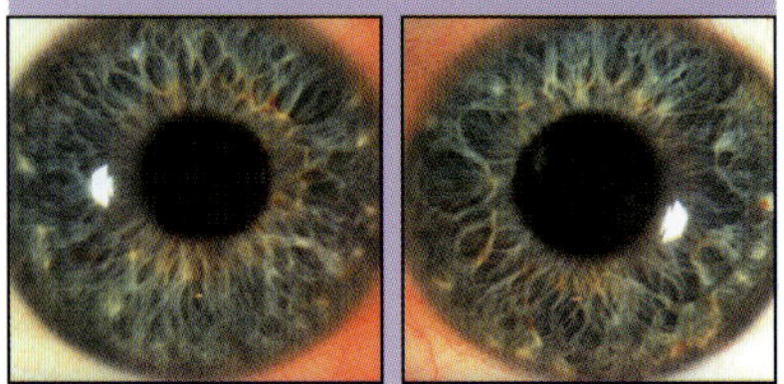

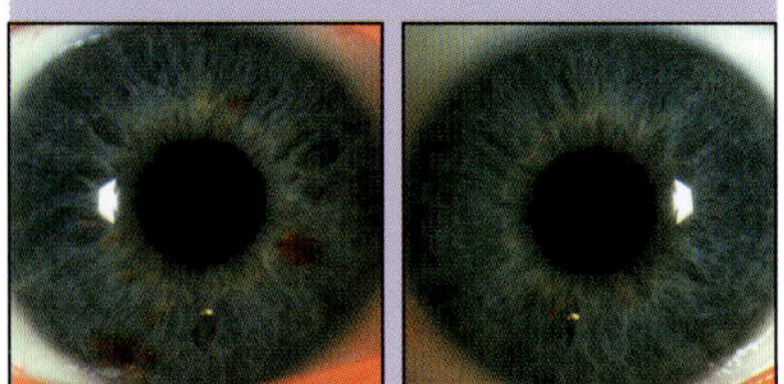

Left-brain dominance

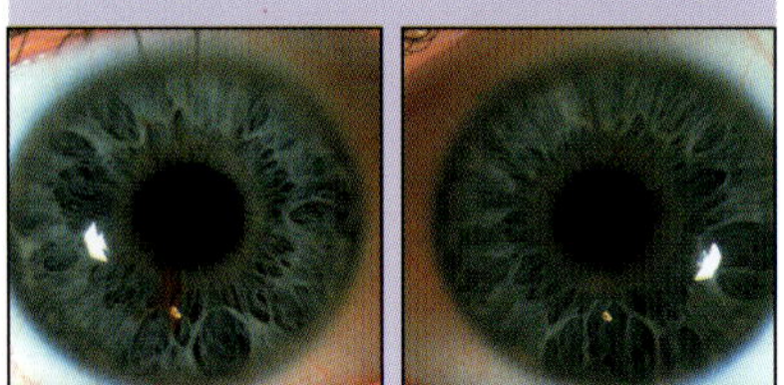

HEMISPHERIC DOMINANCE

Another important polarity system in the Rayid Method is that of hemispheric dominance in the brain.

The cerebrum of the human brain, which regulates conscious processes and behavior, is divided into two large lobes (the cerebral hemispheres), connected by a thick cord of nerves called the corpus callosum. Although they have many gross physical functions in common, the two hemispheres have been found to play significantly different roles in the higher functions of the mind. People tend to favor one hemisphere over the other when processing information, creating distinct and identifiable differences in personality. If they tend to use the left hemisphere more than the right, they are said to be left-brain dominant (or left-brained) if they favor the right hemisphere, they are right-brain dominant (or right-brained).

Its Use in Consultations

Hemispheric dominance has a tremendous impact on behavior and should be a key element of any iris interpretation. People usually have little resistance to acknowledging their hemispheric orientation, so this is often the easiest part of an interpretation about which to get confirmation during a consultation. It is also the area of the Rayid Method that is most readily accepted by allopathic medical practitioners and the conservative, scientific community. In fact, many of our findings about left- and right-brain function have been corroborated by classical psychologists.

Understanding hemispheric dominance enables you, after only a brief glance at the eyes, to give an otherwise complete stranger a synopsis of his postural habits, including which side of the body he sleeps on, to describe his relationships with his parents and his partner, and to outline the main personality differences between his mother and his father.

Masculine and Feminine Polarities

Most of the left side of the body (including the left eye) is connected to the right cerebral hemisphere, while most of the right side of the body is connected to the left hemisphere. Each hemisphere is also genetically linked to a different parent. The left iris (right hemisphere) is linked to the mother, providing information not just about her behavior, but about the feminine qualities of the body and mind in general. It tells us something about the extent to which the individual has accepted and integrated his feminine aspects. The right iris (left hemisphere) provides information about the father and masculinity.

The hemispheres of the brain represent masculine and feminine polarities that influence a person's life experience at every level. Discussions of hemispheric dominance are not just concerned with the brain and physical behavior, but with the interplay between these energies in the personality.

The right brain is more involved in the feminine processes of creative expression, social responsibility, feelings and emotions, artistic endeavor, abstraction and spiritual pursuits of a philosophical nature. Traits in the left iris relate to relationships, attitudes and abilities that are primarily feminine in nature. The primary fear hidden in the right brain (and therefore associated with the mother) is the fear of abandonment.

The left brain is more involved in making decisions about practical issues, gross motor movement, the use of words, and the masculine skills of logic and control. Traits in the right iris relate to masculine personality characteristics and abilities, and to attitudes toward males. The primary fear hidden in the left brain is the fear of criticism. The father is responsible for activating and managing this fear.

Its Influence on the Constitutional Personality

Hemispheric dominance greatly modifies the expression of a person's constitutional structure. The right brain is more flowing, the left brain is more controlled. Being right-brained loosens up the expression of any one of the constitutional patterns. Being left-brained adds a logical, practical quality to the individual's expression.

Hemispheric dominance is usually a compensation for, or an adaptation to, the primary structure. For example, emotional types have a tendency to be left-brained, because left-brain attributes offer the greatest potential to experience control both socially and physically. Control is what the emotional type needs to learn. Similarly, a right-brained person will experience greater degrees of expansiveness, so most mental types have a tendency to go to the right brain. This creates a softening of their natural tendency to be constrictive. While right-brained types do things conceptually or not at all, left-brained types tend to have a practical focus, often to the point of impatience. So while a right-brained Flower might be involved in drawing designs, a left-brained Flower would prefer to actually construct something from those designs. Developing appropriately left-brained or right-brained tendencies is one of the ways in which we compensate for our constitutional personality.

All constitutional types emanate from the interplay of two opposite structures, the Jewel and the Flower. Although they are at opposite ends of the personality spectrum, an individual personality can lie anywhere along the continuum between these two types, being more Jewel-like or more Flower-like, and a person may even move back and forth between these two polar opposites.

Whatever someone's constitutional structure at birth, the *unconscious* personality always tries to attain a state of wholeness. For a Jewel, this means becoming more Flower-like and, for a Flower, it means becoming more Jewel-like. Unless the individual is unusually self-aware, this generally involves the person *shutting down* some facets of the innate personality (the constitutional structure) in order to become its opposite. The unconscious balances the expansiveness of the Flower by shutting down the right hemisphere in order to emphasize the constricted practicality of the left hemisphere.

The elements of personality determined by constitutional structure (Jewel, Flower and combinations) are much deeper than those determined by hemispheric function. They are whole-brain functions, not linked solely to either hemisphere. But this whole-brain expression (the innate, constitutional personality) is inhibited when the unconscious uses hemispheric function to modify the person's expressions and experience. The innate personality is still there, with all of its associated behavior, learning and communication modes, but they are *filtered* through one hemisphere or the other, instead of flowing freely through both. It is therefore not particularly meaningful to think in terms of changing a person's hemispheric function; ideally, the individual will eventually find a way to experience the full depth of his core, constitutional structure – hemispheric preference will then automatically be neutralized.

The Origin of Hemispheric Dominance

Although primarily genetic in origin, hemispheric function appears to be significantly affected by the environment, meaning that a child's genetically predisposed tendency toward left-brain or right-brain dominance can be noticeably altered by experiences after birth. About 40% percent of people start life with one dominant hemisphere and then shift to the the other hemisphere at some point during childhood. It is also possible, however, that hemispheric shifts are more strongly genetically influenced than we are currently able to determine. Environmental experiences which appear to create hemispheric changes may actually be unconscious projections of unfolding patterns in the family tree. The subject of hemispheric shifting is explored later in this chapter in the section entitled *Hemispheric Adaptation.*

The primary influence on hemispheric orientation is the Jewel parent, regardless of the individual's constitutional structure. Because the Jewel structure is denser, it is also gravitationally the most powerful. If your father was a Jewel, you are likely to be pulled toward the left (masculine) hemisphere. If your mother was a Jewel, you are more likely to be right-brained. Your capacity to overcome these forces depends on your degree of personal clarity and self-awareness.

Determining Hemispheric Orientation

When comparing a person's left and right eye, the dominant iris will have a greater number of traits (jewels, flowers or stream characteristics). This is the most important indicator of hemispheric orientation. In addition, the *overall* color of the iris can be helpful; the dominant iris may appear *slightly* darker in color. Being able to distinguish the dominant eye allows you to understand the way in which the individual's constitutional structure is expressed.

There are also a wide variety of behavioral, postural and other physical indicators of hemispheric dominance. These are noted in the tables accompanying the descriptions of hemispheric orientation. The most reliable and useful indicators are the thumb half-moons and the relative droop of the eyelids. The pattern made by interlacing the fingers and sleeping posture are accurate about 70% of the time. When you look closely at the thumbs you will notice that one half-moon is usually higher (longer) than the other. In virtually all cases, right-brained people have a higher left thumb half-moon; they generally interlace their fingers with the right thumb on top and they prefer to sleep with the left cheek down. This usually places the partner on the right, since most couples naturally sleep back-to-back. There are many other indicators, not all of which make sense intuitively; you simply have to memorize them. For example, when walking, the foot connected to the dominant hemisphere will track straighter but, when lying down, that same foot will tilt more to the outside.

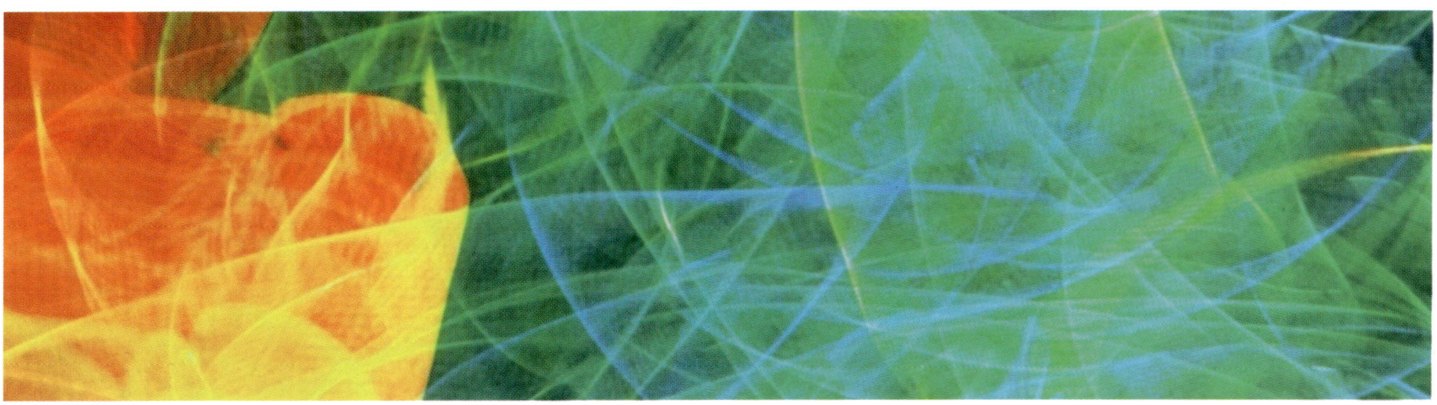

RIGHT-BRAINED TYPES

People with more characteristics in the left iris utilize the right hemisphere of the brain more effectively. The right brain is responsible for creativity, emotions and abstraction. It represents the subconscious personality, the collective consciousness and the past. The right brain is the seat of memory, the part of the brain that holds your self-image and that stores the collective experiences of your ancestors. Traits in the left iris relate to feminine personality characteristics and abilities, and to attitudes toward females.

Right-brained people are usually agreeable, social and creative. Casual, easy-going and informal, they have a tendency to be disorganized and cluttered. Future-oriented and philosophical, they add imagination, originality and spirit to any endeavor. They are usually closer to, and more cooperative with, women and have a greater rapport with their mothers.

Right-brain dominants tend to be more vibrant, flowing and gregarious. They are usually more open to other people, more receptive to new ideas, and their gestures are more open and circular. They have smoother interactions and smoother gestures.

The right brain is the point of access to creative inspiration. The great visionaries behind successful entrepreneurial ventures are invariably right-brained types. In most cutting-edge companies, there are a couple of right-brained "goofballs in the lab" who do the research and development. These creative people come up with all the ideas but leave the implementation to an entire company of troopers who manufacture, market, manage and sell the products that the goofballs invented.

Right-brained types are often impractical and typically lack the skills necessary to manifest their dreams. Many smaller companies that should have been highly successful are hampered by a right-brained creative genius who had the vision necessary to start the venture but then wouldn't hand the managerial reins over to a left-brained implementer. They are often most successful if they are involved in service-oriented businesses, teaching or some other situation that deals with relationships or community.

Right-brained people have a tendency to avoid responsibility, and their laid-back, flowing natures can make them rather rambling and disorganized. They tend to deny material limitation (so don't like to balance the checkbook) and avoid domestic chores (such as cleaning) unless trained by a demanding parent.

Sometimes, right-brained types even use spirituality as a technique for avoiding material responsibility. They are the ascetics and mendicants who believe that, in order to be spiritual, they must give away all their possessions and be impoverished. While left-brained people usually like the organizational nature of religion, right-brained types dislike structures and believe that the necessity of work gets in the way of them getting closer to their concept of God.

Compensatory characteristics visible in the iris may modify these responses for a given individual but they are true in general. Right-brained types need to come to grips with their avoidance patterns by being more focused, more consistent and learning to follow through on their initiatives.

In conversation, right-brained types tend to agree with what you're saying, giving the impression that they are receptive to your ideas. They don't necessarily follow through with cooperative behavior after apparently agreeing with you, however. They also have a tendency to nod their heads up and down and to look like they're saying "Yes" all the time, or to use affirmative responses like "Right, right," "Uh-huh," or "Whatever."

Going right has a tendency to increase the openness and receptivity of a person. The body is often thinner, more angular and flowing – generally more feminine in nature. Because the right brain is feminine, females are usually healthier and feel more comfortable if they have some right-brain qualities. In general, however, right-

Two examples of right-brain dominance (this page and opposite). Notice the greater number of traits in the left iris.

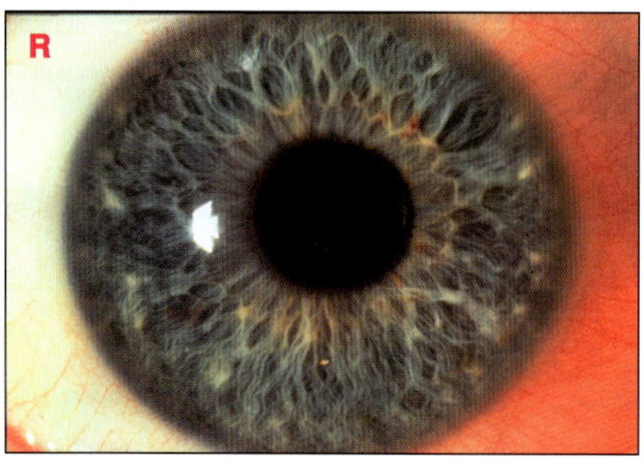

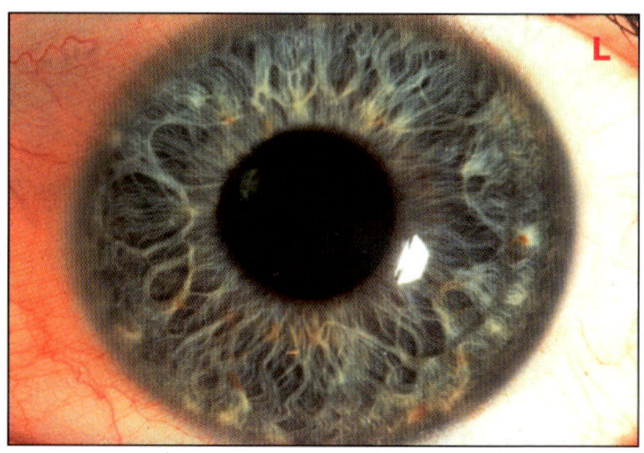

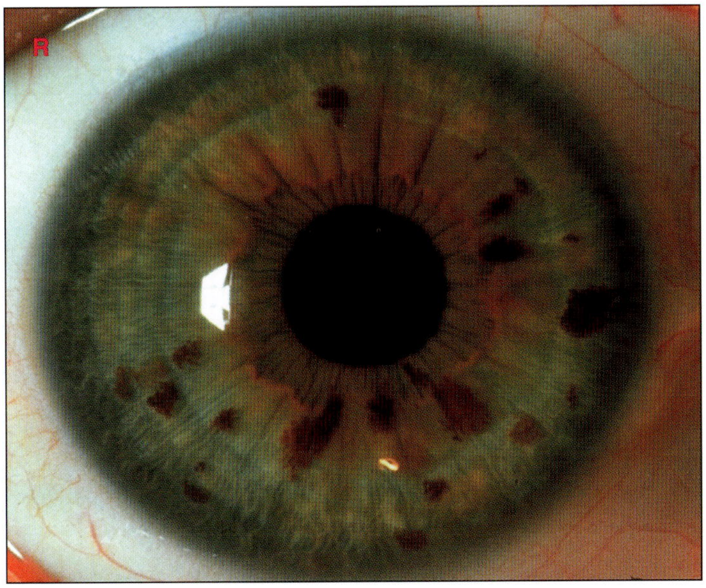

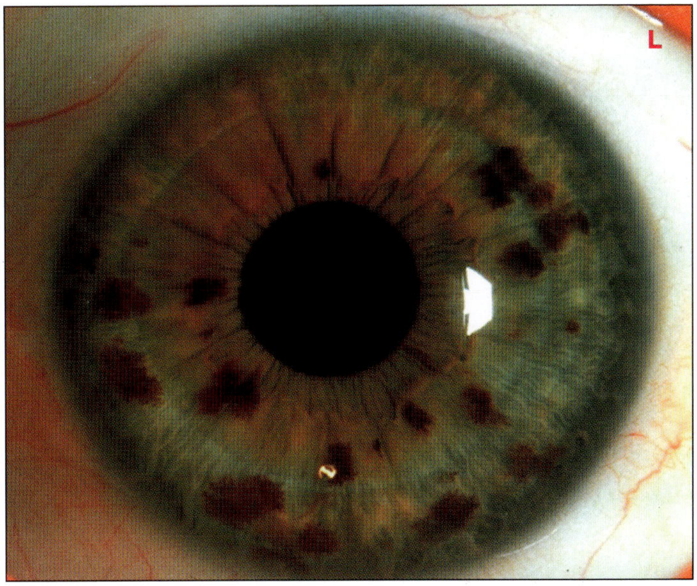

brained people are less physically healthy than left-brained people.

People who are going strongly to the right almost always feel they are from the mother's side of the family, and the overall shape of the face usually resembles the mother's family (not necessarily the mother). Right-brained Jewels usually have an affinity for the grandmother on the mother's side, sometimes even more than for the mother.

Right-brained people attract mates who are moving to the left and who therefore probably had a difficult maternal relationship. If the mate you attract acts like your father at times, you are probably going right. The temperature of the hands is another indicator of hemispheric orientation: cold hands usually indicate a movement to the right, warm hands a movement to the left. Flowers usually have warm hands the degree to which their hands are cooler is the degree to which they are right-brained.

See the table (below) for a summary of all possible physical, postural and behavioral indicators of right-brain orientation. Not all of these indicators will be present at the same time.

Indicators of Right-Brain Dominance

Most iris traits:	Left eye
Most iris color:	Left eye
Thumb half-moons:	Left higher
Upper eyelid droop:	Right eyelid droops more
Interlaced fingers:	Right thumb on top
Stands primarily on:	Left leg
Legs crossed:	Left leg on top
Skin tone:	Smoother, almost glossy skin
Neck/shoulder pain mainly:	Left side
Prostrate, greatest tilt with:	Left foot
Sleeps primarily on:	Left side
Sleeps with partner on:	Right
Partner or self talks more:	Self talks more
Attracts partners who act:	Younger or childlike
Familial rapport:	Mother's side
Difficulties with:	Father or men
Face outline resembles:	Mother's side of family
Oldest child in family is:	Female
Disposition:	Spontaneous, accepting, future-oriented
Energy:	Feminine, creative, imaginative, intuitive
Behavior:	Spacey or casual, easy-going, even sloppy
Orientation:	Group-oriented, sociable, conceptual
Conversational style:	Agreeable yet opinionated
Response time to questions:	Quick to respond
Fear:	Rejection

LEFT-BRAINED TYPES

People with more characteristics in the right iris utilize the left hemisphere of the brain more effectively. The left brain is responsible for verbal communication, voluntary muscular function, precision, logic and choice. It represents the conscious personality and the present. Your ability to be in your left brain determines how well you can process information that is given to you. Traits in the right iris relate to masculine personality characteristics and abilities, and to attitudes toward males.

Left-brained people are usually logical, practical and self-oriented. They ask definitive questions, have specific material goals and prefer to be organized. Valuing formality, and holding traditional values, they add stability and structure to any endeavor. They usually have a greater rapport with their fathers and men in general.

Materially oriented and more concerned with their physical environment, left-brained people tend to be possessive. Interested in structure, function and organization, with a greater attention to detail, they are generally the ones who balance the household checkbook and strive for long-term security. More masculine, more assertive and more grounded, they are better short-term decision-makers than right-brained types.

The left brain crystallizes and clarifies the abstraction of the right brain, and without the practical, grounded quality of the left brain, nothing would get done. Left-brained people are achievers and manifesters, the ones who turn the dreams of the right-brained visionaries into material reality.

Generally skeptical and slow to change, left-brained people resist new concepts until they have been convinced by hard evidence. Engaging you in debate, they make you *prove* your point, challenging your suppositions, insisting that you scientifically test and verify your hypotheses. Being confronted in this way can be very useful it tempers your argument and improves your presentation. It strengthens you and is a useful quality for society as well.

This questioning, doubting nature can, however, make left-brained types prone to cynicism and haughtiness. When cut off from the depth of their own emotions, they tend to be rigid in their views with little appreciation for abstraction and the creative force of inspiration. When this happens, they are only robbing themselves of a fuller, richer experience of life. Left-brained types would do well to develop a greater sensitivity to others, learning to be more open, accepting and flowing.

The left brain is the seat of language, and left-brained people are generally precise, verbal communicators. (Left-brained Jewels are also logical and analytical.) They tend to use short sentences, and their conversational style can sometimes seem quite choppy. They tend to interrupt with phrases such as "Wait. Wait. Wait." or with challenges such as "Prove it to me," "Why?" or "What do you mean by that?" They tend to phrase things in questions, rather than statements, and often favor the past tense. They tend to use words that end in -ed, -ly or -ing. They typically offer resistance to what they hear, with furrowed brow, unconsciously tilting the head or shaking it from side to side.

More controlled and physically contained, left-brained types tend to sit erect, using sharp gestures that are held relatively close to the body. They have a tendency to point at you, or to wave a fist at you when angered. Their energy is more focused, which sometimes makes them seem more energetic and powerful. Being more physical in nature, they are also likely to be more aggressive. Left-brained types seem to be more driven by testosterone and males are often subject to balding.

Going left has a tendency to increase the constriction and density of a person. Because the left brain is masculine, males are usually healthier and feel more comfortable if they have some left-brain qualities. However, going *too* far left can be unhealthy for anyone, especially men. One of the functions of the right brain is

Two examples of left-brain dominance (this page and opposite). Notice the greater number of traits in the right iris.

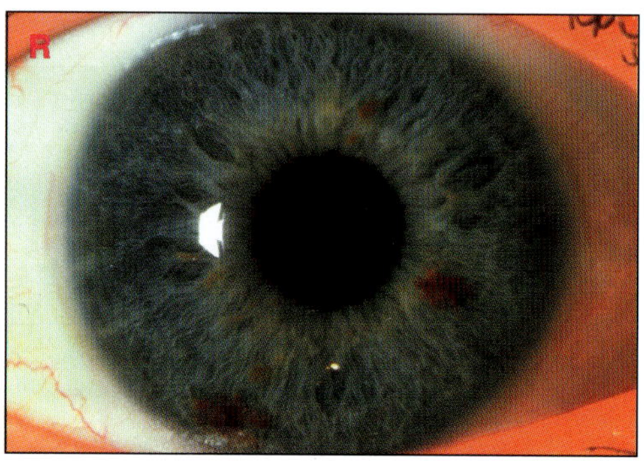

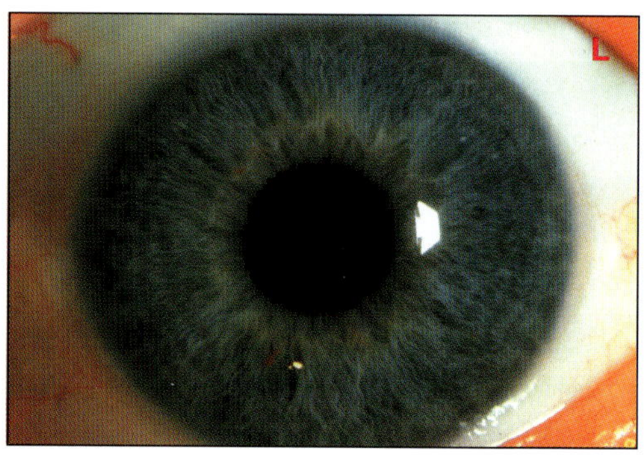

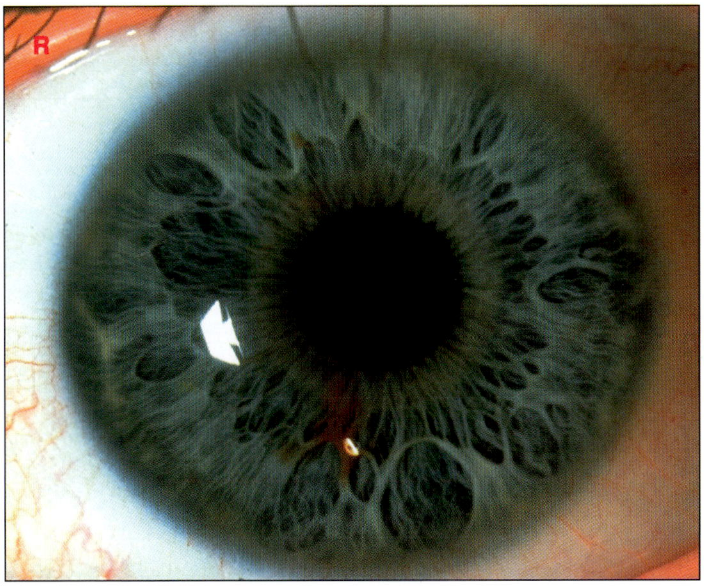

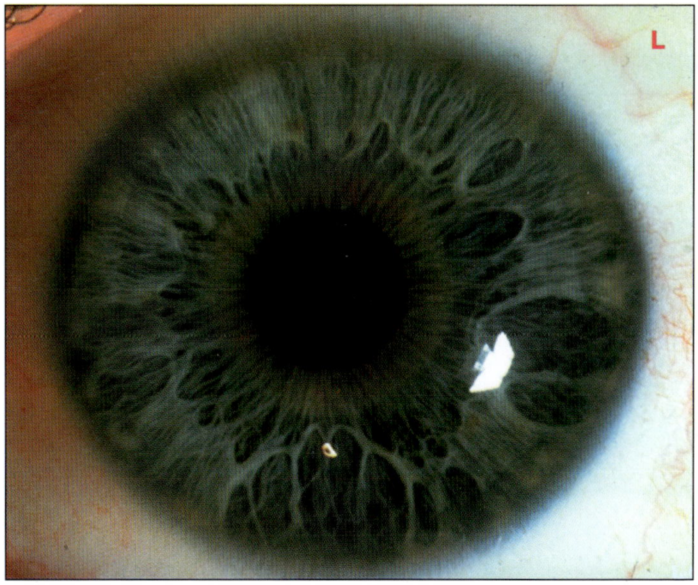

release, which is equivalent to emotional cleansing. When someone is stressed, tense or emotionally upset on the inside, those feelings act like a kind of toxicity if they are not released. If a male goes too far left, he doesn't get a chance to release there is too much constriction, too much retention and not enough elimination. This can lead to a sudden, shocking or aggressive release.

People who are going left almost always feel they are from the father's side of the family. They often speak their minds and then apologize for it. However, the further to the left they are, the slower their speech patterns and the less likely they are to do this. Left-brained types are materially self-oriented, and are often bigger than right-brained types. Flowers going left often choose older partners or partners who act older, more mature and who dominate in the relationship. They usually have an affinity for the grandfather on the father's side.

See the table (below) for a summary of all possible physical, postural and behavioral indicators of left-brain orientation. Not all of these indicators will be present at the same time.

Indicators of Left-Brain Dominance

Most iris traits:	Right eye
Most iris color:	Right eye
Thumb half-moons:	Right higher
Upper eyelid droop:	Left eyelid droops more
Interlaced fingers:	Left thumb on top
Stands primarily on:	Right leg
Legs crossed:	Right leg on top
Skin tone:	Coarser, rougher skin
Neck/shoulder pain mainly:	Right side
Prostrate, greatest tilt with:	Right foot
Sleeps primarily on:	Right side
Sleeps with partner on:	Left
Partner or self talks more:	Partner talks more
Attracts partners who act:	Older, more secure
Familial rapport:	Father's side
Difficulties with:	Mother
Face outline resembles:	Father's side of family
Oldest child in family is:	Male
Disposition:	Fixed, doubtful, traditional, slow to change
Energy:	Masculine, logical, practical, factual
Behavior:	Compulsively ordered, restless
Orientation:	Self- and achievement-oriented, materialistic
Conversational style:	Questioning, contradictory, interruptive
Response time to questions:	Slow to respond
Fear:	Being alone

HEMISPHERIC ADAPTATION

"Adaptation" is the term used to describe those cases when a Flower behaves like a Jewel, or a Jewel behaves like a Flower. The notion of adaptation is closely related to that of core structures (see *Introduction to Rayid Therapies*). As an individual moves closer to his true self, or core nature, he displays fewer and fewer personality traits, eventually reaching a point of stillness and harmony where you cannot tell by his behavior, posture or gesture what structure he is. This point of stillness is where a Jewel experiences pure, inner knowing and a Flower experiences true peace.

As the individual moves further away from his core essence, toward the right hemisphere if he is a Jewel, or toward the left hemisphere if he is a Flower, he will behave more and more like the opposite structure. This does not happen with a Jewel who is truly left-brained or a Flower who is truly right-brained, so these personality types are not said to be in adaptation; such cases, however, are unusual, representing less than 10% of people.

Most people, therefore, are in some form of adaptation to their primary iris structure. As was mentioned in the introduction, hemispheric adaptation is actually an attempt to balance the primary constitutional structure. Flowers tend to go left in order to control, contain and focus their natural expressiveness, and Jewels tend to go right in order to find release from their innate constriction.

The strongest factor determining hemispheric orientation is the Jewel parent. Although this subject is covered in detail in *The 16 Vibratory Channels*, a brief description of the process would be useful here. It is interesting to note that both one's constitutional structure, and the means to compensate for it, are primarily genetically determined.

If your father was a Jewel, you will be pulled toward the left (masculine) hemisphere. If *his* father was also a Jewel, this tendency will be compounded, and you will be even more left-brained, even more so if your grandfather's father was also a Jewel. Just one Jewel woman in your paternal line (e.g. a Jewel grandmother) would substantially diminish this tendency. Similarly, succeeding generations of ancestral Jewel *women*, starting with your mother, would pull you more and more into your *right* hemisphere.

This shows you how the degree of hemispheric adaptation is determined by the transgenerational influence of the accumulated personality patterns of the three preceding generations of ancestors. In a sense, the term "adaptation" is inaccurate, in that it implies a conscious response or some element of will on the part of the individual. This is rarely the case. Most instances of hemispheric adaptation are caused by a pull from someone in an earlier generation. However, environmental factors *can* change hemispheric orientation, most noticeably in instances of hemispheric switching (see below).

As Jewels move away from their core essence, they develop the anxiety associated with a restless desire to understand. Instead of just "knowing," they start analyzing things more and more, and experience frustration. As they move even further away from core, the flow of blood is increasingly constricted, cooling the hands and extremities, and restricting the flow of blood to the brain. This can cause a noticeable dizziness and "spaciness." If pronounced, a Jewel far away from core will act like a clumsy, emotional Flower, and can even find himself caught in the nightmare of schizophrenia.

Similarly, you may encounter a controlling, bossy Flower who behaves exactly like a Jewel because he has gone so far left that he has "solidified" his emotions. He may be demanding, selfish and, in extreme cases, exhibit psychopathic tendencies.

Switch Patterns

Hemispheric switching is a not uncommon form of adaptation in which the individual actually changes dominant hemispheres. Such people have an iris structure indicating an affinity to one hemisphere yet they manifest behavior associated with the other. This crossing over can result from mental, emotional or physical pain, as a defense to further suffering. Switch patterns generally have made a complete break with the parent linked to the originally dominant hemisphere (right hemisphere – father, left hemisphere – mother), usually because of some traumatic event in childhood that pushed the individual away.

Hemispheric shifts create dramatic changes in the personality and in the intensity with which the personality is expressed. Someone who has switched to the right hemisphere, for example, will be much more radically right-brained than someone who naturally originated in that hemisphere. People with a switch pattern are essentially suppressing their natural tendencies. This can bring balance and

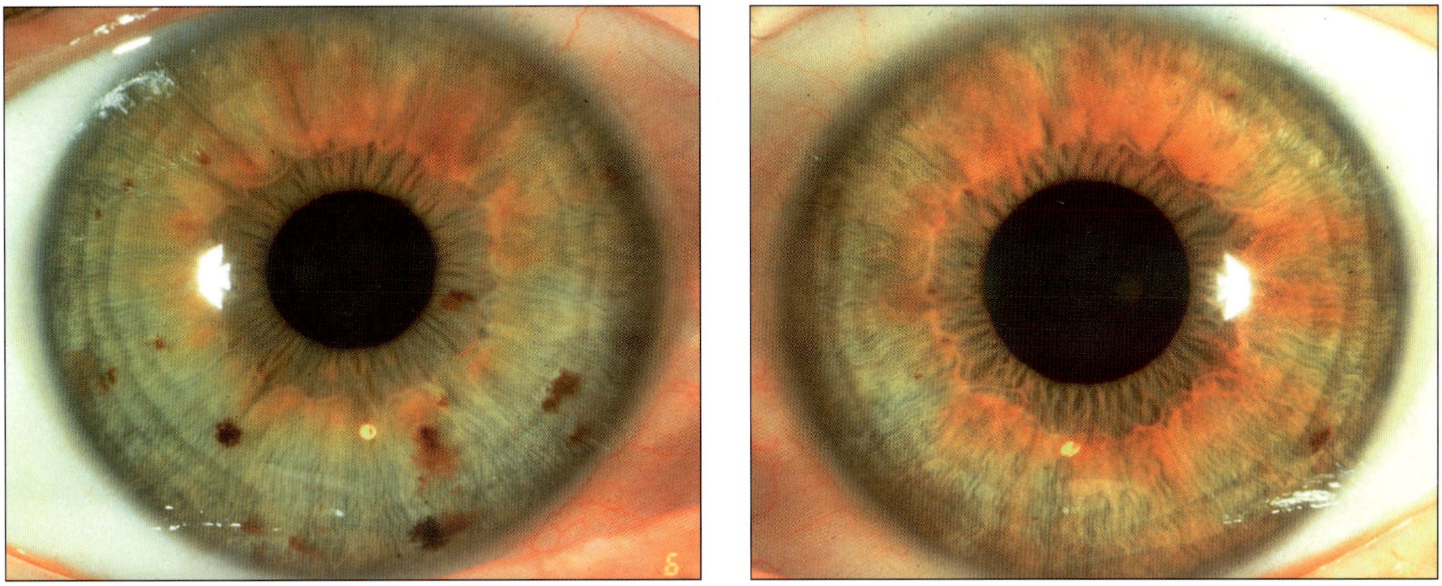

Two examples of hemispheric switching. The top iris pair shows a person who has gone from left to right; the bottom pair shows someone who has gone right to left.

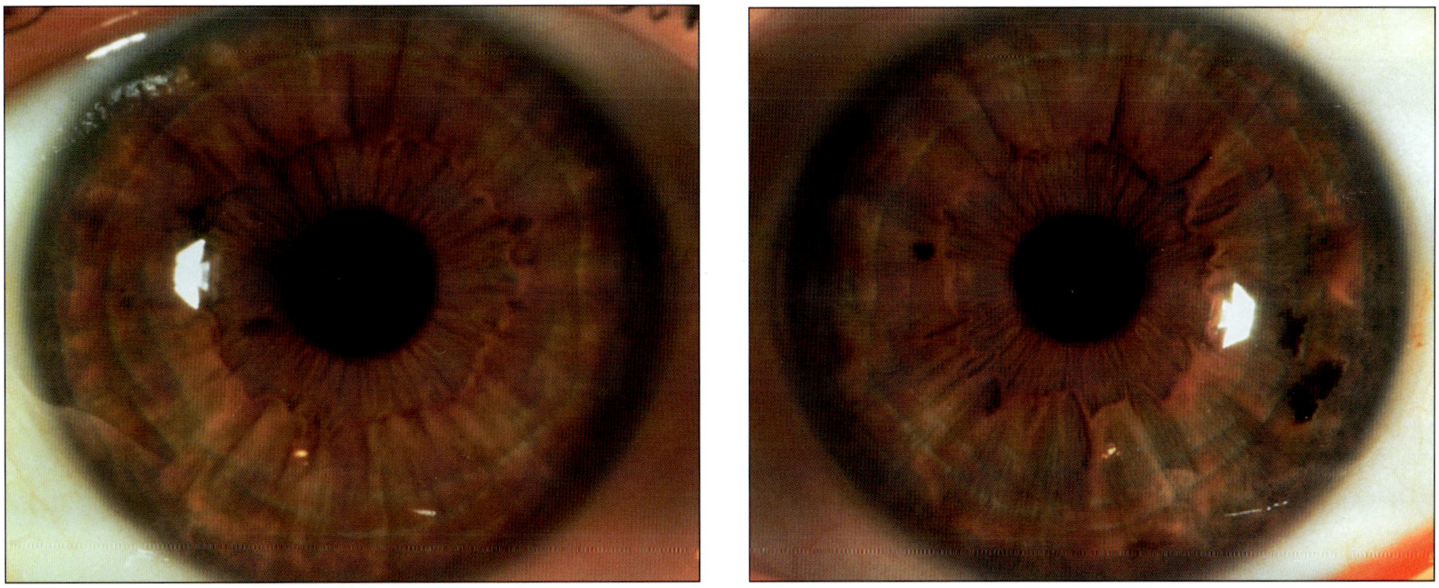

integration, or create confusion, frustration or irrationality when unresolved. For such people, true self-knowing and forgiveness are necessary to heal the wounds of the past.

Determining a switch pattern in the iris can be a challenge. Typically, such people have a greater number of traits in one iris but with more evident color in the *top* quadrant of the *other* eye. There may be a particularly large Anger or Resentment issue in the apparently dominant iris (see *Positions in the Iris*) but, other than that, the practitioner may have to rely on asking questions.

The best indication of a switch pattern is when someone's behavior is clearly inconsistent with the interpretation. For example, a person with more traits in the left iris (indicating a right-brain orientation) but who exhibits other distinctly left-brained behavior patterns (such as sleeping predominantly on the right side) has probably switched left. In order to spot switch patterns in a consultation, it is important to be attentive to such discrepancies between physiological indicators of hemispheric dominance and what the eye reveals.

With advanced training in the Rayid Method, it is actually possible to determine the age at which the hemispheric shift took place. For example, because the contour of the face is determined quite early on, the face of someone who has switched from right to left after the age of one will still resemble the mother (right hemisphere), even though the other body signs indicate a left-brain orientation. If the person switched left before the age of one, the outline of the face will resemble the father's side of the family, and the only indication of a switch pattern in such instances may be the predominance of iris traits in the left eye (indicating a right-brain orientation at birth). Similarly, patterns of interlacing the fingers are usually determined around the age of two, so if the switch to the left hemisphere occurred before the age of two, the hands will be interlaced with the left thumb on top; if the switch happened after the age of two, they will be interlaced with the right thumb on top.

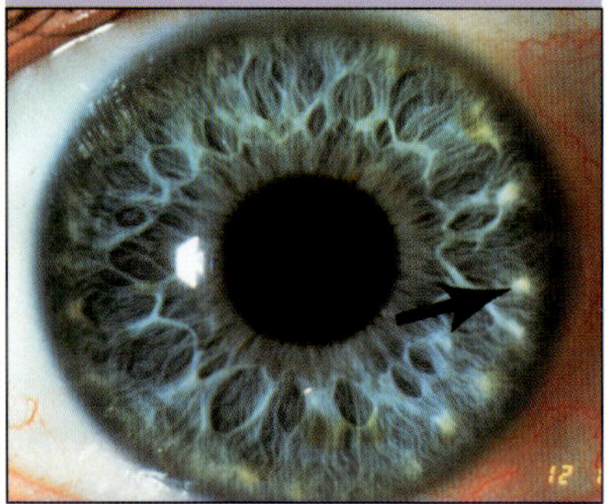

Ring of Harmony

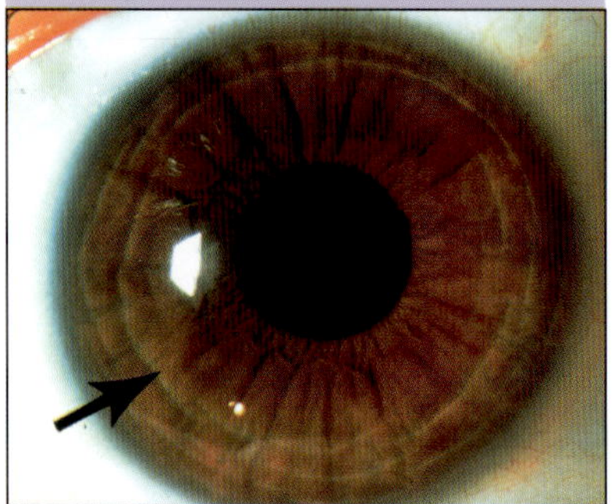

Ring of Freedom

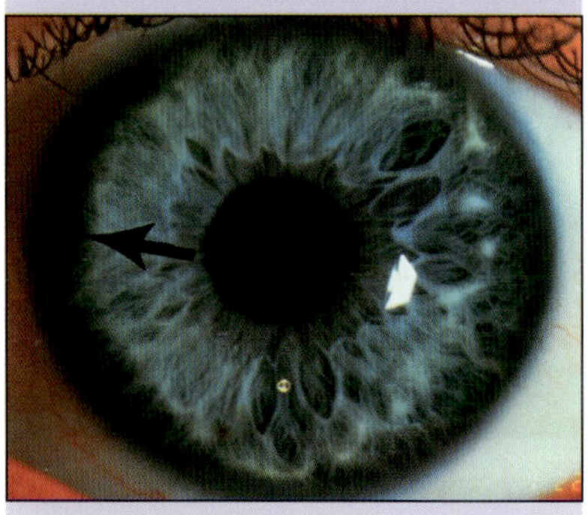

Ring of Purpose

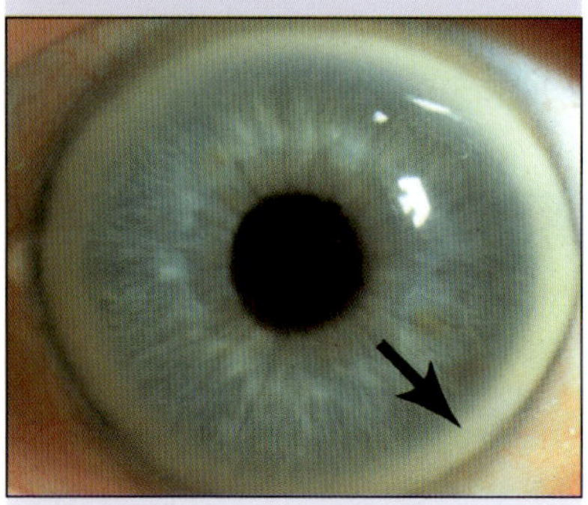

Ring of Determination

Rings in the Iris

Rings in the iris are often easier to recognize and easier to interpret than the primary iris structures. This is because they are easy to identify – there are hardly ever any "borderline" cases – and they are generally not influenced by the individual's iris structure. A beginning Rayid student can therefore expect to be fairly accurate when describing the personality of someone with a ring pattern. Iris structure, on the other hand, is heavily modified by hemispheric adaptation. Most Flowers, for example, are so left-brained and constricted on the outside that they actually behave in many ways like Jewels.

Two of the rings, the Ring of Freedom and the Ring of Purpose, appear to be primarily determined by genetics; they are usually as well-developed by birth as they ever will be. Although the Ring of Harmony is also present in newborn infants, it can become more distinct as the person gets older. The Ring of Determination, on the other hand, is never seen in children. It develops during life, apparently in response to the individual's experiences, and is rare in people below the age of 50.

If you notice a ring forming in a child, please don't think in terms of preventing the ring from fully developing. It is not as productive to think in terms of preventing the ring from evolving as it is to think in terms of creating a positive counterbalance in the child's life that would nullify the adaptive behavior associated with the ring.

RINGS IN COMBINATION

When the Harmony and Freedom rings are found in the same eye, the person will have a quality similar to that of a Shaker but more physical and personal in nature. The feeling function of the Harmony pattern, when combined with the piercing nature of the Freedom ring, electrifies (animates) yet binds (constricts) the individual's full character expression. All in all, it creates great intensity and an urge to achieve the ultimate goal, with compassion.

When a Harmony pattern exists with the Ring of Purpose, there is a softening and slowing of the outer expression of the personality and a subtle movement toward individuality and intellect. The Purpose ring makes the person more detached and mutes the reactiveness of the Harmony pattern. This movement increases the person's ability to observe in a mental state.

When Freedom and Purpose are found in the same eye, it heightens the sense of specialness and deepens the sense of urgency to achieve a mysterious outcome. These two rings in combination can create a restless anxiety which must lead to internal conflict or ultimate resolution. It is difficult for a person who has both of these patterns to sit on the fence.

THE RING OF HARMONY

The Ring of Harmony is a pattern of soft, cloudy white and/or yellow dots forming a circular ring around the pupil, usually toward the outer periphery of the iris. People with this pattern tend to have high ideals about social and environmental issues. They dislike disorder and strive to maintain balance. Self-denial and unvocalized expectations of others can cause these sensitive individuals to feel used or let down by other people. Their disappointment can then result in cynicism and self-imposed isolation. Manifesting personal harmony when faced with disorder allows this personality type to be effectively involved in life without becoming cynical.

The key to understanding the Harmony pattern is that it generally indicates an absence of Stream qualities in the individual; hence the significance of the personal quest for harmony, which is an innate Stream characteristic. Family-oriented, they strive for togetherness. The appearance of this ring indicates a loss of bonding and communication *between generations*. Hence they feel a deep call to action, to bring people together, even if they destroy themselves in the process.

Unlike many iris characteristics, the Ring of Harmony can be observed in people of any age, even in newly born infants. It is also quite common; 25-30% of the population have some degree of Harmony pattern. Although it will be more difficult to see in someone with brown eyes, the pattern is there in people with all iris colors.

The Essence

At their innermost core, people with Harmony patterns are motivated by a yearning for tranquility, peace and harmony, and by a deep desire for environmental purification and stability. They also have an underlying desire for brotherhood and crave the experience of the whole human family in communion. Although this can be interpreted as an idealistic desire for a utopian perfection, it is actually a sincere and heartfelt need. The Ring of Harmony indicates a powerful urge for constitutional stability (Stream qualities). Harmony patterns therefore have a deep desire for a sense of support between people around them.

Their need for stability makes Harmony patterns extremely sensitive (both emotionally and physically) to any form of physical or social breakdown in their environment. Because of their sensitivity, combined with a tendency to take personal responsibility for events, people with a Harmony pattern exhibit a kind of "white blood-cell consciousness."

Like a white blood cell in the human immune system, Harmony patterns cannot tolerate any form of challenge to, or sensory disturbance of, the tranquility in their environment. They are very sensitive to loud sounds such as crying, or to any form of suffering, and react strongly to conflict, familial breakdowns or any other kind of environmental distress. All of these disturbances are perceived as intrusions into the natural, harmonious state and, like a white blood cell, the Harmony pattern will see it as his responsibility to step in and restore harmony.

Their extreme sensitivity makes Harmony patterns acutely empathetic, and they have a deep desire to take care of the environment, to heal its wounds. The fact that Harmony patterns often seem to attract the refuse of life is perhaps an inevitable byproduct of their willingness to clean up the world's garbage.

Another key to understanding the Harmony pattern is to see that it is really excessively expansive, seeking stability by creating kinesthetic connections between people and families. What people with Harmony patterns do before they wake up to their power is to expand at the expense of their own capacity to be in their bodies. They are usually chronically tired.

Although it is quite common for people with Harmony patterns to feel driven to do something about the world, they often don't recognize their own power or understand how to use it. They generally have a noble and idealistic desire for a better world, but tend to feel let down and overwhelmed by the realities of the world .

Interpretation

Depending on where the clumps of the Ring of Harmony appear, the individual's idealism will be expressed in different ways. The portion of the iris with the greatest density of clumps will indicate whether the pattern is most likely to be visible in the area of society and outer relationships, philosophical idealism, intimacy and personal relationships, a disappointment with home, family, touch or any of the other specific possibilities (see the map of iris regions in *Positions in the Iris*).

For example, if the clumps indicating a Ring of Harmony occur just outside the Ring of Expression, in the emotional region, there is a great desire for social experiences, for a feeling of communion, of wanting to be loved. The Harmony pattern will be apparent more as an emotional longing than as a direct and focused desire to take care of other people, trees or baby seals. This is an unusual place for the Ring of Harmony to be found, but it does occur.

The Challenge

The Ring of Harmony can have a powerful impact on an individual's personality and experiences in life. Many of those experiences are far from easy, although they all have something to teach.

Not knowing where to draw the boundaries between themselves and the world, Harmony patterns have a tendency to take on more than they can handle. Even when ridiculously overburdened, Harmony patterns will continue trying to help, frequently leading themselves into a state of physical deterioration and exhaustion. Their behavior can seem to other people to be quite frantic at times. The image which perhaps best encapsulates the Harmony pattern is that of an underpaid, perpetually burnt-out social worker.

Harmony patterns are the most exhausted structures, even more so than Flower types, because their feeling sensitivity is compounded by an impossible desire for perfection. They exhaust themselves trying to overcome the limitations of earthly reality.

A Flower with a Harmony pattern is therefore even more likely to become exhausted, because his innate tendency toward exhaustion is amplified. Both are empathetic, both have a tendency to give and both are particularly reactive to sounds. A Jewel structure with a Harmony pattern, on the other hand, has some constrictiveness to help hold him together.

The origin of the Harmony pattern lies in the lack of integrated transgenerational support. It is most likely to result from the absence of a feeling of family or support while the individual was in utero, but could be traced back to a preceding generation. The individual's tendency to create exhausting situations is a direct consequence of this original lack of support.

Harmony patterns tend to be hyperactive, rushing about from one place to the next and from one activity to another. The reason for this is that they are avoiding the accumulation of pain in the central nervous system which originated with their initial abandonment, during gestation.

It actually hurts to stop, because it brings up all the pain from the unconscious. At some level, someone with a Harmony pattern knows that slowing down will entail re-experiencing the pain that was there when his mother did not feel supported by his father – and he wants to avoid this at all costs. Hence the self-sabotaging technique of staying so busy that he doesn't have to face the pain.

Adults with a Harmony pattern often go out and try to heal all the bonds in their environment, either between people, or else between people and the planet: saving the trees, defending baby seals, etc., depending on their specific primary structural type.

People with a Ring of Harmony are always looking for a cause to champion, a banner to raise; they are fighters. But they usually end up feeling broken-hearted when the cause doesn't succeed, or when they feel they have been misled by the leader of the cause. They have a tendency to be disappointed in the outcome of their initiatives. They become bitter, depressed and antisocial when they are thoroughly exhausted by this life pattern.

When they are strong, they go out and defend the weak. When they are not strong, taking on all of the world's problems eventually makes them feel weak; they feel used and typically react by withdrawing into antisocial isolation. They may complain that they are always working for other people but they never get anything back: "Why won't the world support me?" they ask.

Harmony patterns want a type of support and environmental peace that at our level of social evolution is simply not there yet.

Some people with Harmony patterns have to go

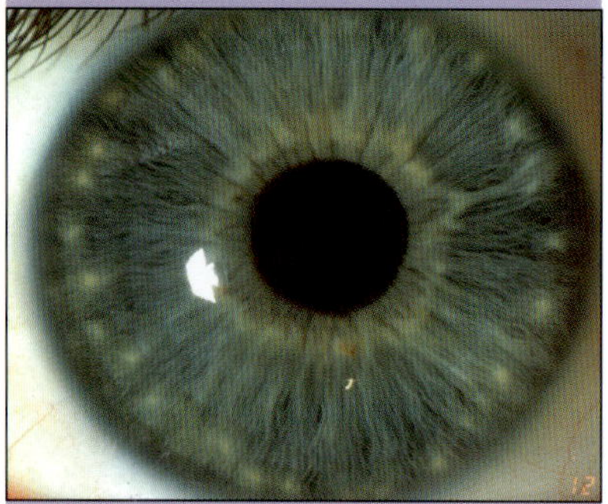

Examples of the Ring of Harmony

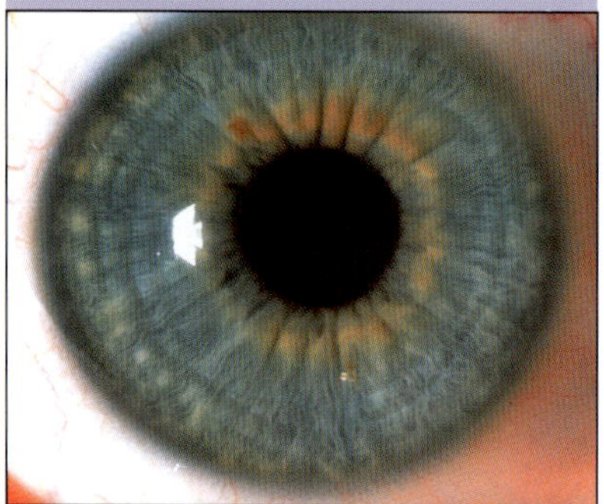

through the experience of being burnt out so many times in their lives that they eventually realize that they don't actually accomplish much when they try to do too much, when they burn themselves out like that. It's futile.

Feeling abandoned and unsupported, people with Harmony patterns eventually respond by becoming bitter and negative. They begin to create the very isolated and unconnected environment that they hate so much, and may even hate themselves for withdrawing. In other words, their antisocial, isolationist behavior comes about because of their sensitivity and desire for harmony.

They can become cynical, going inside themselves in reaction to their disappointment with the world not living up to their ideals. Unlike a positively-motivated inner quest for meaning, this type of reaction is unlikely to lead them back out again into a new and healthy relationship with the world. They may still express concern for the environment, but it is less likely to be emotionally empathetic and more likely to take the form of bitter, angry attacks on the state of the world. Their deepest desire is for environmental peace, purity and harmony, yet a cynical Harmony pattern will be aggressive, attacking and distinctly unharmonious. His body will show the signs of this emotional strain.

Someone in this state of mind would do well to explore possible solutions instead of just emphasizing the problems with the world. We all create our own experience of life to some extent, and need to see our experience in terms of choices.

Case Study

A woman conceived a child out of wedlock. She told the father, who said he didn't want a child and thought the woman should have an abortion. Immediately, the mother and developing embryo were in an unsupported situation. The woman decided she wanted to have the child, but kept her pregnancy hidden from her family for a while, as she had serious doubts about whether her family would provide her with any support. The mother was therefore essentially alone throughout her pregnancy.

When the baby was born, it had a strong Harmony pattern, and also a virtual absence of fiber density in the iris. The density of fiber that we observe so clearly in classical Stream structure is indicative of a sense of connectedness and support.

People with Harmony patterns have a greater than normal sensitivity to sensory stimulation. The baby in this case had an ongoing reactiveness to sound, taking the form of a frequent, jerky reflex.

The woman then became involved in a relationship with another man (not the biological father of the child) who her family thought was unlikely to support the child adequately. About three or four months after the relationship began, the infant contracted a severe form of spinal meningitis and nearly died.

Spinal meningitis is a bacterial or viral attack on the lining of the brain and spinal cord, the very core of the person. Problems with the central nervous system are often linked to a need for community or family support, and for the individual to be integrated into the environment. Furthermore, a child with a Harmony pattern is quite likely to get sick if it senses a disturbance between the parents; by doing so it is reacting to a sense of breakdown in its environment.

It seems that the child's illness actually created the mechanism for overcoming the lack of support in its environment, since the family then pulled together to support the infant in the hospital.

The Gift

When Harmony patterns awaken to their true creative potential, the personality characteristics that previously seemed so difficult now become a source of inspiration and strength.

People with Harmony patterns are acutely sensitive to the world around them. When they become awake, conscious of their otherwise subconscious behavioral mechanisms, they reverse the direction of that flow; instead of being a walking psychic and emotional vacuum cleaner, exhausting themselves by absorbing the world's rubbish, their empathetic connection to the world around them gives Harmony patterns the ability to influence other people wordlessly – they have a powerful effect on people just by their presence.

If he's feeling good, an awake Harmony pattern walking into a room full of people will infuse everyone in that room with a positive attitude. They react to his presence unconsciously but, because he isn't sounding a fanfare to draw attention to his actions, they won't consciously be aware of his power. For this reason, someone with a Harmony pattern can be thought of as something of a "Trojan Horse." His profound capacity to influence people is hidden within.

People with Harmony patterns play the role of the Trojan Horse in the transformation of consciousness. Whether they recognize it or not, their personal evolution is intimately linked with the evolution of human consciousness in general. When they become aware of this, and act on it, the effect is similar to the impact on the body of stimulating an acupuncture point. The whole body of humanity is healed when the Harmony pattern feels better.

Their extremely open energy allows them to overcome every resistance; they have the ability to encounter the densest form of consciousness and alter it without saying a word.

This ability gives the person with a Harmony pattern quite a responsibility. He must take care of his personal needs so that he can amplify his capacity to deliver his message: harmony, peace, joy and brotherhood. In order to do that, he must carry that message within him. He cannot possibly be as effective at spreading the message if he goes out into the world exhausted, sickly and weak.

Unlike straight Jewel types, for example, who deliver their message auditorily, through the mind, people with Harmony patterns deliver their message through a sense of unconscious empathy which, on a feeling level, can be *simultaneously* transmitted to many people at once.

Transformation

Before venturing out into the world again, disillusioned Harmony patterns must become joyfully enlivened with personal health. Before they can heal other families and transform the mass mind, they must first heal their own fragmentation. The key to their transformation is rest and *stillness*, if only they will take the advice.

Harmony patterns have a strong tendency to lose their energy to the world, but they also have the ability to rapidly rejuvenate themselves. Periods of intense, exhausted rest can keep them going for a while it just isn't a very healthy way to live.

It can be extremely difficult to get this type of person to slow down. Even when you tell them that their primary therapy has to do with being still. They may acknowledge that their health requires that they rest, they may even take a few days off work, but they still don't get the kind of rest that they need. Instead, they tend to collapse into states of consciousness in which the body itself is not being rejuvenated (such as exhausted sleep).

People with a Harmony pattern need to take the time to create a sense of support within their bodies. Once they achieve this, they no longer need to run around taking care of people one at a time and getting exhausted by it; their transformational consciousness can be applied to large groups at a time.

Luckily, Harmony patterns generally respond well to a call to duty. They wake up fast. But they also have a tendency to want to run out and change everything at once. They must slow down, rest and rejuvenate, or they'll just burn themselves out with their newly rediscovered enthusiasm. When they start to feel good is the time to lay down again to build up their ability to hold energy. Otherwise they just discharge their power before it has built up to its full potential.

Constitutional Weaknesses and Common Ailments

Physiologically, the Ring of Harmony can be the most devastating ring pattern to have. It depletes the person's body, creates social turmoil and depression, and people with this pattern often suffer from immune deficiencies. They don't feel connected to their bodies, are drained by the environment and often look emaciated.

People with Harmony patterns can have a tendency toward lymphatic cancer because their immune system suffers from their social role as an absorbent "white blood cell" – they take on lymphatic consciousness on behalf of the whole of humanity. A lot of Harmony patterns have allergies, which are often unconscious signs of wanting to throw up some inner garbage.

Another characteristic trait of people with Harmony patterns is hyperactivity in the sympathetic nervous system, usually accompanied by an apparently contradictory glandular underactivity, especially in the pancreas, pituitary, adrenal and thyroid. They have a tendency to be hypoglycemic because of overactivity in the pancreas, and hyperadrenal and hypothyroid because they don't relax.

Like a horse that has been ridden too hard for too long, the glands have been overstimulated for so long that there isn't much energy left for another burst of activity when it is needed. Just as the horse will eventually drop if it is ridden like this, so the person's ability to resist disease and adapt to the environment gets stifled. The normal hormonal control mechanism can't function any more.

The glands need to be fed: light for

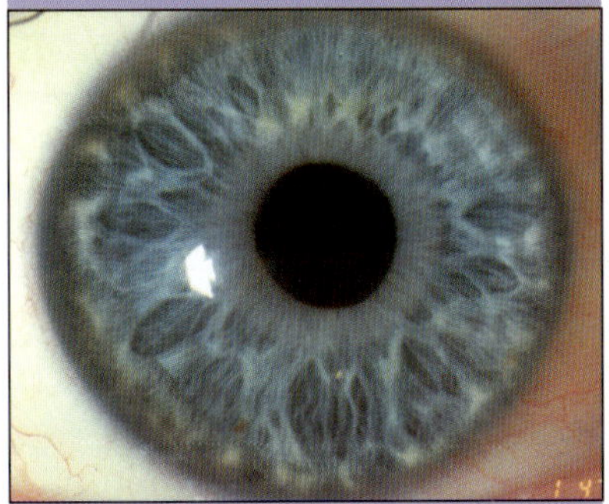

Examples of the Ring of Harmony

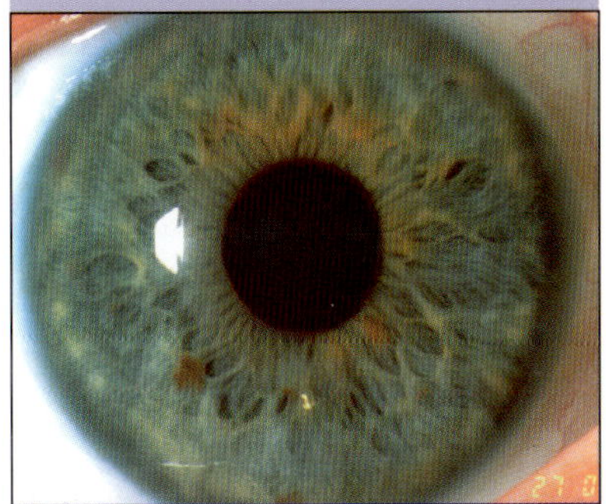

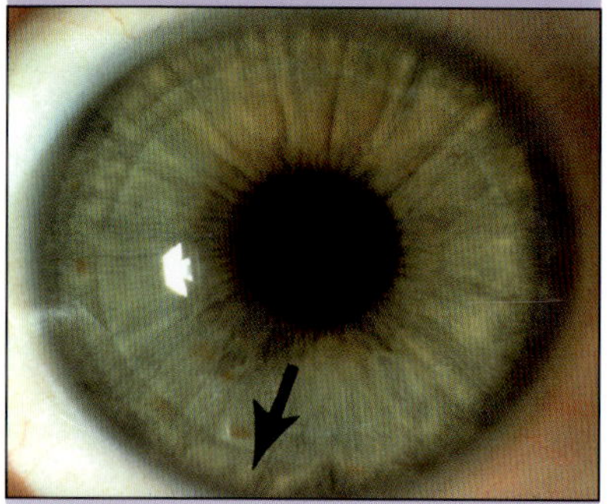

Examples of the Ring of Harmony

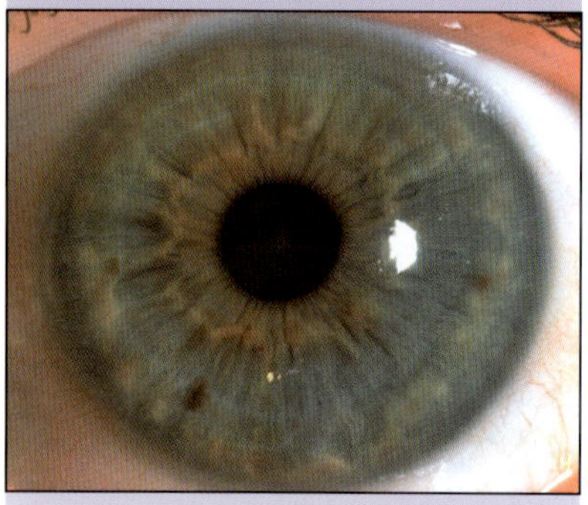

the pineal, voice for the pituitary, touch for the thymus, breathing for the thyroid and for the whole electrical system of the body (the nervous system).

Recommended Therapies

There are two key therapies for the Harmony pattern: stillness and singing.

Rayid practitioners should follow the same therapeutic sequence as they would to strengthen Stream qualities in a person, adding to it an essential ingredient: the need for a constant feeling in the body of indwelling *joy.* Strengthen the central nervous system and do what you can to increase their capacity to retain joy in their bodies. They need to *laugh.*

If you found the Harmony pattern in a Jewel, the Ring of Harmony would override the way that you would normally treat a Jewel and the therapies that you would prescribe. But remember that a Jewel with a Harmony pattern is most likely a Shaker-Jewel – the primary needs of this individual are still kinesthetic, related to a need for social integration, romance and creating a feeling of connectedness. The Jewel's need for intimacy is still being addressed, just targeted at the level of intercellular connections first.

People with this eye structure are somewhat addicted to movement, trying to move everything and everyone, all the time. They would prefer to have a therapy that would put them into motion, rather than one that would bring them toward stillness. It is important to give them a therapy (such as Chi Kung) that creates stillness first; after they have mastered that (quite a challenge!), they can move on to other therapies.

The most effective "nonmovement" exercise for a Harmony pattern is alpha-meditation (see the *Therapies* chapter for details). It is a simple meditation technique involving breathing and stillness. Because they are so depleted, Harmony patterns need to do this exercise at least three times a day in order to rejuvenate their bodies; four times a day to really heal themselves.

There is no quick way to break free of the self-imposed bonds of this structure. The individual will say "Heavens! Lay down for 20 minutes three times a day? I haven't got time for that!" He will clutch at any means to maintain his manic tendency to take care of the world, without beginning to take care of himself, until he can no longer bear the pain.

One way for Harmony patterns to create harmony in their own bodies is to use the healing power of sound. They should sing to their inner being. Singing is one of the most important therapies for a Harmony pattern, since it directly stimulates the myelin sheath surrounding the nerve fibers, particularly those in the spinal cord. Imagine that this sheath is like a drum skin that you vibrate with harmonious sound, particularly voice.

Sing for at least 15 minutes every day and listen to joyful, uplifting music. Keep the following image in your mind: when a Harmony pattern is awake and vibrating with joy, he can walk across a barren meadow and flowers will blossom in front of him. For some people, chanting is even more effective than singing. Try different voice techniques and see what works for you. This therapy is of great benefit for everyone, whether they have a Harmony pattern or not.

Good exercise and a clean, macrobiotic diet with plenty of protein would also be beneficial, but be careful always to maintain a sense of building and stillness. Harmony patterns should be *nurtured* back into a yang state, rather than doing a fast. Whatever therapies are used, it is important that they do not deplete the individual's energy further by overburdening them with too many things to do.

If Harmony patterns feel stressed, they can obtain short-term relief by taking time out from their schedule to concentrate on their breathing for a while. They should inhale the words "strength" and "peace." This is what the Harmony pattern needs; strength to overcome the insanity of the world and a sense of peace to be able to do it with a loving heart. They should exhale the word "harmony." But it is important not to let this little breathing exercise be an excuse to avoid doing the crucial relaxation and meditation work. The breathing is a stop-gap measure, a way to discharge tension and not, by itself, enough to produce significant change.

People with a Harmony pattern need kinesthetic stimulation. For Flowers with a Harmony pattern, use a gentle, peripheral massage technique with soft strokes. For Jewels, it is appropriate to use deeper strokes, getting into the underlying tissues.

Although nutrition is vital for strengthening the system, it is not enough. Once the Harmony pattern starts to feel better, he will be tempted to expend all his newly acquired energy on the world around him, with a tendency to deplete himself just as much as before. Cleansing herbs such as Burdock root should be taken. Chlorophyll is also useful because, having a similar

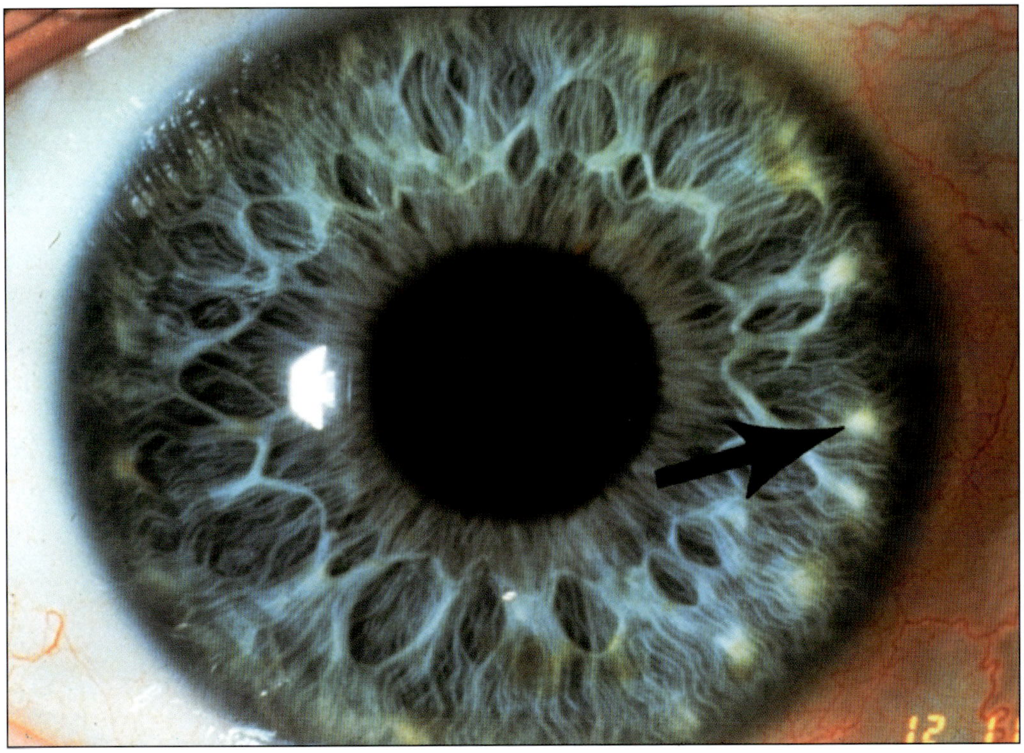

The Ring of Harmony is identified by a series of white, yellow or brown dots forming a circular pattern around the iris, usually toward the periphery.

The Ring of Harmony at a Glance

Iris trait:	Ring of white or gold dots/clusters
Key personality trait:	High ideals of people and environment
Greatest strength:	Influencing others
When imbalanced, they are:	Easily taken advantage of/influenced Cynical, disappointed Depleted, overwhelmed
Achieve balance by learning:	To slow down, rest, rejuvenate Honest and faithful expression To build personal harmony and knowing

structure to hemoglobin, it carries oxygen, helping to oxygenate the system and purify the blood. Iron and folic acid also nurture this pattern.

Be careful when considering movement therapies. Harmony patterns are attracted to endurance exercises but this is not what they need. Metaphorically, they are the sort of people who do aerobics three times a week, work out at the gym and run marathons on the weekend. It is almost impossible to get them to go inside, to rest. They won't take on the effortless responsibility of just stopping. Chi Kung is such a useful therapy for this structure because it simultaneously creates a sense of stillness while focusing attention on inner movement. It also strengthens the central nervous system (the trunk of the person) and develops fine motor skills. It teaches the individual about "holding," about containment.

So what is the key advice for someone with a Ring of Harmony who is tired of being disappointed, who has made the decision to change?

Picture yourself as a fountain of life purifying all of Creation. It's easy. All you have to do is sing and laugh all the time because you know that by putting your own house in order, by being happy and healing your own relationships, you are healing families all over the world. It is your very presence on the planet that has such power; you don't even need to come into direct contact with people to help them, just as you don't have to be consciously acknowledged when you walk into a room in order to have a profound impact on the atmosphere.

Remember that you're a Trojan Horse – you don't always look like what you are, and that can make you even more effective at changing the course of history. This may be hard to understand, but you don't need to understand it in order to make it work!

THE RING OF FREEDOM

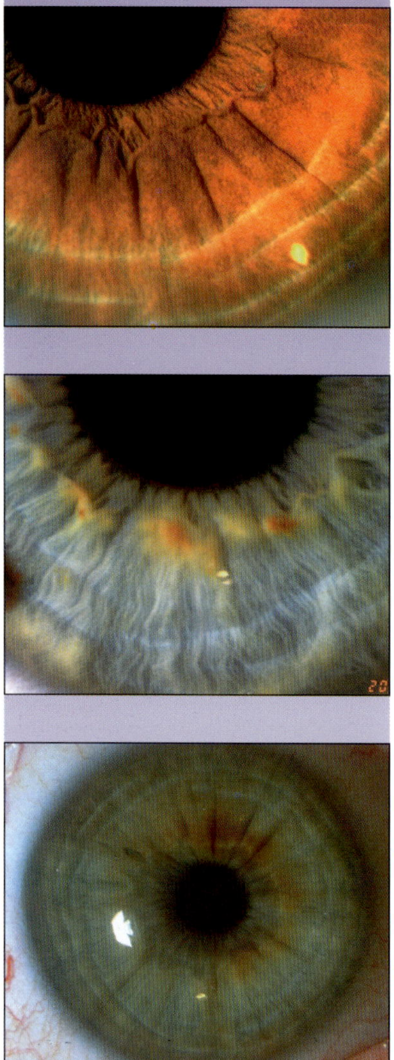

Three examples of the Ring of Freedom.

Sometimes called Rings of Achievement, concentric ridges encircling the pupil suggest an accomplishment-oriented nature. Hyperachievers, these frenetic people have a sense of urgency about them and need to be continuously occupied. Possessed by revolving mental chatter, they live in a state of nearly constant anxiety. They achieve most by channeling their restless energy into specific action and seeing their initiatives through to completion.

In their quest for a more ideal environment, people with an Freedom pattern have a drive to pierce and break up the polarized imbalances in the world around them. Quietly restless, they disturb and dissolve what isn't working. These impatient perfectionists won't accept procrastination or indecisiveness in others and tend to be particularly intolerant of their partners.

Although the Ring of Freedom is more common in irises with some kind of density, such as Jewels or Streams, it can be found in all of the constitutional iris structures and appears to be fully developed by birth. Having photographed the eyes of the same individuals as very young babies and then again several years later, we have not observed the slightest change in the shape or width of any of these lines. They seem to be just as permanent as flowers and jewels which, once formed, do not appear to change either.

People with this structure are extremely sensitive and seem to be constantly in search of something. The greater the number of rings, the greater the effect of the pattern on the personality. They tend to have a lot of dreams, are prone to neuroticism, and are also prone to nervous stress and muscular tension. That does not mean, however, that this ring is a reflection of current stress in the person's life. It reflects something much deeper.

In general, the sensitivity of people with Freedom patterns is associated with an absence of bonding and communication *within this generation*, often characterized by the disintegration of the family unit, particularly the breakup of two-parent families. This ring tends to be found in people who, as children, seldom saw love and kindness between their parents, and so deeply desire it now. But they generally have great difficulty with achieving lasting relationships because of their idealism and perfectionism. If they are disappointed in a relationship, if it doesn't live up to their expectations, they tend to leave quickly. Seekers of the truth, they may insist that their partners also confront the "truth" in their relationship. Lacking in empathy, they are a clear opposite to people with Harmony patterns who generally have too much empathy and self-pity. These two structures generally form complementary relationships and it is possible that the Freedom/Harmony combination represents another paired opposite in the Rayid system.

Children with this structure are less beholden to their genetic patterning, and so are more likely to move beyond the limitations of preceding generations. Their nervous dispositions and stress symptoms seem to be a consequence also of their core-level rebellion, arising from the conflict between their inner knowing and their social programming. This is a conflict that people with a Ring of Freedom must resolve before they can achieve balance; they must learn to focus their energy and act on the basis of their inner knowing.

Breathing meditations and therapies are useful tools for helping people with a Freedom pattern to feel less anxious. They are also deeply affected by smell, which means that aromatherapy is particularly effective. People have little conscious capacity to regulate their sense of smell, so aromas can quickly penetrate deep down into the core of the central nervous system. One's state of consciousness can be instantly altered and enlivened with scents.

Nowadays, 40% of babies have these concentric circles, whereas they are very rare in people over the age of 60. This pattern is now so common that it could represent a new primary iris structure, a fifth structural type that is indicative of our times. This ring appears to represent a new type of personality that has been growing rapidly in importance during the past 30 to 40 years; perhaps a new kind of consciousness is developing on the planet in order to effect social change.

If the Jewel, Flower, Stream and Shaker represent the polarization of direction into north, south, east and west, the Ring of Freedom metaphorically represents that which is unpolarized. People with this ring have a tendency to destroy polarization. They dislike any system that divides, categorizes or labels, especially if it tries to label *them.*

People with a Freedom pattern do not want anybody to have control in a situation, not even themselves. When

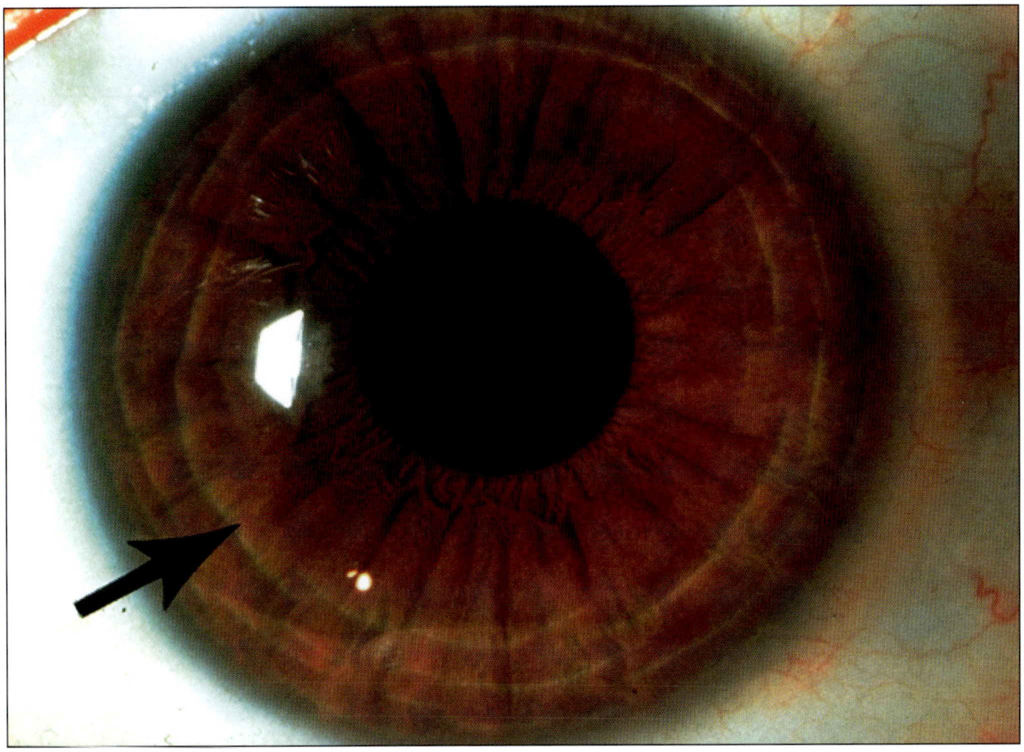

The Ring of Freedom consists of light, concentric lines encircling the pupil.

The Ring of Freedom at a Glance

Iris trait:	Complete or broken concentric lines
Key personality trait:	Achievement-oriented
Greatest strength:	Motivation to produce
When imbalanced, they are:	Frenetic, have an undirected urgency Anxious Helpless
Achieve balance by learning:	Appropriate, focused action Giving

there is control, there might be confinement and limitation, and that would conflict with their preference for remaining in a dynamic state of unrest. At the very deepest level, however, they yearn for oneness.

They don't have any aversion to groups per se but they don't like it when people follow the herd. They are most comfortable in a cohesive group of dynamic individuals who are all appreciative of each other's qualities and who are all self-responsible – a leaderless group. They do not do well in a hierarchical situation. They are disobedient, reactive and simply refuse to follow orders. For this reason, they make *very* poor soldiers.

People with a Ring of Freedom are nonconformists. When they find themselves in a conformist situation, they destroy it. They don't like to learn from teachers. They prefer to have a direct experience of whatever it is that they are trying to understand.

Despite being in a state of constant agitation, they are none the less highly productive because they are always striving to create something. But their productivity does not bring contentment. They are usually uncomfortable with their creations, especially if they obey a system of rules. As artists they tend to be subversive, challenging the accepted norms of structure and form. Whenever people with this pattern try to accomplish something using an established system, they quickly become frustrated with its limitations. These are the reformers and transformers of society. In their search for the experience of oneness and perfection, they constantly destroy and rebuild.

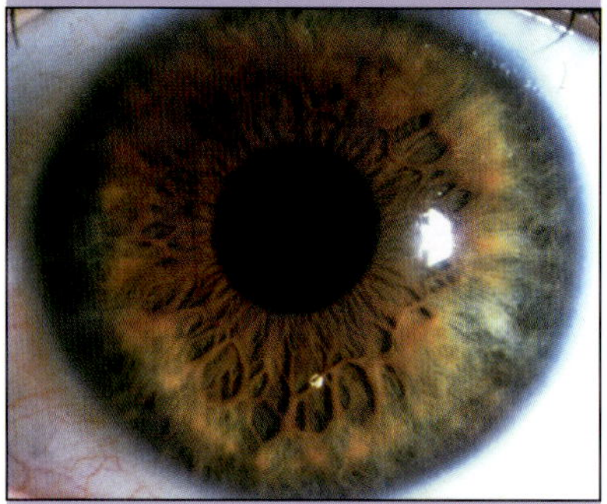

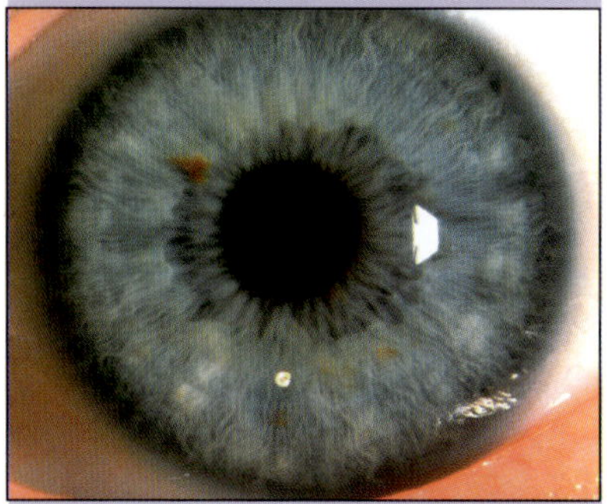

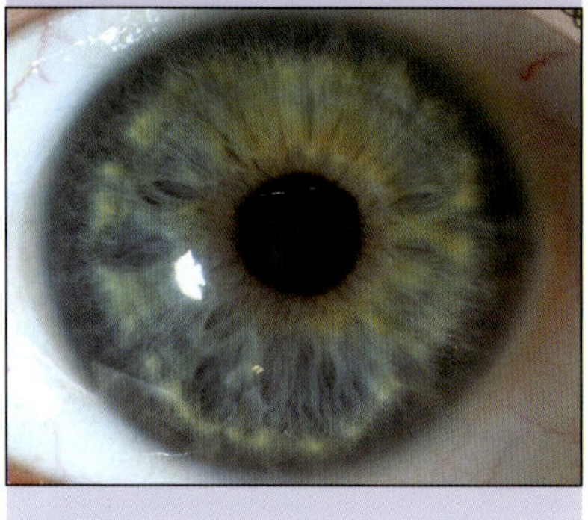

Three examples of the Ring of Purpose.

THE RING OF PURPOSE

A blue or dark ring at the periphery of the iris indicates a sense of special purpose. People with this ring are constantly searching for their mission in life. Through diligence and commitment, they are capable of anything. Unclear about how to accomplish their objectives and focus their action, however, they can experience indecisiveness or stagnation. Through hard work and focused action, this personality can experience all of life as having a special purpose.

The Ring of Purpose, sometimes called the Specialist Ring, is created by an absence of fiber at the periphery of the iris. This is relevant because the periphery of the iris represents the kinesthetic, the physical aspects of life. People with this ring have a highly conceptual nature and so have difficulty manifesting their efforts in the physical world. They are the kind of people who say, "Yes, I could do anything!" But when you try to get them to be more specific about what they want to do, they resist. They don't want to get trapped by anything so they prefer to keep their plans nebulous. They typically assert that, sometime in the future, when it's appropriate, they will get a clear signal from a place of inner knowing and inspiration telling them what to do – a kind of divine telegram.

Soft, quiet, not outwardly opinionated nor anxious about life, people with a Ring of Purpose can, however, seem a little smug and satisfied with their own sense of specialness, implying that it is only a matter of time before their virtue is recognized; inwardly, however, at a subconscious level, they are often deeply dissatisfied. Although they tend to feel inwardly confident, they also know, at a subtle level, that they could risk losing that sense of confidence if they were to experience failure. They usually have a fear of failure, and therefore have a tendency to dissolve risky initiatives before they produce or create anything. That way they're safe from possible adverse outcomes.

People with this iris structure also tend to be idealistic, and are sometimes the head of a special cause. Knowing that their time is coming, and not prepared to accept less than their ideal, they would rather wait a lifetime than take action to change their situation *now,* to implement the steps that would transform their ideal into a reality. They are prone to procrastination and, while feeling like they could certainly handle power if it came to them, they prefer not to actually do anything about it for the moment. Generally outwardly allowing, this reluctance to act can make them intrinsically fixated to the point of inertia.

Often displeased in relationships, they usually fail to communicate it. They prefer to "Live and let live." This laissez faire attitude is a reflection of their preference not to examine what does and doesn't work in their lives in general. They avoid calls to action in their relationships, in stark contrast to people with a Ring of Determination, who will usually tell you more than you want to know about the ways in which they are dissatisfied. At the root of this difference may be their general sense of optimism that things will work out; people with Determination patterns tend to be rather cynical and pessimistic about life.

Apart from their tendency toward procrastination, and a propensity for arterial constriction, cold hands and feet, there are no particularly negative manifestations associated with this iris structure, either physically or in terms of their social behavior, precisely because they tend to be so self-contained.

The Ring of Purpose can be discerned as readily in newborn babies as in adults. There doesn't seem to be a higher incidence of the ring in a particular age group, nor do we have any photographic evidence of it changing permanently. It appears to be exclusively genetically determined, since environmental experiences don't appear to have any effect on it. Apparent changes have been photographed but are due to the fact that the size of the iris is not fixed. At varying stages of development the outer portions of the iris seems to become slightly "submerged" in the sclera, and at other times to rise out of the sclera which makes the band of the Ring of Purpose appear broader. This effect, however, is transitory and the iris always comes back again later.

People who have a Ring of Purpose are fun to deal with. If you are a practitioner, you will find that they are very easy to reach. If you help them, they are most appreciative, making you feel like God's favorite child, which is exactly how *they* feel most of the time. They feel special, blessed, chosen. And they keep waiting for some kind of directive from on high to tell them what to do. They know that they are on a special mission; they just haven't been given their orders yet. They feel capable of doing anything, but they wait. There

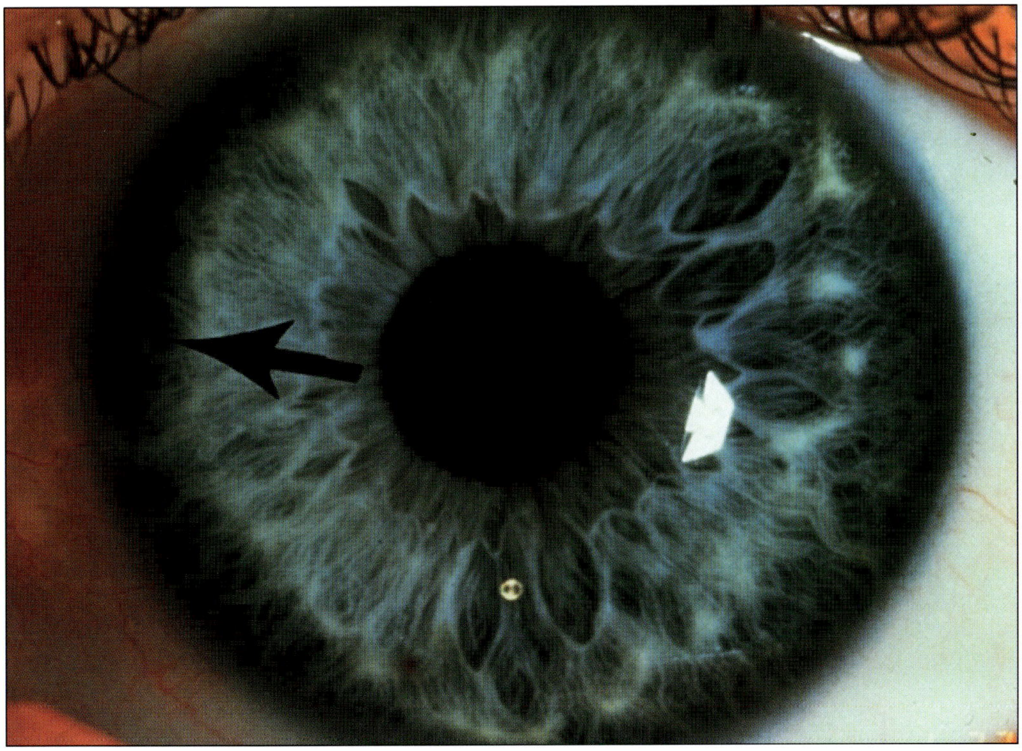

The Ring of Purpose is a blue or dark ring at the periphery of the iris.

The Ring of Purpose at a Glance

Iris trait:	Continuous, blue or dark peripheral band
Key personality trait:	Sense of specialness or mission
Greatest strength:	Poise, calmness
When imbalanced, they are:	Confused Indecisive, stagnant Quietly smug
Achieve balance by learning:	Diligence Commitment Alertness

is a conceptual, abstract, future-oriented quality about their lives. It is the indecisiveness which stems from this abstraction that is their biggest challenge.

Achieving Balance

With an aversion for the grounding experience of physical reality, people with this structure commonly avoid touch. This avoidance brings with it a tendency for them to lack connections with other people. Being touched is a very tangible experience and they generally prefer to live in the etheric realms. When approached sensitively, they can actually benefit greatly from some type of physical stimulation: a skin brush or light massage to improve circulation at the periphery of their bodies, for example. But the real issue is their habitual process of keeping things conceptual.

As with almost all of the rings, the Ring of Purpose invariably appears in the outer third of the iris, which represents physical actualization. For people with this ring, the lack of fiber at the periphery of the iris metaphorically represents their limited presence in the physical world. They need to actualize physical contact or actualize physical commitment. If they keep focusing their experience on conceptual reality, they are unlikely to free themselves of their procrastination, doubt, confusion and inward orientation.

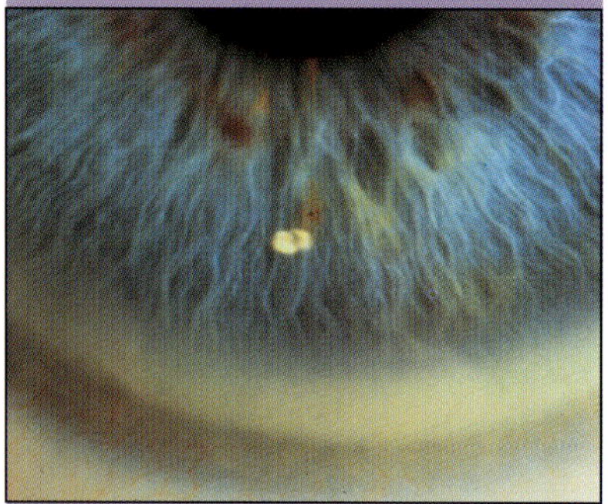

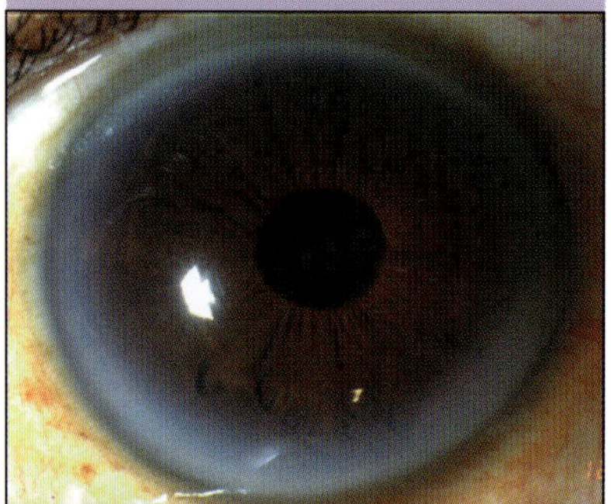

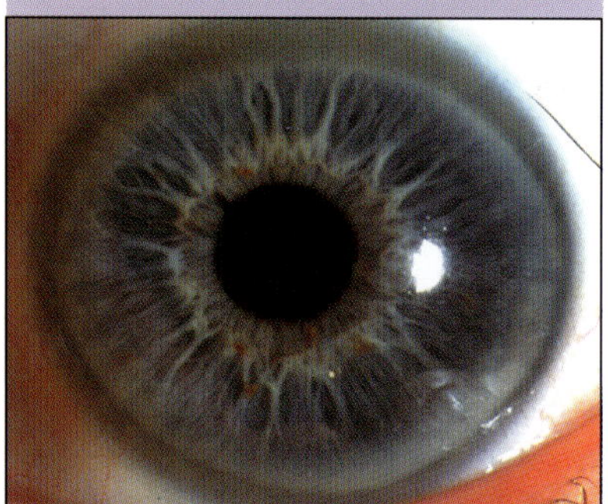

Three examples of the Ring of Determination.

THE RING OF DETERMINATION

A continuous white band at the periphery of the iris indicates a hardening of the arteries and a hardening of the attitudes. It identifies a determined or decisive nature. Clear about the virtue of their beliefs, people with this ring usually possess strong opinions *and* the skills to accomplish their objectives. Often rigidly single-minded and inflexible, they come across as being opinionated and unwilling to accept another person's point of view. By going inward and developing spiritual certainty, people with a Ring of Determination not only learn flexibility and acceptance of others, they also find inner peace.

A Ring of Determination indicates a tendency toward fixation and intolerance. These personality traits are most noticeable in social situations, when people with this pattern show themselves to be intolerant or fixed about what they want. While they may be operating from an emotional perspective, Flowers with this ring also have the power to control their emotions, so this aspect of their personalities may not be evident.

People with this ring typically have a fixation with the past, always dwelling on the way it was. They generally resist anything new, and if someone else in the group wants to talk about change, or something progressive, they often react with scorn. When you get two of them together, they *love* to talk about the past together.

Called the Sodium Ring by iridologists, this white band usually takes 50 to 60 years to form, and is rare in people below the age of 40. It commonly forms from the top of the iris down, although it can occasionally be found at the bottom without being visible at the top. When only partially developed, the general region of its formation seems to indicate the area of life that the person is most hardened about: social relationships, intimacy, philosophical ideas, etc. Refer to the maps of iris regions (see *Positions in the Iris*) when interpreting any partially developed iris ring.

The latter quarter of one's life is usually a time of both physiological and sociological decline, especially for people with a Ring of Determination. As their physical strength wanes, they tend to ignore their bodies and also to withdraw from their families and social situations. This is usually an unconscious attempt to create isolation. This process of withdrawal can appear to be involuntary. Some older people with this ring simply become so reactive and intolerant that nobody wants to deal with them. This creates a separation from their family members as predictably as if they were actively withdrawing by not talking or refusing to come out of their rooms.

With the decline of social connection comes an increase in individuality and a sense of separateness. This, in turn, is a preparation for that last great journey in life, which must always be undergone alone. In the anticipation of death comes the beginning of isolation. If people are afraid of the future, afraid of going down that tunnel into the unknown, they are likely to develop a fixation with the past. This fixation can cause them to literally shut down their fear and consequent constriction shuts off the blood circulation, hardens them and makes them go inward. Such people typically develop a Ring of Determination.

Achieving Balance

There are a number of ways to counteract the fear and reactiveness typical of an elderly person with a Ring of Determination. Taking steps to raise the blood-sugar level, sometimes just by improving the person's ability to assimilate nutrients in general, and stimulating the person's intellectual processes are simple but effective measures.

The mind serves to maintain your self-image; in a sense, it stores the blueprints for your own psychological development. If the template of the mind is fixed, it cannot help but begin to create external fixations. When the mind is being actively stimulated and challenged, when it is growing, developing and learning, the individual is much less likely to have fixed and intolerant opinions, and it is highly unlikely that this white band will develop. Mental stimulation is all that many elderly people need.

Physical stimulation of specific parts of the body can also be valuable, especially those areas that are associated with the constrictive Jewel mentality – the fingers, toes, soles of the feet, the head and the neck, for example – the peripheral parts of the body that are involved in fine motor function and control. Brushing the surface of the skin to improve blood circulation and toxin elimination is also an effective remedy. If you are familiar enough with it, stimulating the parasympathetic nervous system with the fingers will also

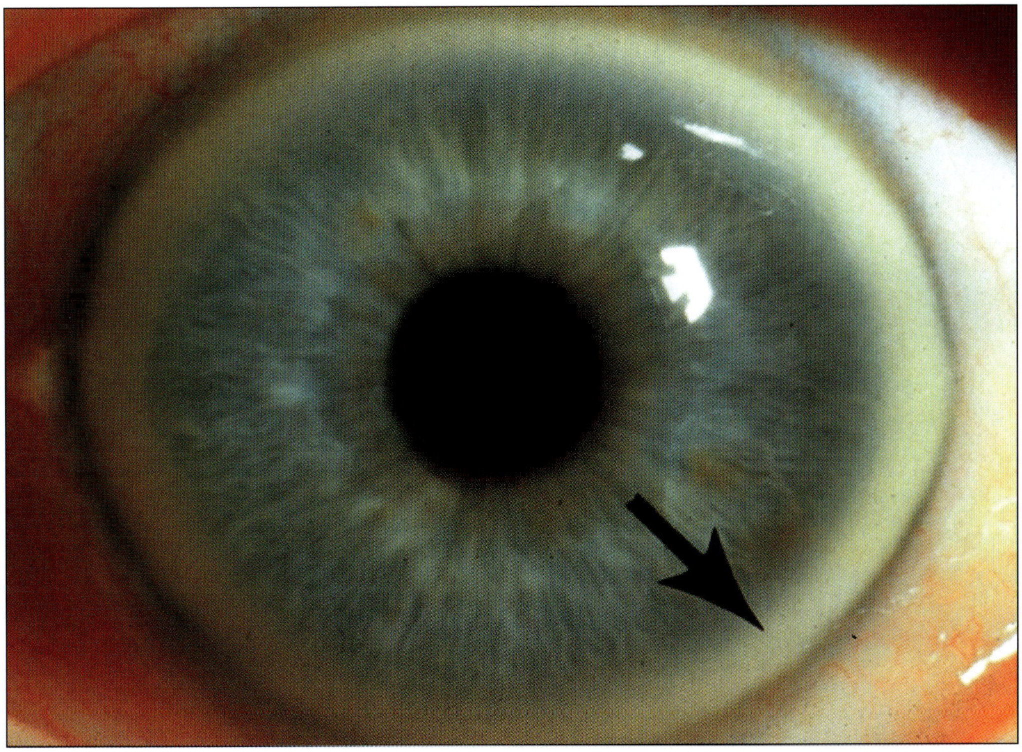

The Ring of Determination is a continuous white band at the periphery of the iris.

The Ring of Determination at a Glance

Iris trait:	Continuous, white peripheral band
Key personality trait:	Decisive certainty of self
Greatest strength:	Determination, boldness
When imbalanced, they are:	Out of touch
	Defensive
	Unyielding
Achieve balance by learning:	Acceptance
	Inner attentiveness, spiritual direction
	To slow down, be still

improve the flow of blood to the brain and around the body. All of these remedies help to develop dexterity and improve the function and clarity of the mind in people with a Ring of Determination.

Have you ever noticed how much older people love sugar? Please don't try to take it away from them. Instead, encourage them to eat a better quality of sugar, such as honey or some other, healthier alternative to processed sugar. The primary thing they're after is blood sugar. In elderly people with a Ring of Determination, the digestive function is typically so weakened that it is difficult for them to break down complex carbohydrates and proteins, so they crave sugars instead.

When a person with this ring is overweight, it is usually in response to an unconscious fear of being fully present in all aspects of his being, particularly the mental realms. By gaining weight, he focuses his own and everyone else's attention on his body. If they can overcome this fear, people with a Ring of Determination are capable of extraordinary creative vision and even psychic experiences.

The experience of spiritual openness is one of the best remedies for those who have a Ring of Determination. If they are spiritually open and allowing, if they are able to be in the present and to contemplate the future with openness and confidence, they are much less likely to develop a reactive tendency to become fixated on the past.

Positions in the Iris

In addition to the behavioral insights that can be gained from an understanding of the overall iris structure and rings, much can be learned by examining the specific location of traits (jewels, flowers and streams) in the iris.

Each area of the iris is associated with different thoughts, feelings and attitudes. The presence of a jewel, flower or stream characteristic in any position activates and intensifies the release of a distinct behavioral temperament. The majority of these behavioral tendencies are genetically inherited from our parents. By using the Positions chart (see p. 58, also available separately) as a map and looking into the eyes, you can determine specific personality characteristics with a greater degree of accuracy than a simple understanding of the primary structural types would allow.

The nature of the trait (i.e. whether it is a flower or a jewel) changes the nature of the interpretation. For example, a jewel in the area of Will (No. 43) would indicate an outward conflict with the eye parent; a flower in the same area would indicate that the individual consents and answers to the will of the parent. In some areas of the iris, a trait will occur only as a jewel, in others only as a flower.

This chapter provides an overview of specific behavioral trigger positions in the iris. It explains key elements of their relationship to the long-term personality pattern of the individual, concentrating on the most important positions.

THE BIG PICTURE

DNA as Puppeteer

When studying the message revealed by individual iris positions, it is important that you understand the factors that determine and modify their effects.

Every position in the iris affects every other position, and every position is affected by whichever of the four primary energies is dominant in the personality: Jewel, Flower, Stream or Shaker. The primary personality is in turn also affected by traits in each iris position. These complex interrelationships make it important to remain aware of the overall message contained in the eye when doing an iris interpretation. Maintaining a clear image of the big picture will improve your effectiveness in consultations and help prevent you from getting lost in the details.

To use an analogy, the primary iris structure describes the particular vibration of the individual as a standing wave pattern, and indicates how he will interact with other people. Jewels operate from a mental perspective, Flowers are more emotional, Streams have a stabilizing frequency and Shakers embody change. These basic patterns are genetically determined.

Each specific trait in the iris represents a modification of this basic structural pattern, vibrational adjustments that speed up or slow down the base vibration of the overall personality type in particular areas of behavior. These modifications to the overall personality, visible as individual jewels and flowers in the iris, are also genetically determined.

In a sense, DNA is the master puppeteer that controls a person's behavior. Individual flowers and jewels in the iris indicate the points of attachment of the puppet strings that determine the variations in someone's personality. At the other end, deep in the unconscious, these puppet strings are attached to the two opposing strands of the double helix of DNA.

The overall effect of this subconscious mechanism of control is far more important than the details of how and why a person exhibits a specific behavioral trait. In other words, it is more important to understand the overwhelming power of the puppeteer than it is to go into detail about the location of the points of attachment of the strings on the puppet. Remember: don't get lost in the details!

Long-term Structural Balance

Having spent several years developing specific therapies to remedy the personality difficulties associated with each individual iris position, it was quite a reawakening to realize that they are all there to fulfill a purpose; when that purpose is achieved, the need for the therapy automatically vanishes and the positive expression associated with the position becomes dominant.

This long-term purpose is the alignment of the personality structure in the experience of wholeness. For example, excessively Flower-oriented people normally have an Anger, Nurturing or Resentment issue in the left eye (right hemisphere) that would push them more into the left hemisphere. This shift allows them to develop some degree of self-control, individuality and emotional constriction, thereby helping to balance their Flowerness.

Your structural type is not your true self. It simply gives an indication of how you will behave when you are out of touch with your core nature. What we describe as "Jewel characteristics" or "Flower traits" are different personality responses to an inner distress, symptomatic of someone who is not experiencing his true essence. When they are consciously connected to their core natures, Jewels and Flowers behave in similar ways, and all overt personality symptoms of distress are gone. That is the wholeness we seek.

Life is a balancing experience. We set up patterns in our relationships and interactions without realizing that they lead to the outcome of balancing our structure. It is more important to seek an overall balance for the whole person than it is to balance individual personality traits revealed in the iris. Look past the current behavioral issues to see what an observed pattern is teaching. Bear in mind that, wherever patterns exist, they are there to facilitate a change in structure.

For example, if someone has an issue with an absence of nurturing, your goal is not to have them initiate more touch and more bonding in their lives, but to look at what the absence of nurturing is leading them toward. Oftentimes a flower in the area of Nurturing can indicate a tendency toward withdrawn, stand-offish behavior. To suggest that such a person go out and initiate touch, when he is not a natural initiator, could be construed as rather haughty and insensitive. It could also be taking the person away from the long-term lesson of that positional trait. The trait may be there to facilitate a movement inward, or a shift in hemispheres.

An Anger issue in the left eye indicates an anger pattern with women. With therapeutic techniques such as suggestion or psychotherapy, you can change a person's reactions to women without realizing that this issue was there to facilitate a hemispheric shift that would ultimately change the very character of the person and facilitate his long-term movement toward wholeness.

Every position in the eye is a gift; don't think in terms of "getting rid" of an area's influence. Regard all traits as positive attributes. They are not just some transgenerational garbage that is there simply to be weeded out. They are not just problems to be coped with; they are pointers to how we can grow and change. They are there to facilitate a long-term evolution of consciousness.

There is an unconscious mechanism that automatically gives us the lessons we need in order to move toward wholeness. If we find these lessons uncomfortable, we can choose to understand their value and to learn them in a conscious way instead.

INTERPRETING POSITIONAL TRAITS

In addition to position, there are several other factors that must be considered when interpreting traits in the eyes: the size of any jewels relative to other jewels, their shape, and the intensity of their color; the density of fibers in a Stream; and the size of flowers and how closed they are. For example, tightly enclosed flowers indicate a more contained type of expression in any particular position than you might otherwise expect. When determining the behavioral impact of any position, it must also be considered in the light of other key positions.

It is difficult to make a transparent overlay of the location of positions and place it over a photograph of the eye to speed up the interpretation of positions, since the trigger points move a little bit from person to person. For this reason, it is just as important to learn the usual shape of an area as its location. Use the positions indicated on the Positions chart as a guide, all the while understanding that they are not necessarily in precisely the same location for all people. If you are uncertain about the precise meaning of a location, ask your client! As long as you know approximately what is going on in a given region, it can be very productive to approach your client with some humility and say, "You know, this is a challenging position for me. Let me ask you some questions about what it might be and then you tell me what it is." The client's case history then adds to your understanding of that area, giving you excellent information about the meaning of the position.

Any trait right on the Ring of Expression (see p 32) and extending into the emotional region is much more readily expressed. If the Ring of Expression in a Stream is very jagged, regard the "star points" coming out from the ring as traits.

The outcome of having a trait in a particular position may sometimes be the opposite to what you would expect. For example, an Anger issue in the left eye of a Flower may move the person out of the right hemisphere toward the left, making him appear more mental and *less* emotional, but be aware that he is only *pretending* to be nonemotional.

The text refers only to flowers and jewels. Stream characteristics should be interpreted as flowers if the fibers are loose, open or even absent from an area (expansive); as jewels if the fibers are dense and tightly-knit in an area (constrictive). Be aware that someone with a Stream personality won't necessarily be aware of an issue where there is no fiber, precisely because there is an "absence" there.

The Seven Major Triggers

There are seven major trigger points in the iris that are most useful in a consultation. These are the positions that are most likely to create a hemispheric shift affecting the individual's current behavior. The effects of the other positions are generally minor, although there are a few others that can be important, e.g. No. 42 (Authority).

The seven major trigger positions are: No. 1 (Nurturing), No. 2 (Resentment), No. 3 (Anger), No. 14 (Impatience), No. 16 (Self-esteem), No. 43 (Will) and No. 45 (Heart). With only one exception, a jewel or flower in any one of these seven positions will tend to move the person to the hemisphere associated with the *opposite* eye. For example, a flower in Anger in the left iris (associated with the right brain) indicates that the person is or will be moving toward the *left* hemisphere.

The only exception to this general rule is that a jewel in Nurturing *pulls* the individual toward the hemisphere associated with the iris in which the trait is found, e.g. a Nurturing jewel in the left iris will pull the individual toward the right hemisphere.

In most cases, if there is a trait in one or more of the major trigger positions in the left eye, you would not expect to find triggers activated in the right eye. The triggers tend to compound each other in effect, and it is unusual to find significant traits in the major trigger positions of both eyes.

REGIONS OF THE IRIS

The iris can be divided up into regions in a number of different ways that aid in-depth analysis.

1. Vertical Axis

The upper half of the eye does not seem to have as much effect on the personality as the lower half, and there are almost always more traits in the bottom half of the eye than in the top. There is a great accumulation of *transgenerational* patterns in the lower part of the eye. At the top of the eye, traits will not have such a dramatic impact because they are newer. There is an energetic movement from the top of the eye to the bottom, just as there is a movement from the pupil to the periphery of the iris.

Auditory/Mental: The top third of the eye provides information primarily about auditory, mental, philosophical, individuality and will issues. No matter what our primary iris structure, we all have iris traits that reflect our mental (Jewel), kinesthetic (Stream) and emotional (Flower) characteristics. This area of the iris gives insights into the Jewel aspects of the individual personality.

Kinesthetic: This is the area across the horizontal axis on both sides of the pupil, including positions 1 , 45, 46, 27, 28, 29 and 30. Other positions also have kinesthetic applications but this is the primary area. The kinesthetic (Stream) region relates to body movement, movement in relationships, family and home, and inward journeys.

Emotional/Creative: The lower third of the eye relates mainly to emotional and creative personality traits, group dynamics and flow. These are the Flower aspects of the personality.

2. Horizontal Axis

If you knew only the lateral region of the eye, you could successfully diagnose the majority of people.

Lateral region: The outer portion of the iris is primarily related to social interaction, one-to-many relationships and emotional experience. This is the region of social dynamics, your interactions with people at large, providing insights into how you bond, express yourself and create in a social context. This is also the more conscious half of the eye, relating to the front part of the body. As this region is the most easily accessible to the conscious memory of the individual, it is here that the initial part of a consultation should be directed, since it is relatively easy to get confirmation from the client of your interpretations in this region.

Medial region: The half of the iris toward the nose is primarily related to inner dynamics. Although all positions in the iris are concerned with how the individual relates to other people, this half of the iris reflects his interactions one-to-one.

This region also gives insight into the unconscious part of the personality

Right iris:
Left-brain/ Masculine traits

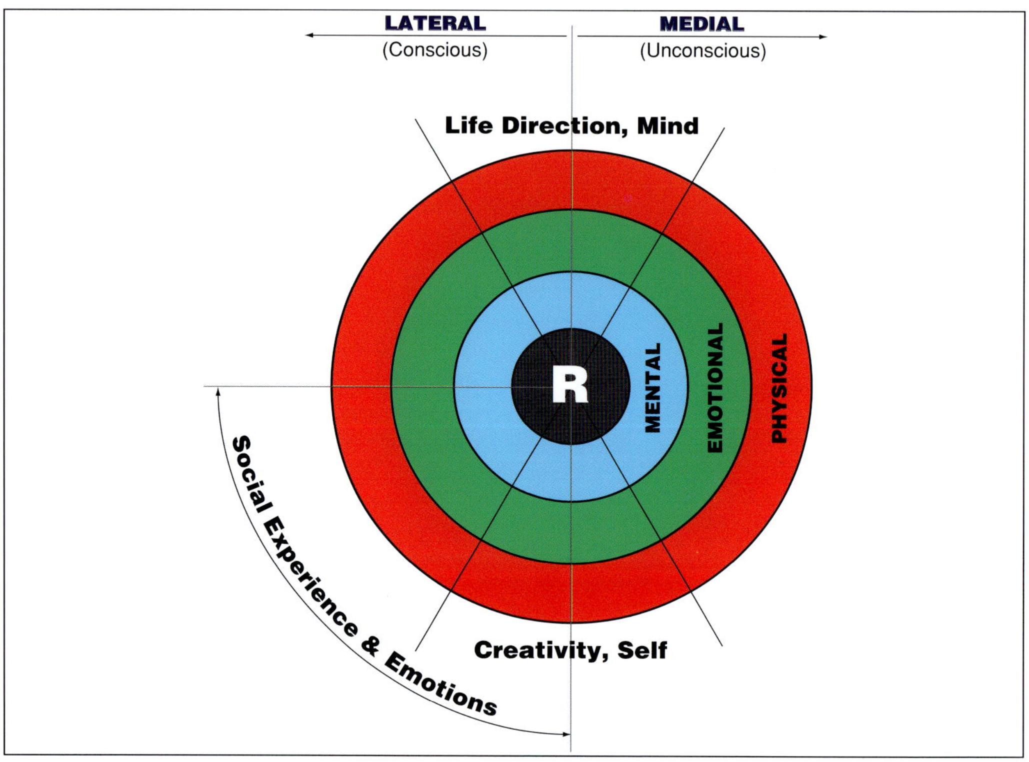

and represents the (hidden) back half of the body.

3. Moving Out from the Pupil

The zone closest to the pupil indicates the condition of the mental body; the physical body is reflected in traits around the periphery of the iris; and the emotional body is the area sandwiched in between.

Some interpretive areas, such as No. 1 (Nurturing), span two or more of these radial regions. In such cases, if a trait within the area is found closer to the pupil, it should be interpreted in the light of its mental or emotional aspects; if it is found toward the periphery of the iris, it will be more likely that the individual has had a physical experience associated with the issue.

All traits found closer to the pupil (deeper into the iris) are more subtle in nature, so it is harder to get a confirmation on these traits from the client. They are less easily confirmed since the individual is generally less aware of them.

Any time you have a jewel trait in one of the mental body positions (No. 7 through No. 21 on the inner part of the iris, toward the pupil), it will manifest as some type of worry. That worry is a constant regurgitation and repetition of a situation or relationship pattern that once caused the individual to experience insecurity. They also manifest as control issues. The most likely trait you will find on this inner part of the iris is a jewel, and a jewel is a control-oriented pattern because of the tightness and constriction associated with it.

Jewel traits are also the most likely to appear at the periphery of the iris.

4. Iris "Petals" and "Wedges"

Adjacent areas in the iris are also related to each other. If you change position slightly within a given region of the iris, you are picking up variations of a particular frequency of thought. Positions 7, 6 and 5, for example, are all similar ways of acting out a particular frequency of emotion. Similar, yet different.

To help you to group together related positions in the eye, imagine that the iris is a flower composed of about ten large petals, each of which is about the size of areas 14, 15 and 16 together. These petals represent the ten major regions of personality-affected behavior.

Just as positions in the upper part of the eye are more mental, those in the middle are more kinesthetic, and those in the lower part of the eye are more emotional, so the same pattern is repeated holographically around the eye. This insight can be used to understand the relationship between positions that are grouped together in a particular region.

Many of the regional iris petals can be further subdivided into neighboring sections shaped like a wedge or slice of pie. For example, if the area bounded by positions 1, 7, 5 and 8 is one iris petal, then positions 1 and 7 form one wedge within that region.

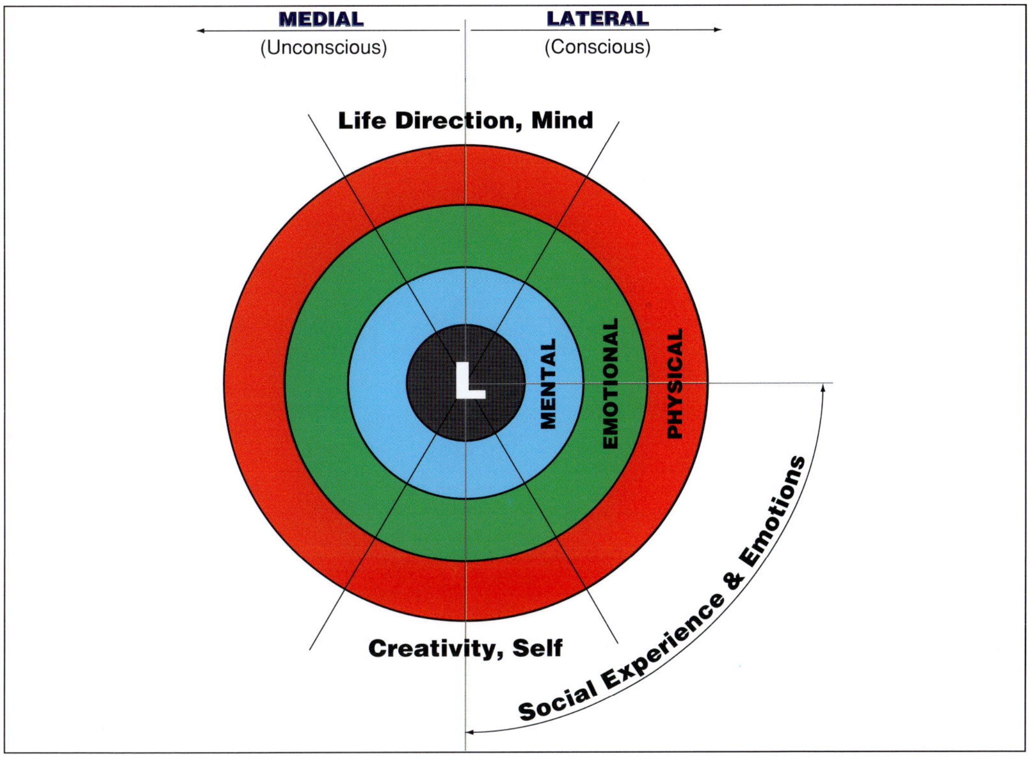

Left iris:
Right-brain/ Feminine traits

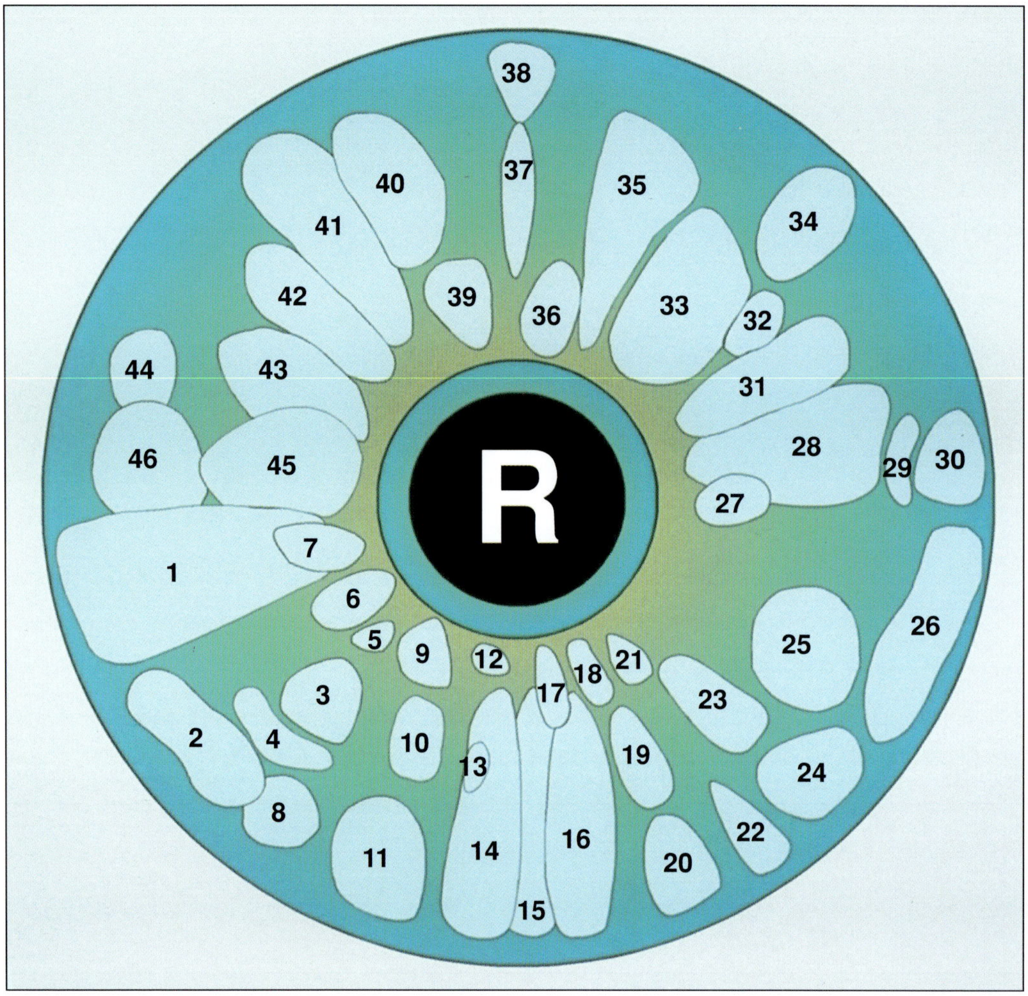

Iris positions, right eye

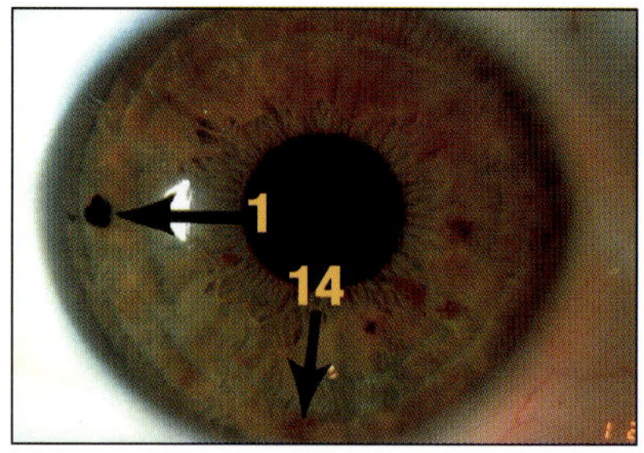

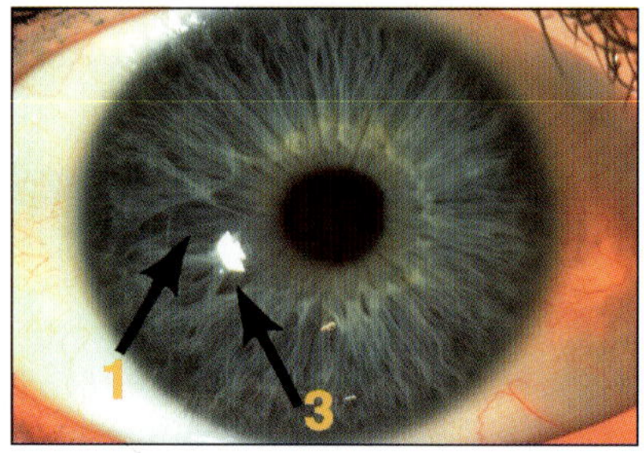

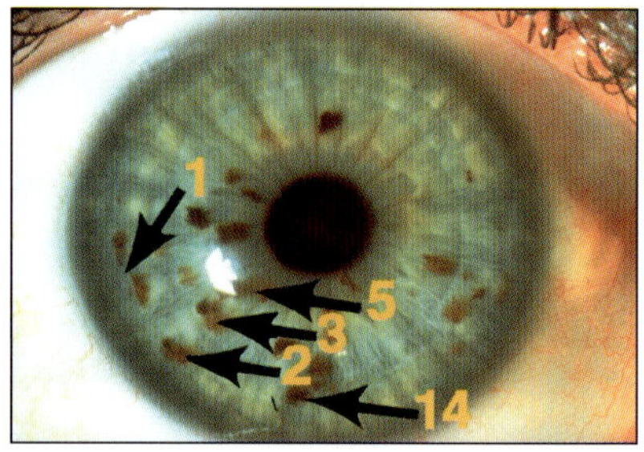

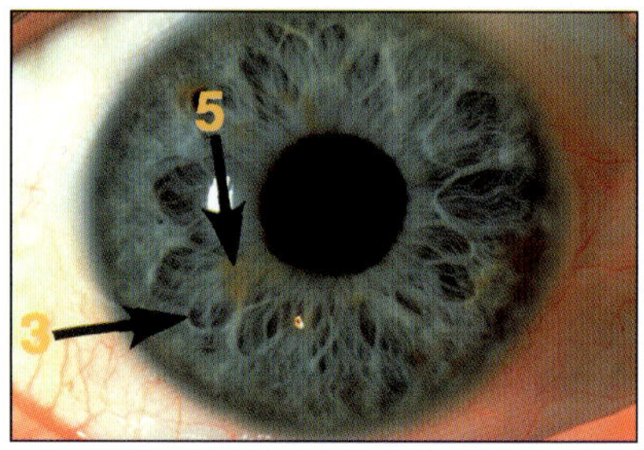

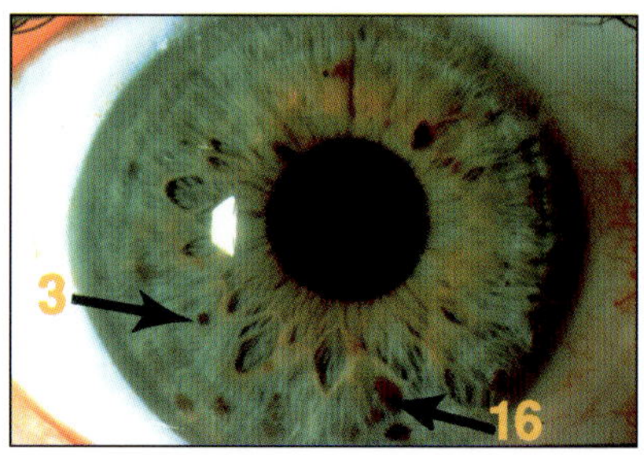

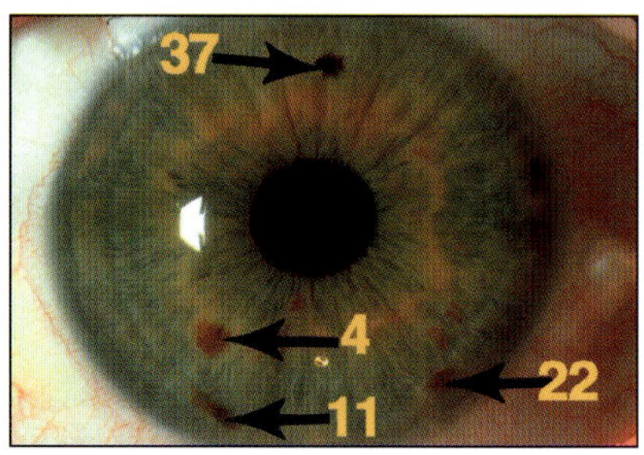

Throughout this section, irises are placed as they would be if you were looking at someone. Imagine that the gutter between the two pages is a person's nose. The left iris is to the right of this gutter, and the right iris is to the left of it.

Petal 1 - 8

This region is concerned with the nature of control: the control of one's movements, emotions, expression, bonding, giving, receiving and sex. It describes inner dynamics and relationships.

1. Nurturing

This area has a lot to do with kinesthetic *motivation.* It is about physical expression and physical involvement. A flower in Nurturing indicates internalization and a desire for independence. A jewel in Nurturing indicates externalization and a person who works for approval and/or love. It is more common to find a flower in this position than a jewel. The lesson associated with a Nurturing trait could be to develop individuality or to de-emphasize the person's material nature.

Jewels in this position are primarily an environmental or present-generational trait, while flowers are usually a sequential follow-through of a jewel trait from a previous generation. In either case, the pattern can stem from issues between the parent and the child, or between the parents, or between the parents and their parents.

Nurturing issues may be reflected in difficulty with the initiation of projects it is a difficult area in relationships because people with Nurturing issues are almost always looking for rejection.

For an in-depth study of this position, contact Rayid International for a copy of the *Nurturing* tape or booklet.

Flower: A flower in Nurturing usually has a round shape. It tends to create stand-offish behavior but it also creates independence, self-reliance and individuality. It creates mental

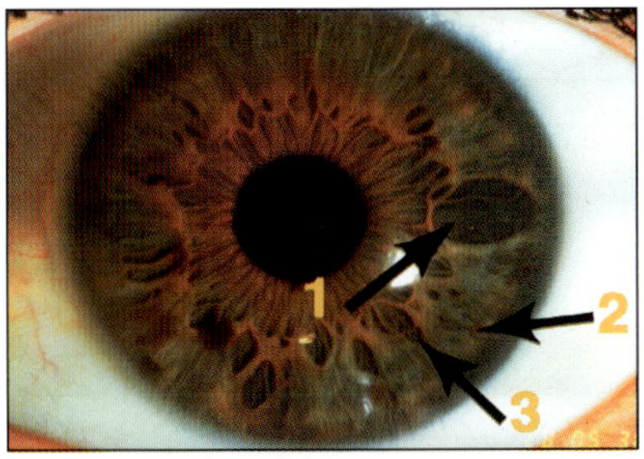

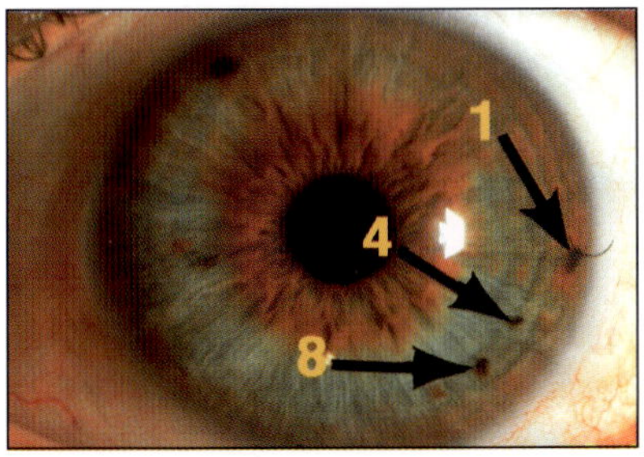

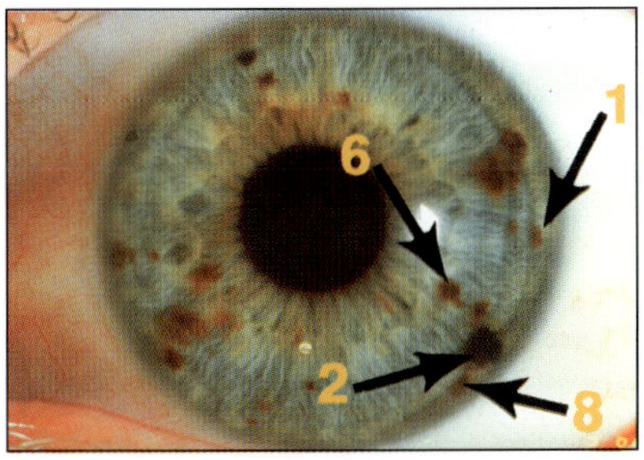

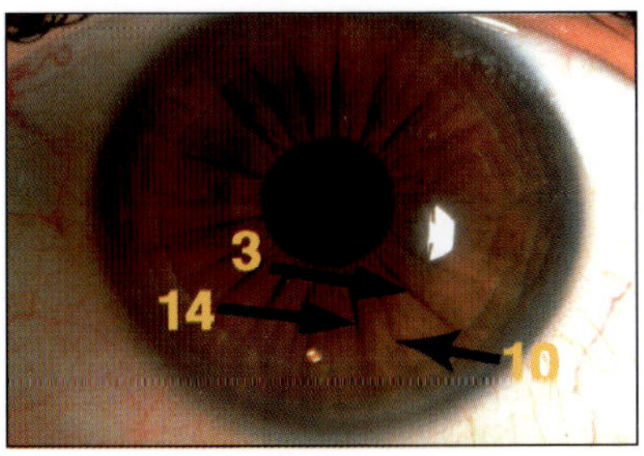

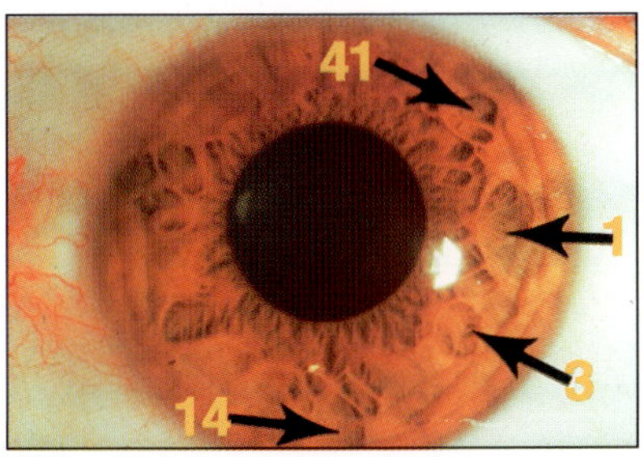

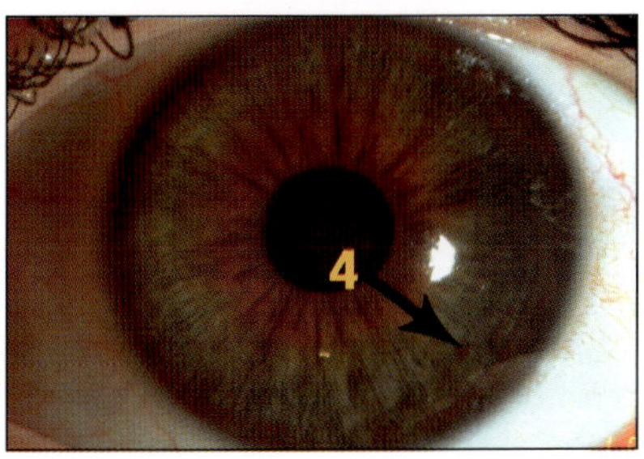

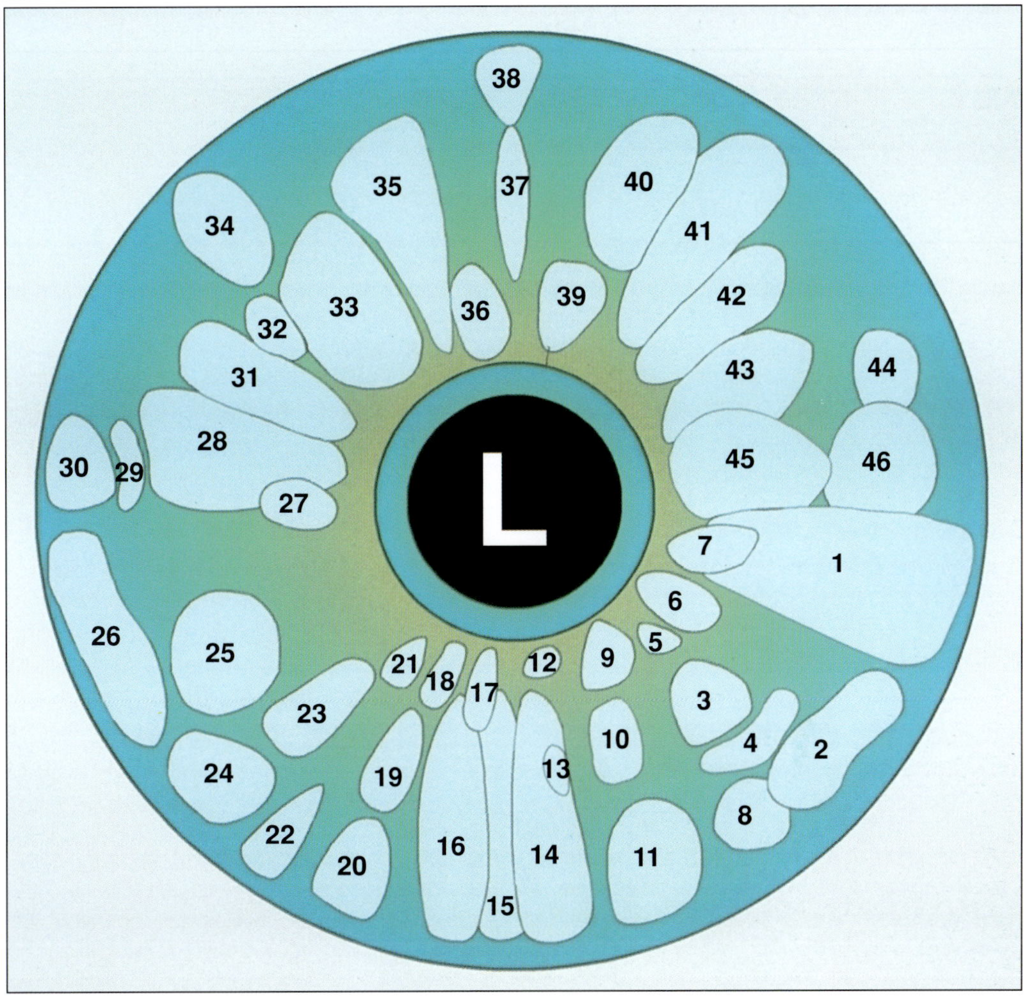

Iris positions, left eye

stimulation and mental expression, and verbal communication is emphasized in favor of kinesthetic communication (the vocabulary increases). A flower in this area acts as if it were blocking the flow of energy to the body, keeping it in the head and increasing the intellect. The effect of a flower trait here is generally to develop the mental body, the will, self-control, philosophical direction and/or spirituality.

If the flower is toward the inside of the Nurturing area (close to the pupil), it indicates a more mental way of expressing the issue. If the flower appears further away from the pupil, the expression will be emotional, or physical if it's out at the periphery.

There is sometimes a tendency for a trait to manifest its opposite form in behavior, e.g. a person with a flower in Nurturing may appear to be dependent, whining and may behave irresponsibly. Such a person is engaged in a process of self-discovery. Once he realizes who he is, there is an opportunity for the behavior to reverse itself and for the positive expression to come out.

A flower in Nurturing usually indicates that the person didn't receive nurturing from the eye parent, or that the eye parent felt a distinct absence of nurturing during his or her own life. That does not necessarily mean that the individual wasn't close to the eye parent, because he may well have nurtured the eye parent himself.

Jewel: With a jewel in this position, a person feels a need for activity, responsibility, movement, the expression of success and performance. It connotes a movement outward, an increase in vitality and energy. The jewel is there to increase movement toward the hemisphere in which it is found. It also indicates someone who is good at team work. Someone with a jewel in Nurturing tends to be very active, tries to please others and is often a workaholic.

A triangularly shaped jewel indicates more of an anger or resentment about issues in that area, whereas a rounder jewel indicates more of an acceptance about the issues.

Double Nurturing issues: People with a double Nurturing flower (i.e. a flower in that position in both eyes) tend to separate themselves from groups. They experience feelings of separation. They are usually easily hurt or may use hurt feelings to attract others.

A double Nurturing jewel really accentuates the associated characteristics. Such a person might appear quite Flower-like because he is trying so hard to please.

With a flower and a jewel in Nurturing, the individual is torn, giving a double message to people, beckoning with one hand, blocking with the other.

2. Resentment/Forgiveness

A powerful position, with a great impact on behavior. It indicates the absence of approval or recognition from the eye parent. (See also No. 8.) A jewel is by far the most common trait to find in this position. Flowers are also found, but this is primarily a kinesthetic position and not directly associated with emotion. It is also more common to have Resentment patterns with the father than with the mother, so this trait is usually found in the right eye. This position and No. 3 are the most likely to bring about a hemispheric shift.

Flower: A flower in this position usually has a triangular shape, and can be found anywhere between 3- and 6 o'clock on the iris. Its shape helps to distinguish it from a Nurturing trait.

Jewel: A jewel trait here usually desocializes the person, giving the impression of an absence of connection with the family. While initially creating withdrawal, a Resentment jewel also sets up the desire for social interaction through humanitarian service or leadership. It most readily creates originality, withdrawal from society and sometimes a tendency toward masochism. But when the positive qualities of the Resentment issue are expressed, it creates a deep desire for the healing of humanity.

If there is an absence of bonding, healing or communication with the parents on a one-to-one basis, the child will convert that lack into a desire for communion through social service. If a child experiences an absence of recognition from the parents, it tends to turn inward, develop originality, and use that originality as a bridge to reconnect with people at large, effectively seeking recognition from thousands or even millions of people. In its most positive attribute, this need can eventually become the mechanism by which a great service is delivered to humanity.

Those with a Resentment jewel in the right eye are likely to seek public recognition and approval, while those with the jewel in the left eye generally feel attacked by society.

As this position indicates a separation between the parent and the child, it has a great impact on hemispheric orientation. It is very difficult to have a jewel Resentment issue in either eye without having a strong movement away from the hemisphere associated with that eye.

3. Anger/Grace
4. Competition/Accomplishment

Positions 3 and 4 are in a sense the same position, and require exceptional care in their interpretation. This is the only area of the iris where there is so much overlap in interpretation between different positions.

There is a distinct difference between a flower and a jewel in this area. If there is a jewel precisely in the area of No. 3, it should be interpreted as No. 4 (present-generational competition), whereas a flower in this area indicates some kind of anger issue. Anger issues are always flower traits. A dark jewel structure in this position almost always indicates competitiveness.

Flower: A flower in this area indicates a transgenerationally acquired tendency for emotional expression directed toward other people: a tendency to blame others, to find fault with them, not to accept personal responsibility for events. When the flower is diamond-shaped, or distinctly closed, it indicates a volatile temper. Any time you see a flower in the general area bounded by positions 6, 2, 11 and 9, there is some quality of emotional anger in the person.

If the flower is closer to position No. 10, the issue might be more to do with communication in early childhood; if it is closer to No. 1, it might reveal itself as anger about material things.

The Anger pattern is a useful tool for verifying the nature of the relationship to, or communication with, the eye parent. For example, if someone has an Anger pattern in the right eye, you can get a pretty accurate description of his father. The person will perceive his own anger issues as coming from his father, or will perceive the father as an emotional man with a temper.

This position is the most likely to generate hemispheric shifts, followed by

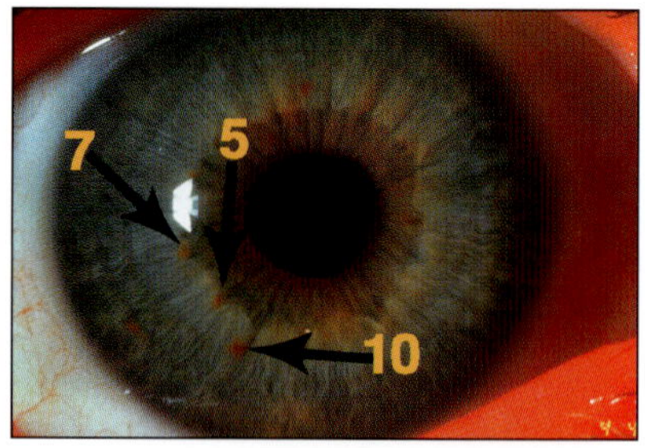

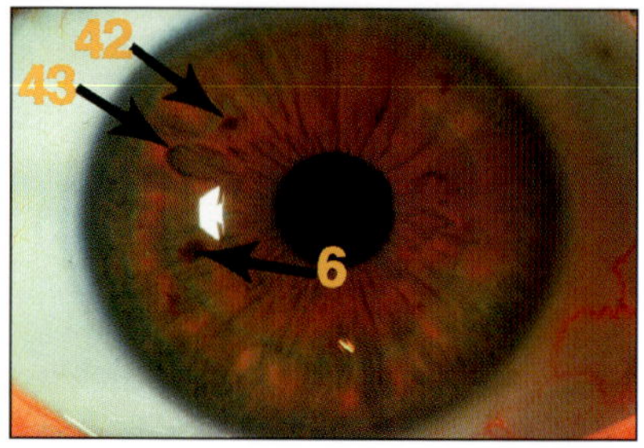

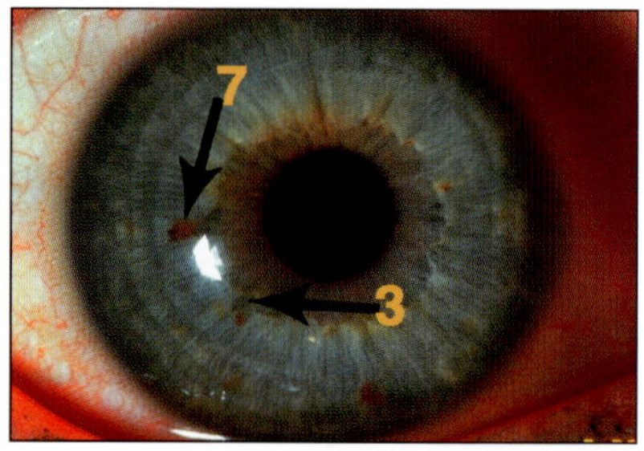

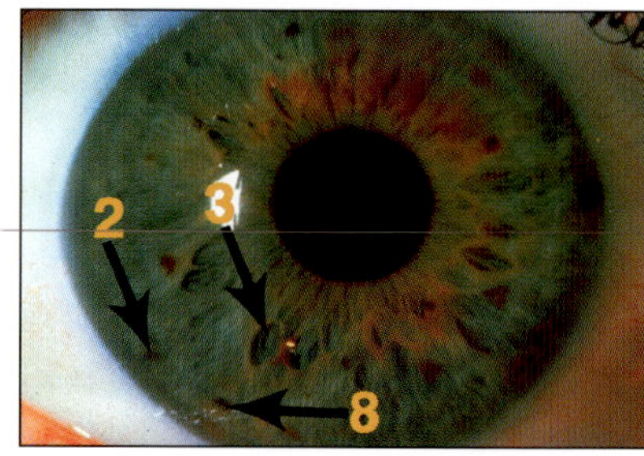

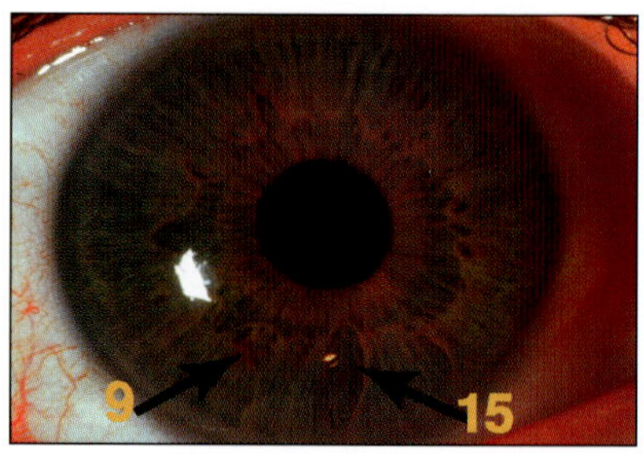

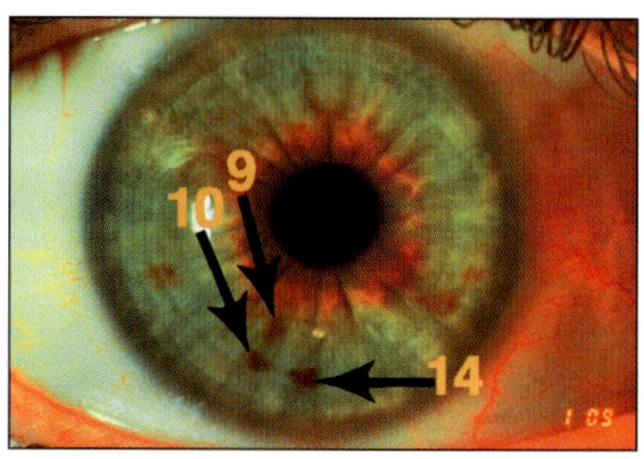

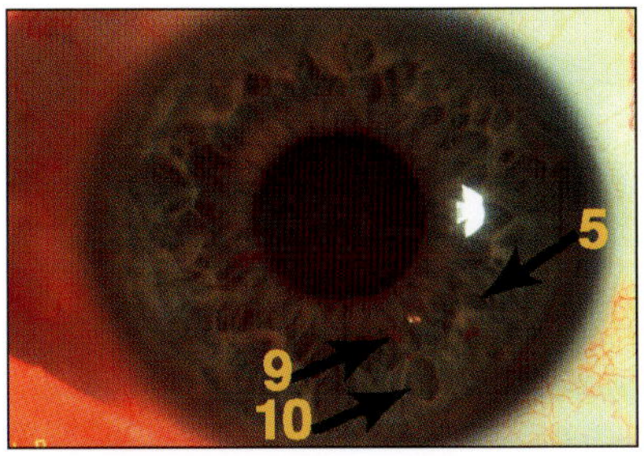

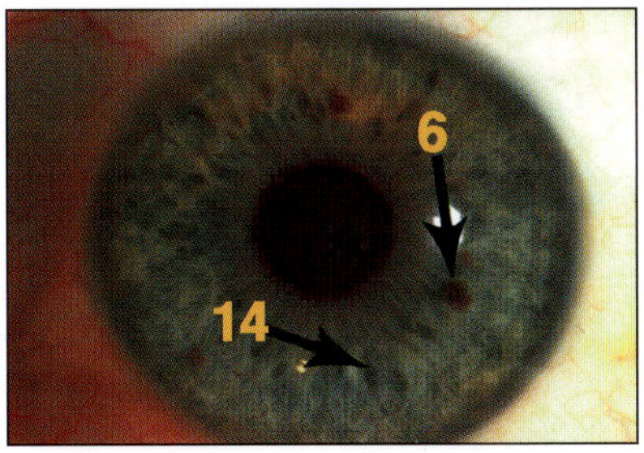

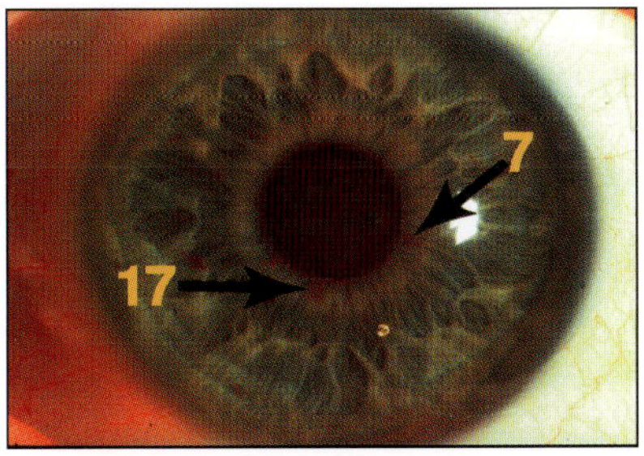

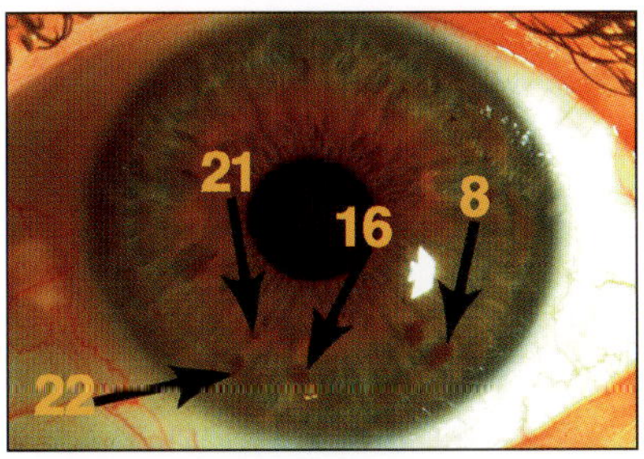

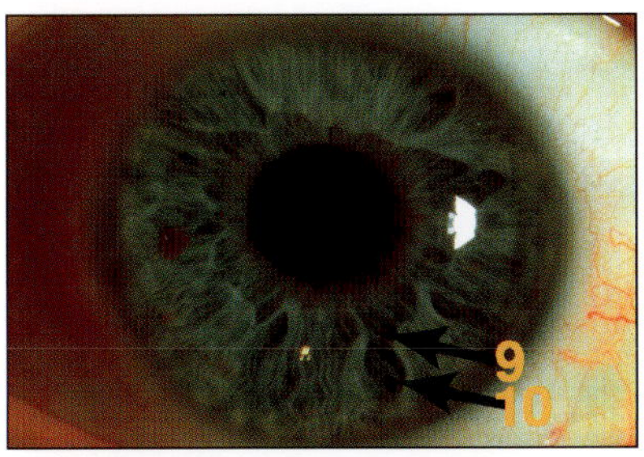

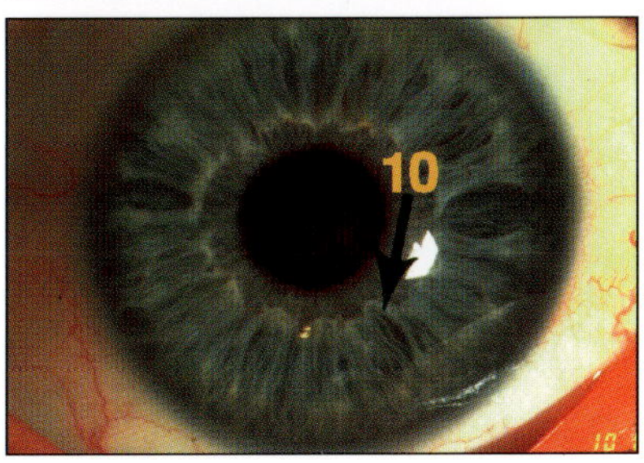

No. 2, followed by the area of gestation (wedge 9/10/11). It even seems as if the Anger pattern is there because of the need to shift hemispheres. An Anger issue in the right eye (i.e. anger with father, authority, bosses, bureaucracy, corporations and masculinity) is there to encourage the person to let go of control and shift hemispheres, moving to the unifying, spatial and feeling qualities of the right hemisphere. An Anger issue with mother (left eye) makes it difficult to trust women in general and even one's own femininity.

A Flower person with an Anger issue in the left eye may move out of the right hemisphere to the left, making him seem more mental, but remember that he is only *pretending* to be nonemotional.

A flower trait in the Anger position can also create a very gracefully moving body, which can make people with this trait romantically appealing.

With a double flower in this position, the person tends to be self-blaming.

Don't forget: If you lose your anger, you may also lose your passion for life.

Jewel: If there is a jewel in the general area of Anger/Competition (Nos. 3 or 4), it suggests the experience of rivalry or competition in the present generation. In 90% of people with a jewel in Anger, there is a sibling involved of the eye sex (left eye – female, right eye – male). It reflects some kind of childhood resentment or rivalry pattern between siblings, perhaps competing for the attention of a parent. Don't confuse this sibling resentment with position No. 2, which reflects resentment toward the parents.

It is unusual to find a jewel in this area if there are no brothers or sisters, since jewel traits are mainly determined by the present generation, in the present environment. The only other way it can occur is if one of the parents is currently engaged in intensely competitive behavior, such as a father who is a particularly aggressive businessman, or if for some reason the child was competing with one of the parents as if it were a sibling. A jewel in this area also has the quality of martyrdom, revealing an excessive tendency to accept personal responsibility for events.

If the Anger jewel appears in position No. 5, closer to the pupil, it indicates jealousy, envy, and subtler emotions; further out from the periphery, for example in position No. 4, it becomes more overt, and can be noticed as a distinct competitiveness and aggressiveness.

In consultation: As No. 3 is a tricky, emotional area, exercise some care when attempting to get confirmation about its impact on the life of your client. It is helpful to address the issue in terms of other people, since that is what the individual will relate to – he likes to blame other people. If the trait is in the right eye, try saying, "It looks to me like you got your emotional disposition from your father." Then move on gently, saying, "Let's see how this emotional disposition affects you and your capacity to bond with others, create intimacy and deal with authority." Consider this area in terms of the lesson or gift acquired from the anger pattern, and you will be more likely to establish a rapport.

5. Jealousy/Sharing

This is an area of great emotional intensity. Although not one of the seven major triggers, this position is also likely to induce a hemispheric shift. The lesson associated with this position is often about learning to share and to accept responsibility for one's emotional reactions.

Jewel: A jewel in this position usually comes from a relationship with a sibling, although it can also indicate jealousy or envy with the eye parent. People with a Jealousy jewel often intellectualize their feelings of jealousy.

Flower: A flower trait occurs so rarely in this position (less than 10% of Jealousy issues) that it is difficult to give a clear generalization of its meaning. It may indicate repressed anger, since it is so deep in the eye. There is some sense of the person not being allowed to expand into the emotional and kinesthetic body. Flowers starting in this position and extending into area No. 3 should be interpreted as Anger traits.

6. Independence/Possessiveness

Generally a very mental position, indicating how closely one is controlled by others, usually the result of a pattern established by the eye parent. A jewel is most common in No. 6.

Jewel: A jewel in this position indicates possessiveness or a mentally controlling nature. The individual will probably exhibit intense self-control, developing an independent nature, and will tend to want to control what other people are doing through mental manipulation.

Flower: A flower indicates self-contained independence. A person with this trait is likely to be quite territorial without directly repelling transgressors. Verbally non-expressive and emotionally detached, people with this trait tend silently to go their own way.

7. Concern

Area No. 1 and No. 7 are closely related. Imagine a pie-shaped wedge with the point of the pie being No. 7, and the wedge being No. 1. In a sense, No. 7 is simply a deeper, more concentrated, but also more subtle aspect of Nurturing. This is another area about which it is easy to get confirmation.

Jewel: A jewel in this position indicates a protective attitude about kinesthetic movements. To get confirmation, tell the client that, "It looks like your [eye parent] tended to be protective and that you now have a concerned, protective, providing nature. You are concerned about the welfare of someone." If the client has a child, he could be excessively protective of his son or daughter (depending on the eye sex).

Flower: A flower in this position is more like a flower in the area of Nurturing, indicating a stand-offish manner. It is similar to the independence of No. 6, but the individual will tend to "push away" anyone who gets too close, rather than just keeping away. This position is more actively repelling than No. 6 because it is closer to the (horizontal) kinesthetic line through the iris.

8. Originality

This position is part of an L-shaped region consisting of positions 9, 10, 11, 8 and 2. It is helpful to consider them in relation to each other.

Flower: It is rare to get a flower out at the periphery of the iris in one of these positions.

Jewel: If there is a fairly large jewel trait in any of the peripheral positions from No. 1 around to No. 11, about the size of area No. 2 on the chart, it represents some kind of resentment issue. There are a few differences between them: No. 11 dates from an earlier age than No. 8, and No. 8 is chronologically younger than No. 2. People with a trait in No. 8 are learning to develop a sense of belonging.

A large jewel in position No. 11 may relate to resentment experienced in the womb, for example if one of the parents felt overwhelmed and resentful about having another mouth to feed.

A large jewel in position No. 8 dates from early childhood (age 0 – 4), for example if the child was resented for making too much noise, crying too much at night or wetting the bed. Resentment associated with unwanted pregnancies could manifest in either position No. 11 or No. 8.

The same characteristic at location No. 2 usually stems from the teen years when the individual first experienced physical independence (a breaking pattern).

It is difficult to get any confirmation from your clients about experiences associated with this position, although they may have the sense of being unwanted as a child. This can in turn create a sense of not belonging in groups or society later on. It generally manifests as a subtle difficulty at the beginning of bonding, a mild antagonism with someone of the eye sex (left – women, right – men) whether in friendships or love relationships. As it relates to early childhood, this trait is usually quite unconscious and covert in expression.

Although related to positions 2 and 4, No. 8 is different because it comes out as a subtle difficulty in communication with people at large. The effects of No. 2 are more conscious and directly associated with a parent; No. 4 is also consciously recognized but is more directly related to competition and interaction with siblings.

Wedge 9/10/11
9. Birthing
10. Communication
11. Decision

This is an extremely significant aperture. There is a cleavage between the medial and lateral regions of the iris running between wedges 3/4/5 and 12/13/14. Wedge 9/10/11 is the bridge that joins these two regions, and has a lot to do with how a person initiates any activity, how he brings his inner creativity into expression. It therefore has special significance for the whole iris.

This grouping of 9/10/11 continues to influence one's life on a nine-month cycle, the period of gestation, and is activated every time one initiates something. If a person has a difficult trait along this wedge, particularly a jewel, then it can stop or hinder the full expression of any activity.

The nine months of an embryo's gestation presents a microcosmic image of the lifetime of the individual from birth to death. That is one of the reasons this position is so significant. If either parent experiences a great trauma while the child is in utero, this will affect the child later in life.

Wedge 9/10/11 is a neutral island that forms the bridge between the emotional qualities of 3/4/5 and the creative functions of 12/13/14. It reflects

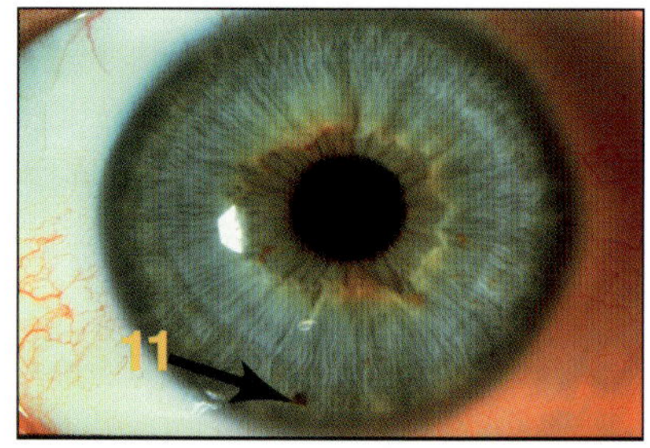

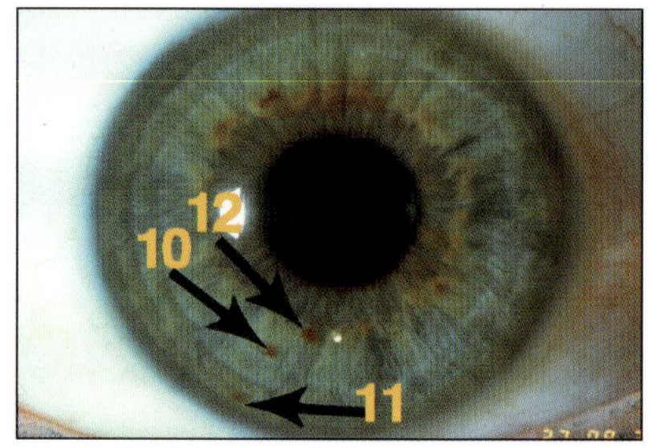

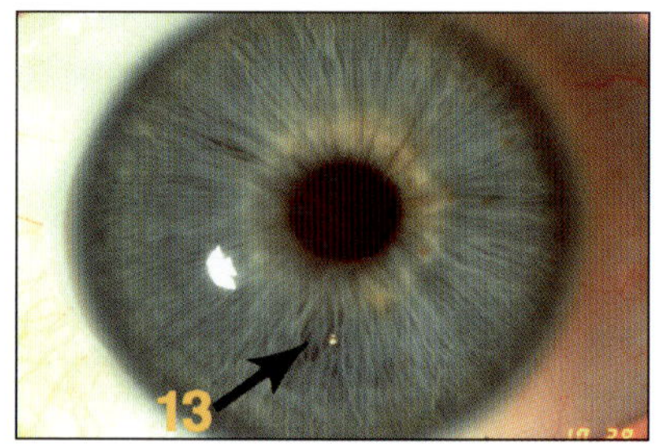

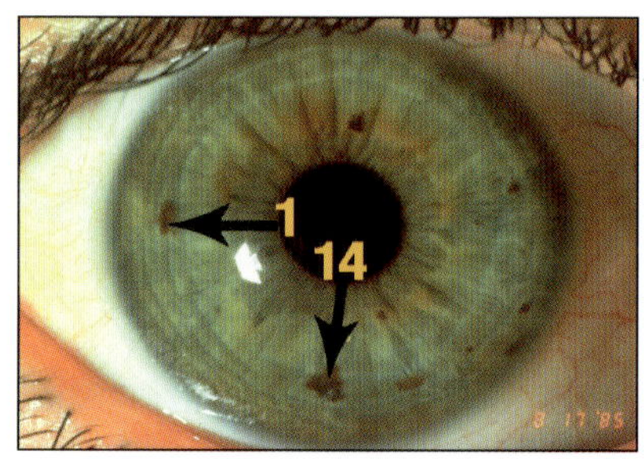

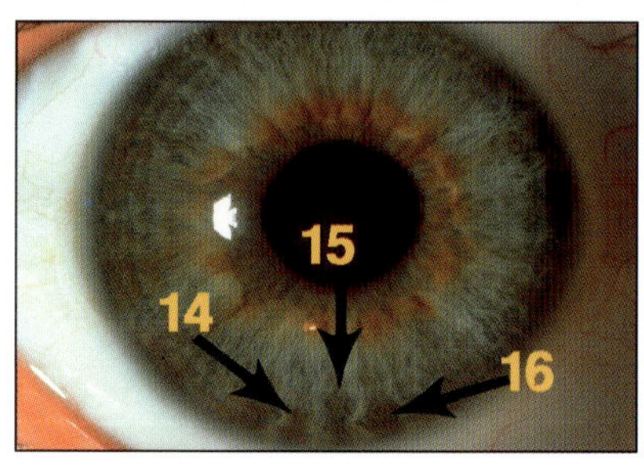

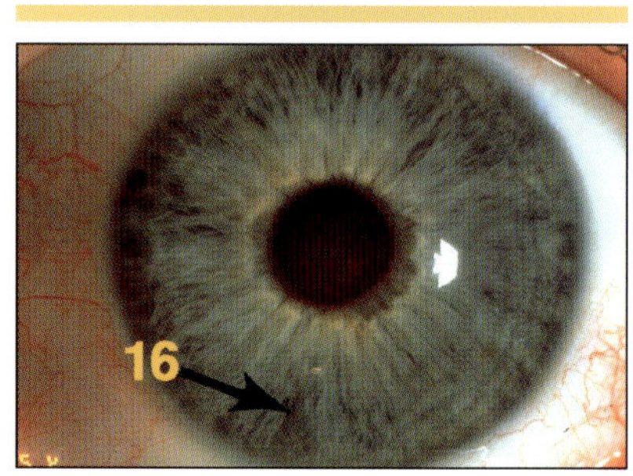

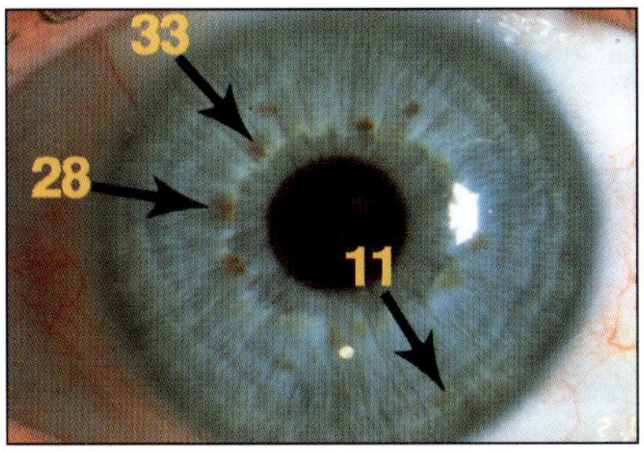

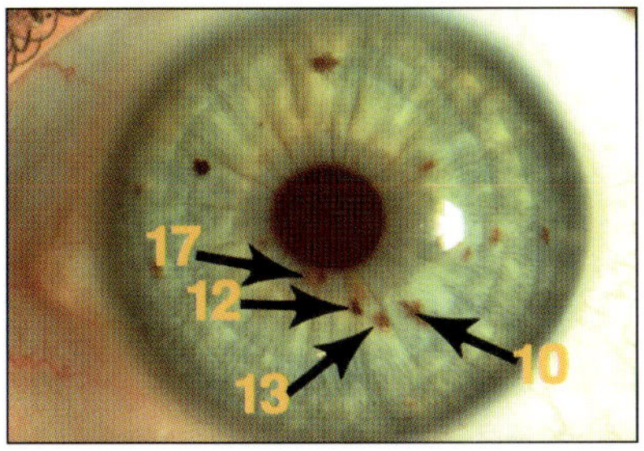

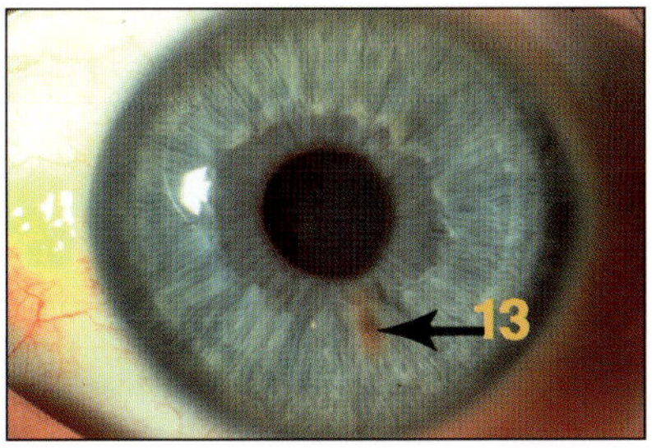

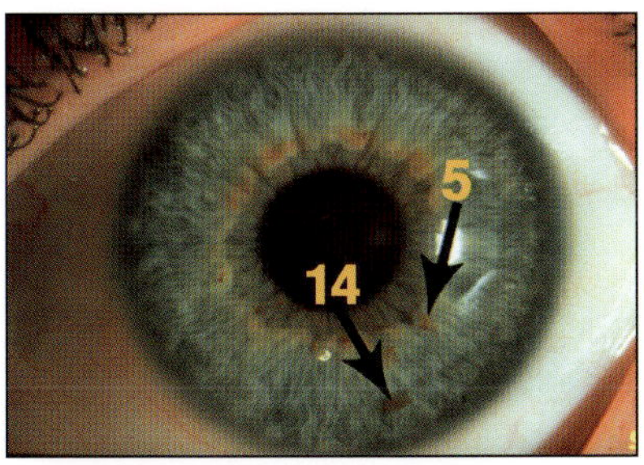

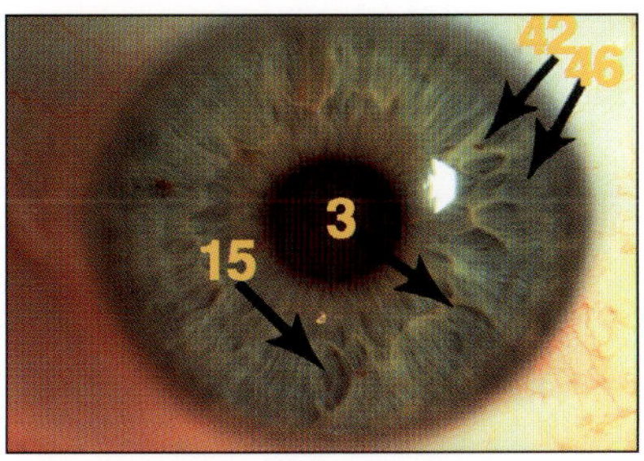

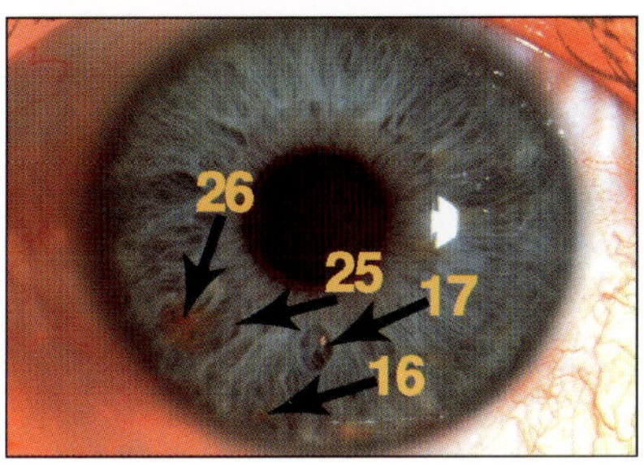

communication patterns established during gestation. Although the effects are generally unconscious, the individual probably recognizes a subtle frustration (jewel) or agonizing difficulty (flower) in communicating with the eye parent, perhaps even a sense of alienation which carries over into his experience of other relationships. He probably has a sense of incompleteness.

There is probably also a sense of frustration with self. It is frustrating to have difficulty communicating your feelings or attitudes about a topic. With a flower this will manifest as more of a volatile frustration.

The likelihood of having a jewel or a flower in this area is about even.

Jewel: A jewel in this wedge could manifest as a difficulty in forming the initial bond in a relationship (No. 9), difficulty in conceiving a child (No. 9), difficulty with expressing a thought in harmonious communication (No. 10), or difficulty with following through with an activity to its full expression (No. 11). Any initiatives will tend to have a mental quality to them and, if the individual has difficulty expressing himself (Communication, No. 10) he will experience frustration when attempting to follow through.

Flower: A flower indicates that the individual finds it easier to initiate, because he experiences an ease of release (a general Flower characteristic), but will find it more difficult to follow through and be successful. The individual probably feels incomplete even after a successful release/initiation because there is a sense of not having done anything. Instead of frustration, a person with a flower in this wedge is more likely to experience a sense of apathy, despair or hopelessness.

Wedge 12/13/14

This wedge has a lot to do with impatience and perfectionism. In some ways it is like 9/10/11 because there is an impatience of expression. While 9/10/11 is more to do with the self in direct relationship to parents and intimates, 12/13/14 indicates impatience with other people and life in general. It is an external impatience, rather than the internal impatience and frustration of 9/10/11.

A trait in this area could manifest as hyperachievement, kinetic hyperactivity or impatience with other people ("Why don't you hurry up?"), but it also manifests as an attraction to very specific types of music or dance, almost a hypersensitivity to some forms (e.g. "I hate Bach.").

A separate booklet about the Creativity region (Nos. 12 – 17) is available from Rayid International.

12. Achievement

With a trait in this position, there is usually concern from the eye parent about the child's outlook on life, its overall direction or its long-term goals. The parent may even express impatience or worry about these issues. The child usually responds by feeling restless or uncertain about the future himself, being indecisive and may be extremely meticulous as a compensation. He will have a tendency to be impatient about the future and to worry about outcomes. This position also concerns immediate choices: "What should I do right now, and how am I going to resolve this?"

Jewel: A trait in this position is almost always a jewel. A jewel in any of the neighboring positions 9, 12 and 17 will increase the mental nature of the person, often as a response to unresolved anxiety. This anxiety may create a restlessness of both mind and body.

Flower: If there is a flower in this area, it usually extends through Nos. 13 and 14 as well.

13. Meticulousness

Most often a jewel with exactly the same shape as the position on the *Positions* diagram. It reveals itself as mental frustration, mental impatience or a tendency to examine things in great detail, and to be very precise. This position definitely has mental qualities, whereas No. 14 tends to be associated with movement. It is also the position directly associated with highly specific tastes in music. If the trait is in the right eye it will tend to manifest as meticulousness with words, a sarcastic wit and a sharp tongue, whereas in the left eye the meticulousness will be more to do with images or music. An individual with this trait tends to be a perfectionist, which can lead to a judgmental attitude toward people of the eye sex.

14. Timing/Patience

A flower is the most common trait in this area. It is a kinesthetic area, concerned with the expression of the body. It is quite easy to get confirmation about this trait. The individual usually is aware of a subtle impatience with someone of the eye sex that is consciously associated with the demanding, perfectionist tendencies of the eye parent. This area is also about external timing, not feeling part of the rhythm of the world.

An individual with this trait is quite likely to be interested in dance. With the trait in the left eye, it would be a more flowing, abstract, musically oriented type of dance; in the right eye it would be a more gymnastic type of dance that required precise physical coordination or physical strength.

15. Perfection

Located exactly at 6 o'clock, this is a pivotal point or fulcrum between Nos. 14 and 16, which are different forms of creativity. While No. 14 has a lot to do with gross motor skills, externalization and other people, No. 16 is related to fine motor skills, internalization, self-esteem and individuality – the self.

Almost always a flower, No. 15 is also an area of creativity in its own right. A trait here usually gives a direct indication of skill with the written word: in the right eye it would indicate a leaning toward technical writing or research in the left eye, fantasy or romance. When the flower extends right out to the periphery of the iris, the creativity is usually more readily available to the person once he is encouraged to engage it. If the flower is closer to the pupil, the individual will have a tendency to start and stop creative projects, or to have expressed himself creatively earlier in life, with a lingering desire to return to that creativity some day.

16. Self-esteem/Spirit

Of all the areas in the iris, this is by far the single most commonly occurring position. It is the focal point for issues about self-esteem, and relates to internal timing: impatience with your own timing (e.g. age). It is about perfection in self.

No. 16 dramatically affects the whole personality. If there is a large flower or jewel in this area, it slows down the function of the associated hemisphere of the brain, and can inhibit the individual's ability to enter fully into behavior associated with that hemisphere (left eye – femininity, right eye – masculinity). It usually stems from the way the eye parent viewed him/herself.

A trait in this position can be either a flower or jewel, although a flower is more common. A jewel would indicate an issue with the individual's physical security; in the left eye it would be more linked to abstract fears (a fear of the dark, for example), and in the right eye it would be more closely associated with a fear of physical phenomena.

Any time you have a trait in No. 16 (either eye), it indicates the capacity for creativity and brings the gift of fine motor skills. If the trait is in the left eye, the gift will be related to feminine qualities and inner expression: abstraction, synthesis and color coordination and combination. If the trait is in the right eye, the expression will be more externalized and the skills will be more masculine, to do with physical dexterity, craftsmanship and building.

The paradox of this position is that the lack of self-esteem blocks the individual's ability to bring the inner creative capacity to fruition. This position is a bridge between the unconscious idea and manifestation. Self-esteem issues must be tackled before it is possible to achieve any significant shift or change in other patterns. The key lesson of this position is about releasing doubt, trusting one's self and allowing that trust to percolate out into one's behavior.

One of the primary ways of dealing with issues associated with this area is to make use of visual imagery, such as painting: If found in the left eye, try working with abstract designs, watercolors, concentrating on color combinations; if found in the right eye, try pen and ink drawings. Regular exercises in creative expression will help overcome a loss of self-esteem.

17. Trust

A jewel is the most common trait in this position. It indicates a great sense of insecurity about people of the eye sex, leading to feelings of mistrust. Subsidiary issues of anger and frustration may also come up. This trait makes it difficult to bond easily with someone of the eye sex, although it is really based on an insecurity about one's self. It is not uncommon for someone with a trait in No. 17 to establish controlling relationships with members of the eye sex, based on dominance and manipulation. With a trait in position No. 17 (mistrust) and one in No. 9 (difficulty with initiating communication), a person would have serious problems forming relationships.

A trait in this position also indicates a fear of death, implying stored doubts and fears. The key lesson of this position is about "letting go," learning to trust others. Once the individual overcomes the fears associated with No. 17, he can exhibit great courage.

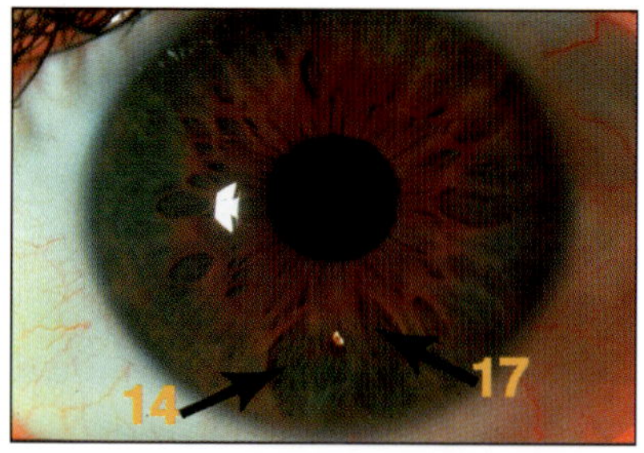

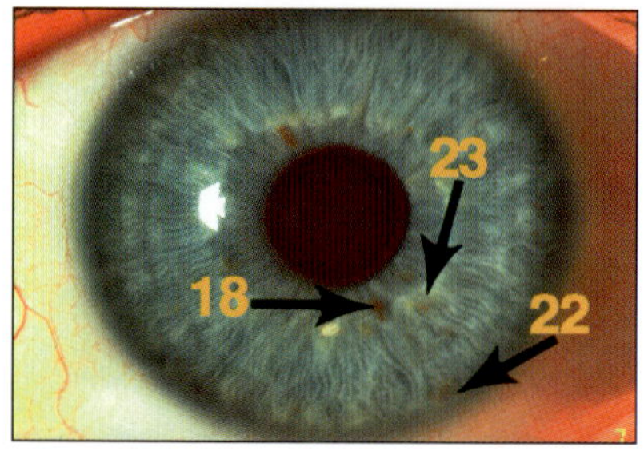

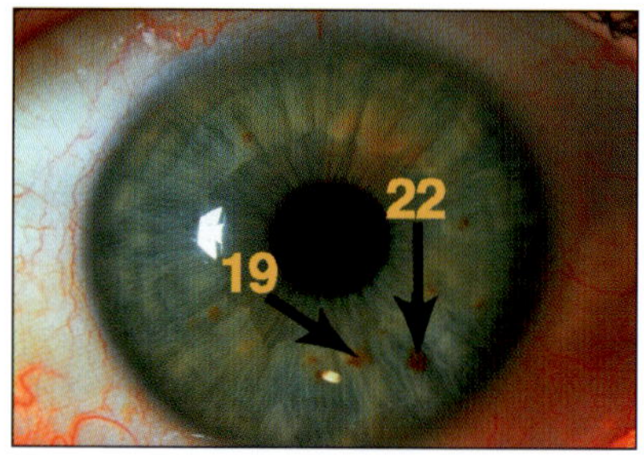

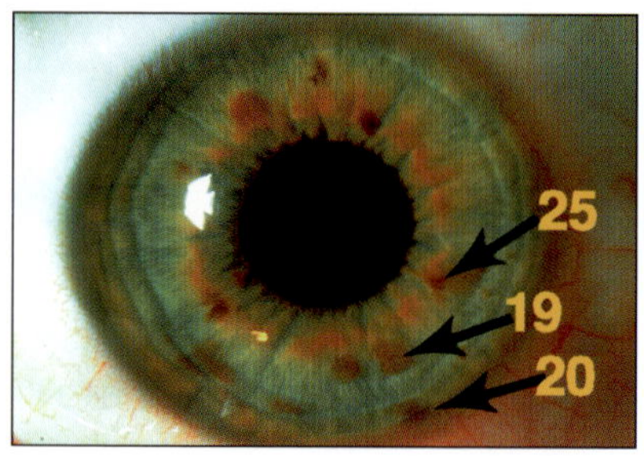

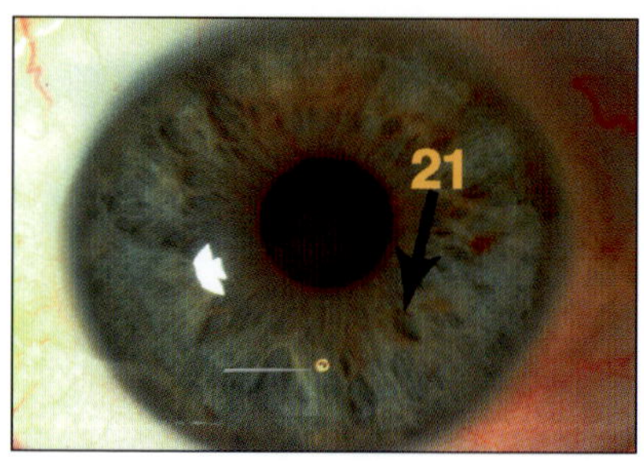

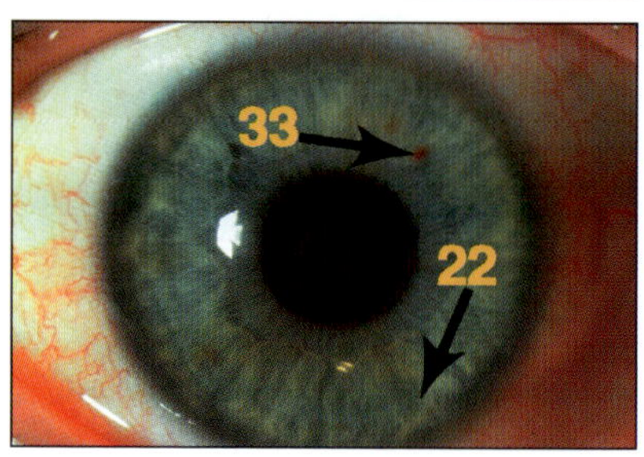

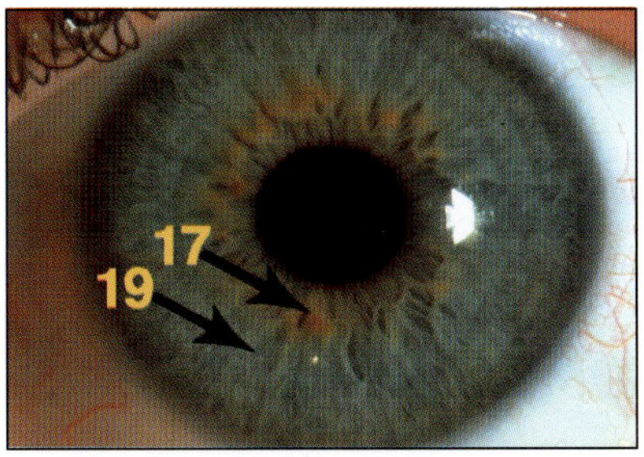

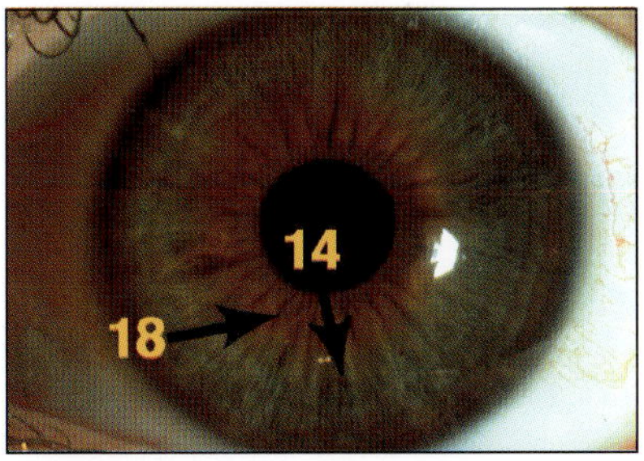

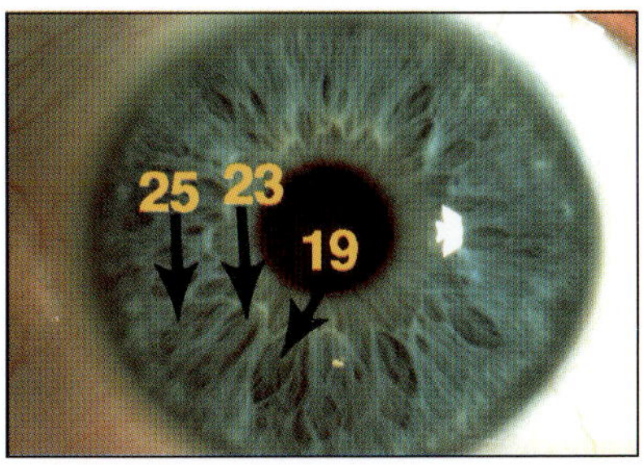

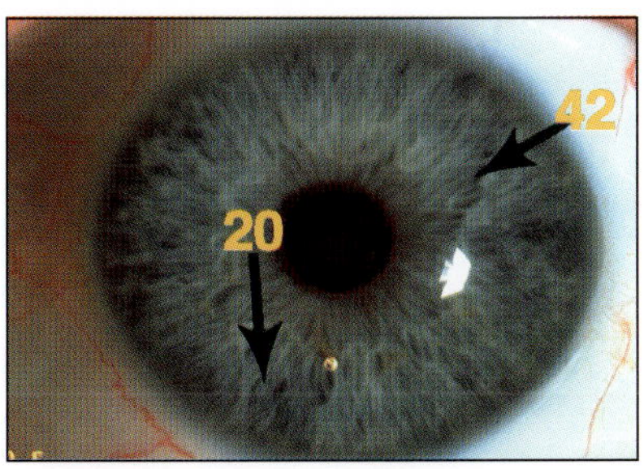

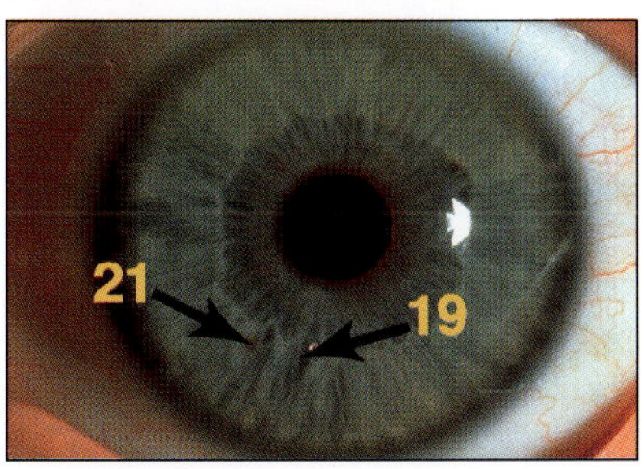

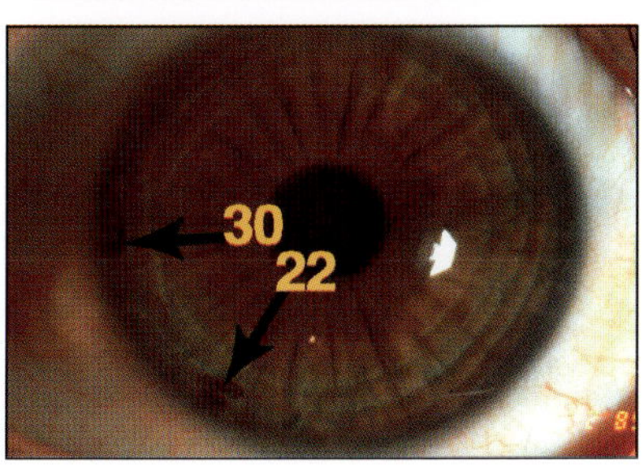

Wedge 18/19/20

Patterns in these areas result from traumas or discipline in childhood which affect the individual's creative self-expression as an adult. They are most commonly linked to fears of death, darkness or abuse. It can be difficult to get confirmation about positions in this area (or any position in the medial part of the eye) because the issues tend to be buried deep in the unconscious. Wedge 18/19/20 could also be called the wedge of enthusiasm. Characteristics along this wedge dramatically diminish the level of enthusiasm in the individual's verbal or kinesthetic expressions. Because 18/19/20 is so close to 16/17, it is also closely linked to issues of self-esteem.

This is one of the few regions of the iris where the positions follow a precise chronological progression. Together, these three positions deal with the childhood years from birth to seven years of age.

Flower: The most common pattern in this wedge is a large flower that runs all the way from No. 18 to No. 20. This pattern usually means that there has been some type of shock to the child, often originating with potty training, and then compounded by some other incident in which the child experienced a loss of control over some aspect of its physical environment, e.g. spilling a glass of milk at a young age or wetting the bed. This affects the child's inner sense of confidence about expressing its creativity. The parents are likely to have repeatedly limited the child's kinetic expressions, for example by saying, "Slow down. Quit acting like a kid. Put that down."

Such early experiences set up long-term patterns. For example, if a child accidentally slams a door and then is severely punished for it, it will forever be careful about how it closes doors, closing them gingerly and quietly for the rest of its life.

Jewel: A jewel trait in this area is often linked to punishment for making too much noise, with reprimands such as, "Shut up. Be quiet." This sort of parental response quite literally deactivates the child's outward expression.

Flower or jewel: The consequence of either trait is that the individual's inherent behavior becomes more withdrawn, perhaps with a sense of fear about retaliation or punishment. People thus affected will come across as quiet, gentle and soft-spoken, which can be quite attractive. That is why this wedge is referred to as Early Childhood/ Serenity/ Innocence.

People with traits in this wedge will readily give you confirmation about the fact that they didn't get a chance to be a child. They feel they didn't have their childhood because they weren't allowed to express themselves fully at that time.

The gift of this area is the quality of serenity and innocence, and also the ability to reconnect with childlike feelings throughout adulthood. If childlike behavior is suppressed when the individual is very young (0 – 7 years), it is not lost but rather is stored internally. It will then return in cycles of seven years beginning around the ages of 30 – 35. It emerges as a playfulness and a deep desire to experience childlike freedom. These feelings are in direct contrast to the individual's actual experience of early childhood, however, so there is a potential source of tension if the person can't allow the feelings to be expressed this time around. This is also the age when the individual is probably raising children of his own, and he may face challenges with allowing his own offspring to experience the childlike freedom he never had.

People with a trait in 18/19/20 usually have youthful physiques and a noble, soft-spoken character. Unlike 9/10/11, which is more to do with difficulty in communication, a trait in 18/19/20 manifests as the absence of a desire or a reticence to communicate.

Lessons: Most often, any trait is there to facilitate a long-term movement toward structural balance. A flower in 18/19/20 is usually found in people with a Flower-extrovert or Shaker-Flower structure. If the overall impression of the iris suggests an outgoing personality, yet the client just sits there looking at you sheepishly, belying his apparent primary structure, take a look at 18/19/20. A flower in this location will deactivate the person's otherwise expressive and animated nature, creating a greater focus on the self and inner realms to balance the overall personality.

Always look for the positive and useful lessons that the individual has gained from characteristics that might otherwise seem purely painful and counterproductive. Once a person with a trait in 18/19/20 acquires the lesson of a more conscious nature then the childlike playfulness will come out automatically.

The primary lessons for people with Flower-extrovert eye structures are to do with the mental body, will, self-development and self-control. They may have acquired the urge for self-control by being raised in a family situation in which their childlike nature and frivolousness was battered out of them.

This area may indicate child abuse if it is found in combination with other positions such as Anger, Nurturing, Rebellion, Authority or Will.

Stated another way, if the experience of pain (abuse) in early childhood is allowed to accumulate as a lesson, and that lesson is realized through the process of searching on inner levels, then there can be a re-emergence of the primary structure, including the childlike behavior. All of the other traits in the eyes can then also be expressed in their positive attributes. But none of this can happen unless a critical level of inward awareness is attained. Until that happens, all of the traits in the eyes will work to establish painful or difficult behavioral and relationship patterns that will draw the extroverted individual into self-analysis and an inward focus. So-called "negative" traits are actually there to encourage people to heal themselves.

18. Early Childhood, Age 0 - 2

Although a flower is still more common, this area is the most likely of the three to have a jewel, since it is so clearly located in the realm of the mental body.

Worries associated with No. 18 are the early childhood fears: fear of the night, fear of being alone, fear of spiders or a fear of going to sleep. The main cause of these worries is the process of potty training. A child does not usually have physical control over its sphincter muscles until after the age of two, and if potty training is initiated before this time, the child can develop fears linked to its initial difficulty with learning that kind of self-control. It can create a fear of defecation, a fear of not being able to control the bladder. The child may tend to stay unconscious longer as a result of criticism associated with potty training, actually disabling its ability to do the very thing it is being punished for.

Issues that surface during early childhood can recur later on in life, setting up a difficulty with encountering new situations on a seven-year cycle.

19. Serenity, Age 2 - 5

A trait in this position generally creates an inner anxiety in the child that diminishes outer movement and increases discomfort in the presence of adults. Often extending into position 16, either a Jewel or a Flower in No. 19 can reduce self-confidence or self-esteem. People with a trait in this position may maintain their outwardly childlike manner throughout life, often as a way to quietly deflect aggression directed toward them. Their method of dealing with other people's anger is to deanimate.

Jewel: A jewel in this position is often associated with childhood anxieties from this period of life, such as a fear of the unknown. It is also associated with repeated warnings from the parent(s) to "Be careful."

Flower: People with a flower in No. 19 generally speak very softly and exhibit conservative gestures and movements, clearly giving the impression that they have been emotionally wounded. They also have a deep humility and genuine innocence.

20. Gentleness/Innocence, Age 5 - 7

Together with No. 19, this area represents coming into consciousness. No. 20 is even more to do with outer/physical functions than No. 19. Worries associated with this position concern the environment rather than inner fears: fear of going outside, fear of physical assault, fear of not locking the doors. Any difficulties a child experiences in emerging into his environment would be manifested in one of positions 19 or 20.

Review of Positions 1 - 20

These areas represent the foundations of the personality. They are the key areas governing the individual's ability to develop a rapport, deal with relationships, establish self-esteem, and a host of other primary personality traits. The remaining areas (Nos. 21 – 46) add their own qualities and direction to the overall personality but their effects tend to be more subtle.

When conducting a consultation, Rayid practitioners are advised to begin their interpretation with the lower-lateral region of the eye (Nos. 1 – 15). Positions in this region are usually consciously recognized, and so are fairly easy to get confirmation on.

Once you move into the medial areas of the iris, beginning with the area of 16/17, and especially with 18/19/20, you are treading much more deeply into unconscious areas of the personality. It is therefore much harder to get confirmation from a client about these areas.

Positions 21 - 26

This region is concerned with the self and with survival, including the survival of the species through procreation. Traits in these positions usually indicate resilience of character. They can be found in some quite unusual people,

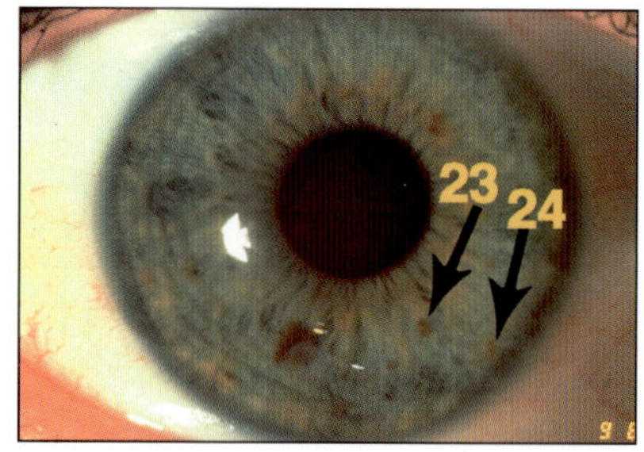

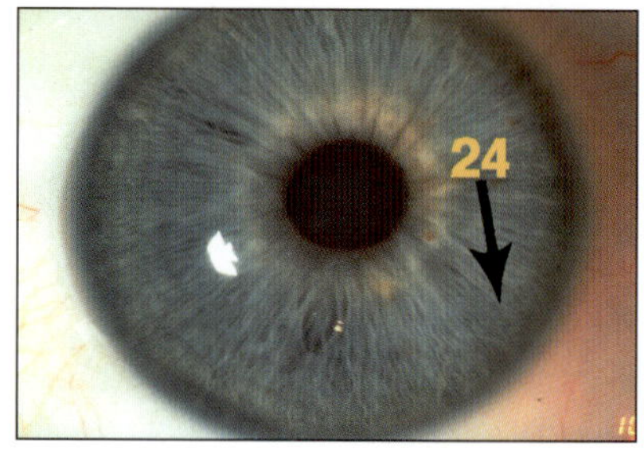

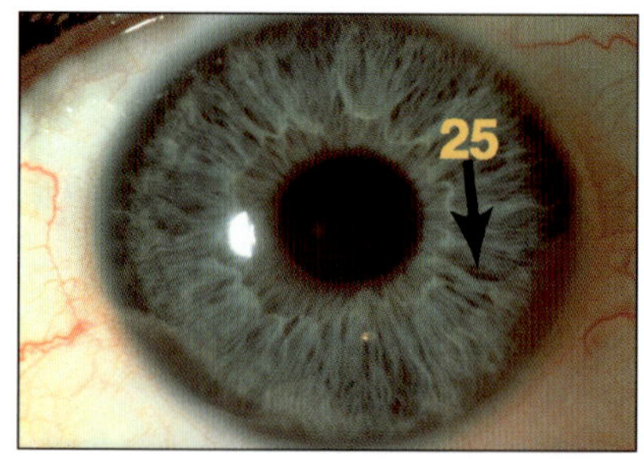

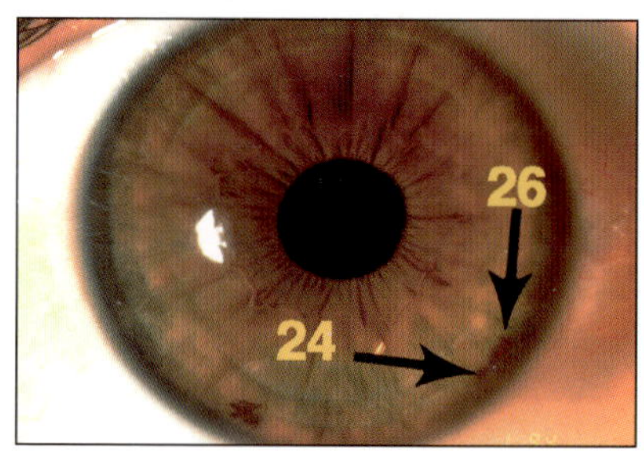

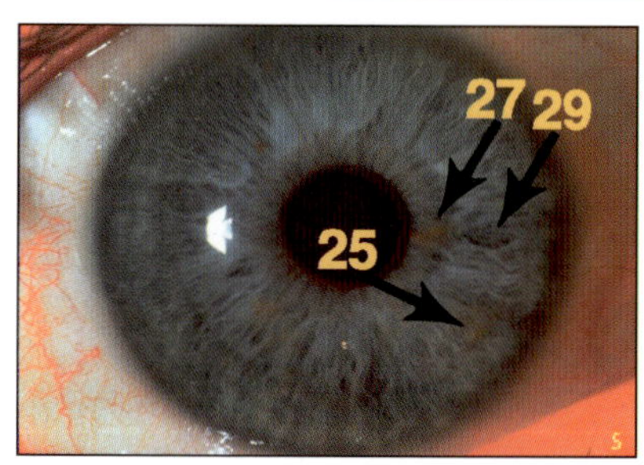

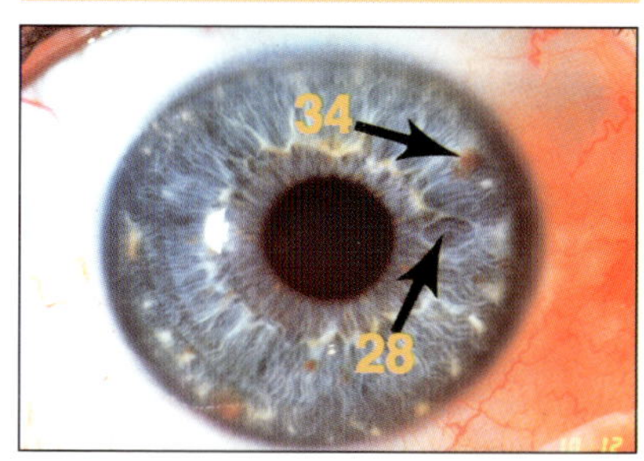

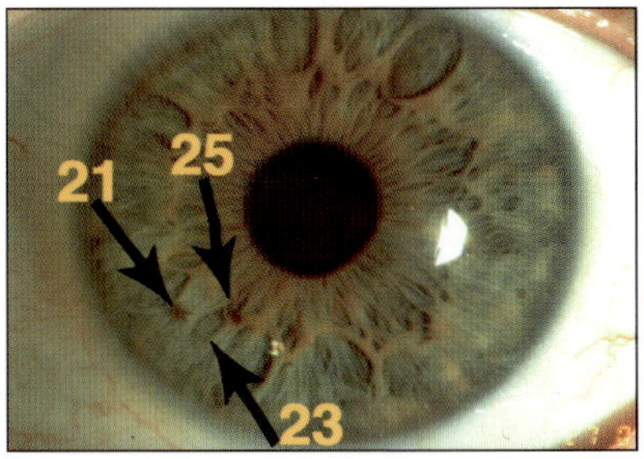

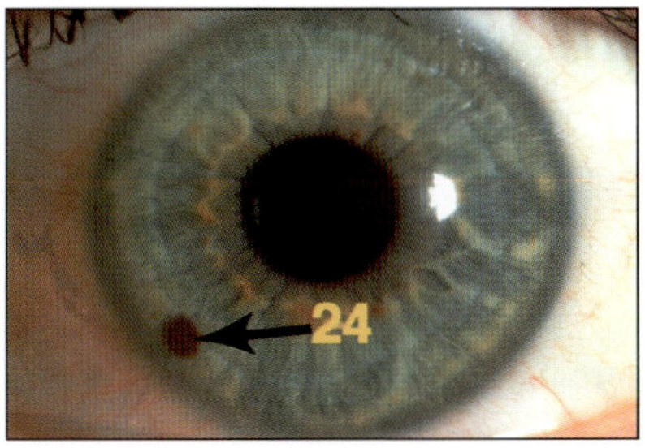

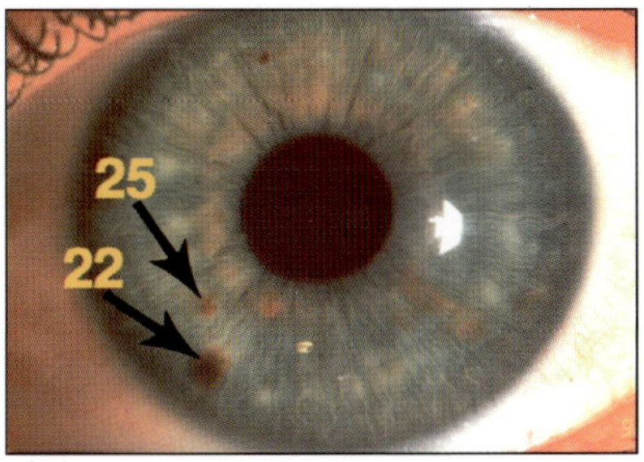

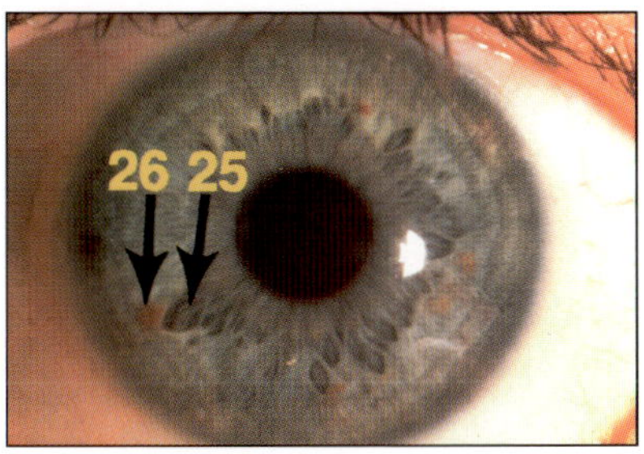

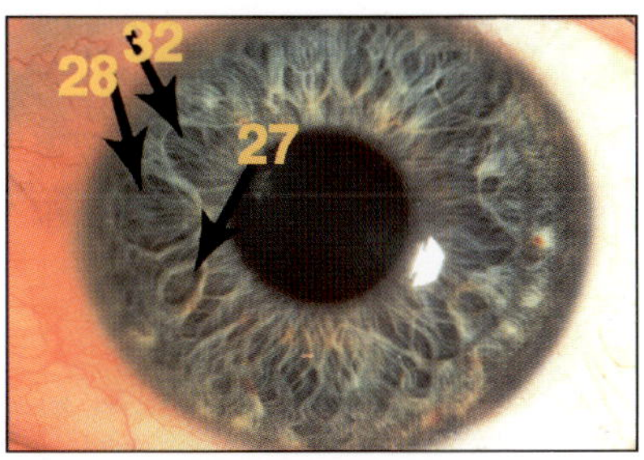

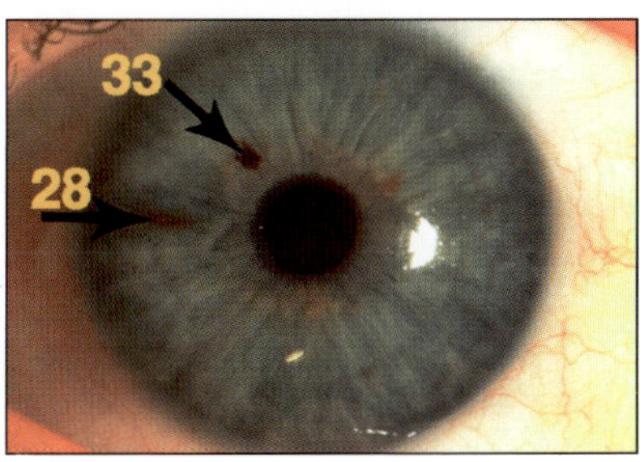

including survivalists, those who are poetically inclined or solitude-oriented, and also in people who are prideful or arrogant. Traits in these positions have a deep impact on the strength and character of the individual. They are usually jewels, although flowers are sometimes found, but this region is really concerned with the mind and its ability to allow feeling in the expression of one's relations to a social group.

21. Knowing
22. Intimacy

Revealing how a person's sexuality is expressed, these are two of the most profound interpersonal positions in the iris. Both of these positions relate to the *physical* expression of sexual intimacy. Traits in these areas can indicate either an overactive or a blocked sexuality. Sexual assault or religious condemnation are the fears most commonly associated with these positions.

A trait in position No. 21 tells you something about the individual's attitudes or beliefs concerning sexual expression and often indicates difficulty with being able to complete the sexual act or with finding personal satisfaction in it. It indicates that, while the individual has the emotional desire for deep levels of intimacy, he is actually unable to deeply relate to another person. A trait in this position suggests that there is some fear, worry, concern or belief system which is interfering with the expression of intimacy, both emotionally and physically.

Position No. 22 indicates a strong need for physical and emotional intimacy. It is most often characterized by a jewel at the periphery of the iris, and can actually be located anywhere between positions 20 through 24. This type of need for intimacy is most often related to the absence of emotional communication, the expression of feelings, in previous generations. This absence creates a profound desire for the *physical release of feeling* through the experience of physical intimacy and sex. This position indicates a deep desire to experience oneness, to know one's true self and one's beloved, through the physical experience of sexual union. It is the position most often associated with the impact of previous generations on one's ability to complete intimacy through the sexual act.

23. Solitude
24. Enlightenment

Closely associated with self-awareness, patterns in either of these areas can indicate an interest in art, nature or spiritual study. When apparent in the right eye, excessive ego-glorification is a likely personality trait, perhaps in connection with psychic abilities or mental instability. When found in the left eye, the individual may be spiritually fanatical.

Position 23 usually indicates someone who is self-responsible or self-taught. Traits in No. 23 or No. 25 are oftentimes linked to an inner sense of pride about one's knowledge – about life, about other people or about things in nature.

No. 24 is similar to No. 22 in some ways except that it is a more concerned with the transcendental experience of one's relationship to groups or to nature. Someone with a trait in position No. 24 in the right eye is likely to be either psychic or self-righteous. He is likely to be a very powerful person whose mind is very strong and who is intolerant of other people's opinions. Position No. 24 is equally likely, paradoxically, to indicate someone who is prideful and arrogant, or who is sensitive to beauty and nature. Interpret it with care!

25. Self-reliance
26. Pride

Patterns in these areas indicate pride, inflexibility or a strong urge for self-reliance. The individual is quite likely to be self-taught and to have a strong will to survive.

No. 26 most often indicates a deep sense of pride concerning the family, the ability to survive financially, and/or pride about the ability to provide for one's own physical needs. In its positive expression, this trait indicates someone who is really capable of taking care of himself; in its negative expression, it indicates a personality that is prone to pride and arrogance.

Unnumbered Position

Between No. 25 and No. 26 and slightly above them is an unlabeled area that merits attention. The presence of a trait in this area indicates that the individual has the ability to compromise and has the willingness to see other people's points of view. This area has a kinesthetic quality which suggests that the person has the ability to successfully balance opposing forces. Someone with a trait in this area is capable of diplomacy and has the capacity to act as a very fair-minded judge, especially if the trait is close to wedge 27/28/29/30.

Wedge 27/28/29/30

This area relates to the capacity for heartfelt self-expression, the ability to express one's innermost feelings through the spoken word. Traits in these positions, particularly in No. 29 and No. 30, also indicate the ability to access a deep, inner knowing and to have profoundly inspiring experiences. They reflect the potential for genius, and for ecstatic states of consciousness.

This wedge is associated with the synthesis of the inspired heart with the ability to persuade others or to heal. An area of great wisdom and purity, where inner knowing is combined with self-expression, this is also the source of great guile, cunning and trickery. To be able to manipulate and direct others with one's heart can bring about great healing, or it can be done for selfish gain. There can sometimes be a fine line between these two forms of manipulation. These positions are associated with the inner character of the individual and his willingness to see beyond the normal limitations of self and to strive for something beyond the norm.

27. Rapture

Representing the inner chamber of the heart, No. 27 indicates a simplicity of approach to life and the ability to express inner revelation in simple, clear and effective terms.

28. Voice

Traits in this area indicate a talent for singing or the use of the spoken word, and can indicate abilities in the area of public speaking. A trait in No. 28 in the right iris reveals the ability to clearly express and enunciate concepts, to communicate with men about material or social phenomena. In the left iris, it is most often linked to musical or emotional expression, particularly with women.

29. Sincerity

In some ways, the precise impact of this position remains a mystery. It is a mystical position, indicating the capacity to access inner genius, to know one's relationship to all life and to express this knowing with clarity. This is the position that most closely relates to the discovery of something beyond the norm. Like all of positions 27 – 30, it often indicates a person who knows more than could be gleaned through conventional education.

30. Discernment

In its positive attribute, this position indicates intelligence, inspiration and wisdom. Someone with a trait in this position is likely to be outwardly observant while also readily connecting with an inner state of ecstasy. This is also a position of genius. In its negative expression, this position can indicate vulgarity, a sense of aristocratic superiority and even a tyrannical nature.

31. Counseling

A trait in position No. 31 indicates the ability to listen, to counsel others and to explain things so that they can easily be understood. It suggests a person who is good at guiding or relating to other people. This position is closely related to position No. 28. A trait in No. 31 or the upper half of No. 28 can be interpreted as showing ability in verbal communication. It is also a link between the inspiration associated with positions 27 – 30 and the inward mental processes associated with the upper portion of the eye.

32. Listening

This is one of the positions that reflects a person's receptivity to others. It is closely linked to No. 31, although it more specifically indicates the capacity to be a silent witness to others, to heal them simply by listening and by being attentive to them.

Positions 32 - 35

This whole area concerns inner seeking and the capacity to be humble and studious. Sometimes saintly and detached (especially with a trait in No. 35) these people can be difficult to engage. They have a tendency to be dreamers (especially with No. 34) or to withdraw from other people without telling them. This withdrawal is in no way reactive or aggressive, however; it tends to be more contemplative and gentle. These upper medial positions are active in people who have an intellectual, spiritual or philosophical quality to their personalities.

Although they may be completely withdrawn, people with traits in these areas also have the ability to let their minds drift off while appearing to be fully present in their bodies. In other words, they can be constantly engaged in imagination or fantasy while still communicating effectively in a normal state of consciousness. People with traits in these positions can have great insights into the meaning of life.

33. Contemplation
34. Meekness

These positions indicate a strong interest in philosophical or meditative pursuits. People with traits in these areas may

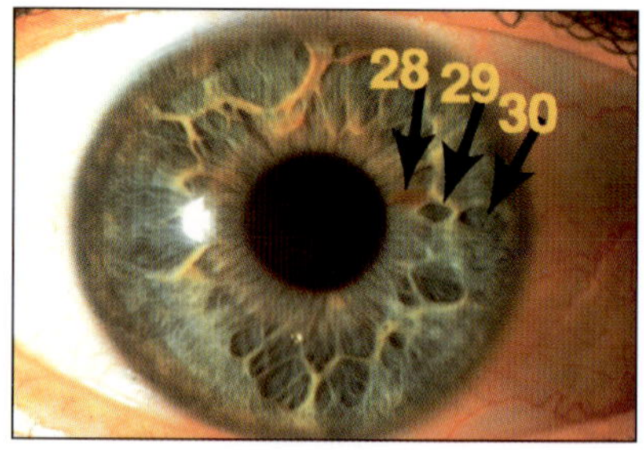

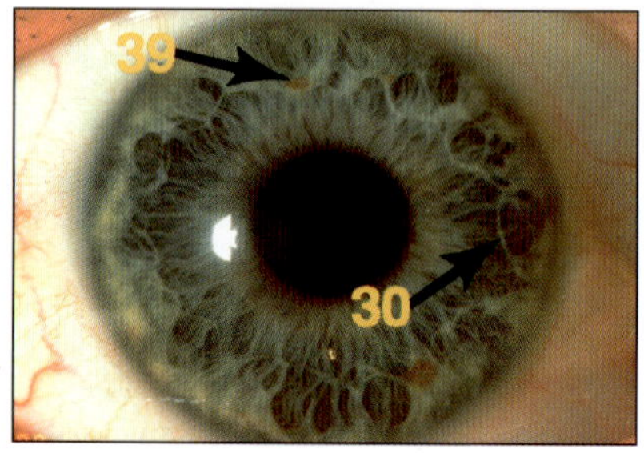

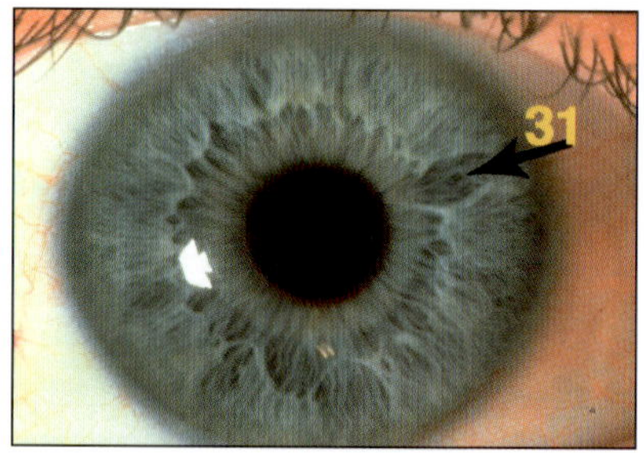

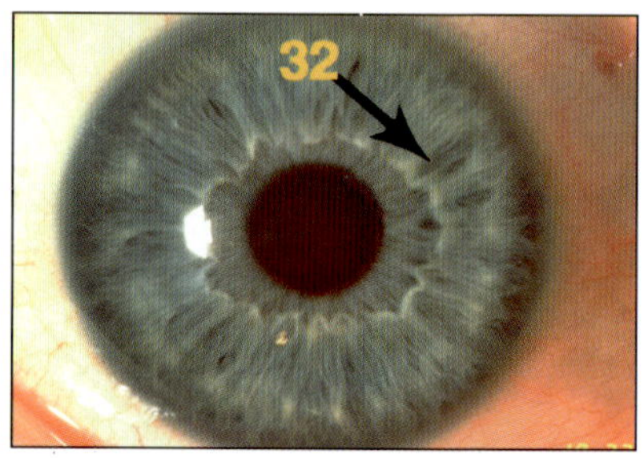

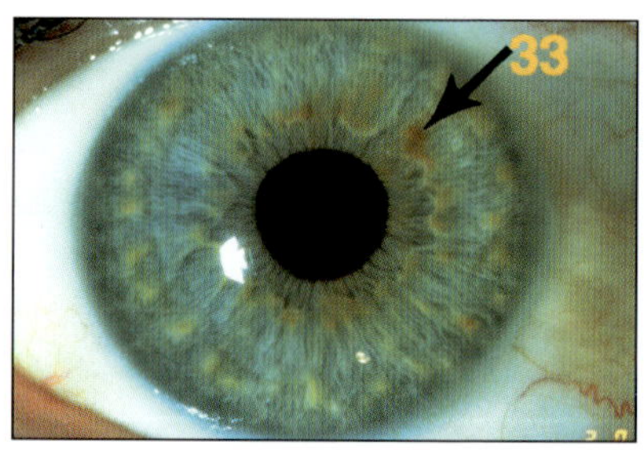

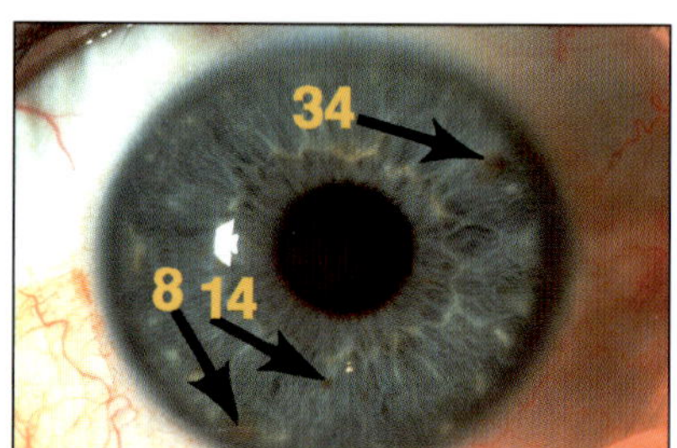

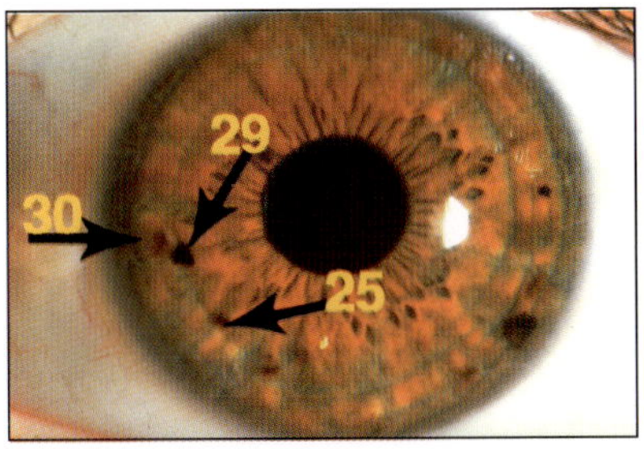

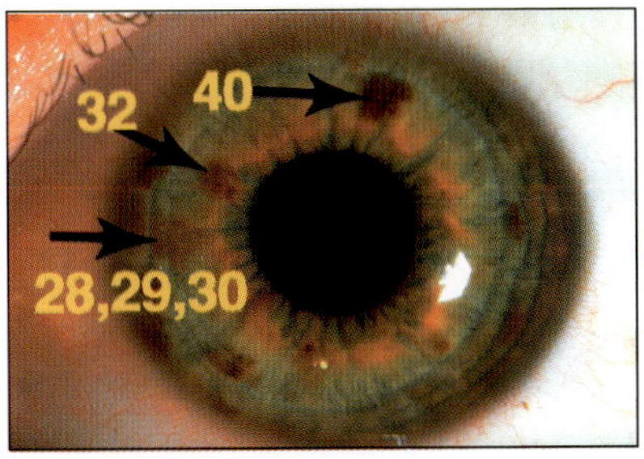

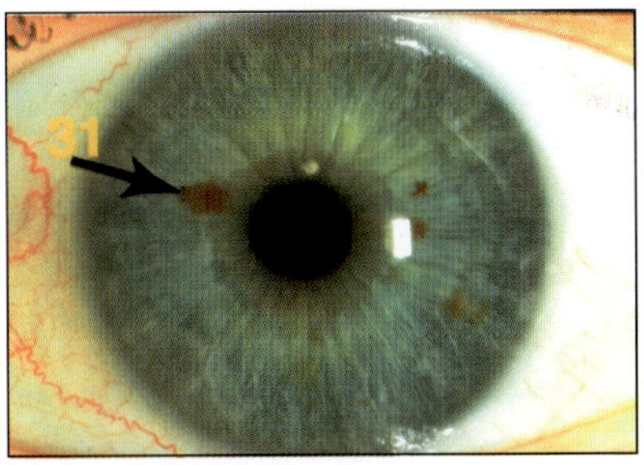

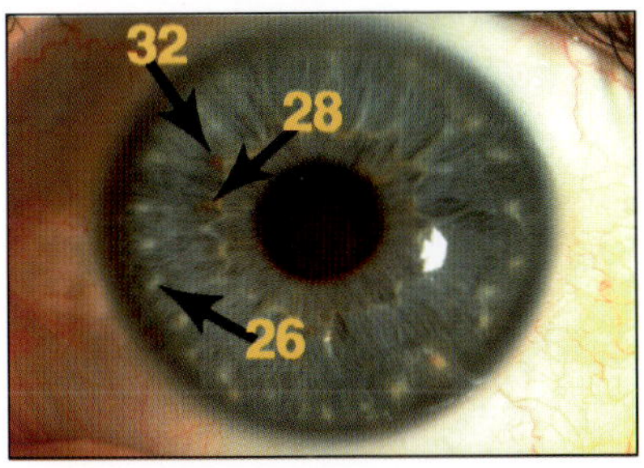

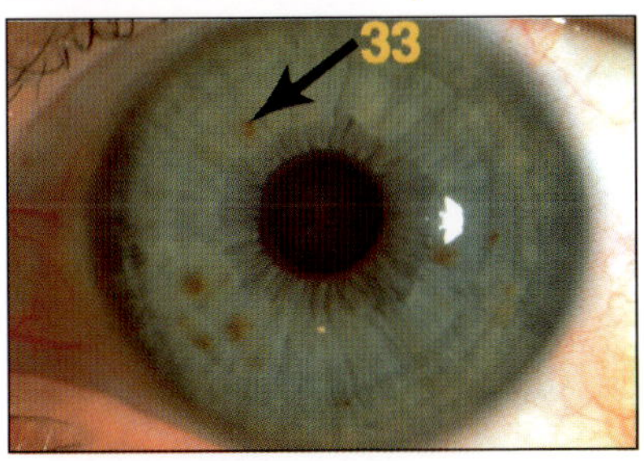

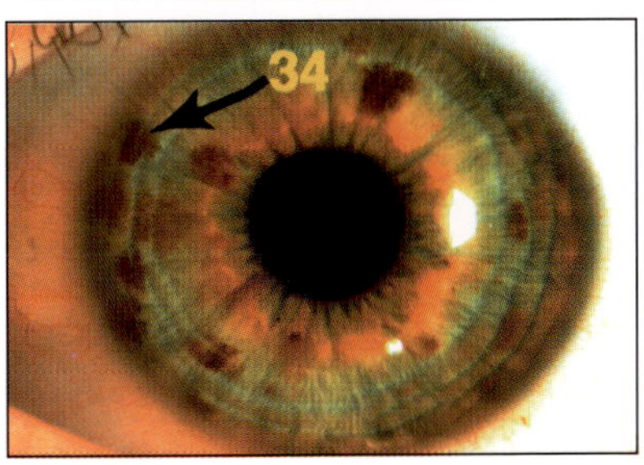

appear to be detached or have a need for grounding. See *Positions 32 - 35*, above.

35. Wisdom
36. Majesty

Traits in these areas often suggest a person who is aloof or distant, and indicate a tendency toward haughtiness or arrogance. Humanitarian insights and farsightedness are also possible with traits in these positions, however. In its positive aspect, No. 36 indicates receptivity to others and a charitable nature, a person who is willing both to give and to receive. With a trait in No. 36, a balanced person may be chivalrous and even altruistic. See *Positions 32 - 35*, above and *Positions 36 - 39*, below.

Positions 36 - 39

In our journey around the iris, it is useful to understand the relationship between adjacent regions. Positions 27 – 30 are about the experience of one's innermost feelings. Nos. 31 and 32 act as pivot points into the higher states of mind, represented by positions 33 – 35. These higher states of mind are then felt and demonstrated in positions 36 through 39. These four upper positions have a lot to do with the mind in its spiritual relationship to others, and indicate the capacity for strength. Characteristics in this region usually show a strong attitude about specific spiritual beliefs.

37. Persistence

In some ways diametrically opposed to No. 36, which often indicates receptivity, No. 37 usually indicates a tendency to be tenacious and persistent or even stubborn and inflexible. Position No. 37 teaches the individual about compromise and diplomacy.

38. Virtue

No. 38 is a position of extremes. Traits in this area are most commonly expressed as self-righteousness and intolerance. In its negative state, position 38 indicates arrogance or hypocrisy, and a tendency to be disrespectful, contemptuous or insulting of others. But these headstrong issues can be expressed positively through integrity and respect for others. When in a state of deep reverence, someone with a trait in this position has a powerful capacity to accelerate the awakening of others.

Positions 39 - 41
39. Self, 40. Philosophy, 41. Ideals

These positions indicate the child's acceptance or rejection of the eye parent's outlook on life. A person with a trait in one of these positions is likely to be outwardly philosophical (especially No. 40) or egotistical (No. 39) in nature. Extreme characteristics associated with this region include utopian attitudes or compulsive behavior.

Positions 39 – 41 indicate the need for an outward expression of the individual's philosophy, unlike positions 33 – 35, which indicate an inwardly philosophical nature that is not easily expressed nor easily understood by others. A trait in No. 40 in the right eye indicates that the father may have been very philosophical, without acting on it, whereas the same trait in No. 41 would indicate that he was more action-oriented.

42. Authority/Rebellion

Providing insight into a person's attitude toward authority, No. 42 often reflects a pattern of rebellion with people of the eye sex. Mirroring the function of positions 31 and 32, No. 42 acts as a pivot point back to the person's emotional self. Positions 42 – 44 all relate to the external expression of emotion. No. 42 and No. 43 both reflect on issues around willfulness, while No. 44 (Understanding) indicates the extent to which a person can combine the heart and the will in the expression of acceptance.

43. Will

This area reveals whether a person is likely to accept or reject direction and guidance from the parents. Patterns of willfulness or submissiveness show up here. A trait in this area usually indicates stubbornness of mind and will, fired with emotion. It can also indicate optimism and the willingness to cooperate with others. Closely related to No. 45, these two positions are a microcosm of the whole personality. No. 43 reflects on the mind and self while No. 45 reflects on the heart in relationship to others. Both No. 43 and No. 45 indicate the ability to express laughter, joy or humor, and the ability to inspire others to experience their feelings, too. All of positions 43 – 46 have a profound influence on the experience of feeling in relationship to others, especially the family and partner.

Jewel: A jewel in this area indicates an outward conflict and a break of the will with a parent.

Flower: A flower indicates that the individual consents and answers to the will of the parent.

Double Will: A double Will issue (e.g. a jewel in No. 43 in each eye) can make an individual very independent but it could also make him really uncertain because he is trying to follow the will of both parents. That can make him feel really "stuck" and confused.

44. Understanding
46. Compassion

Closely related to each other, a trait in either of these positions indicates that the individual readily shows compassion, empathy and sensitivity, and has the ability to cry easily or to express himself through tenderness. Experiences of trauma, grief and separation are also likely. The individual tends to take care of other people while having a great inner sadness, a deep sense of loss that he yearns to have filled. This is especially true with a trait in No. 46. No. 44 indicates more of a quiet sympathy for others, a less animated type of concern and caring.

45. Heart

This position in particular reveals how well one expresses love, joy and laughter. Broken hearts and idealistic attitudes about relationships (especially mate relationships) are quite common. A tendency toward exaggeration or a difficulty with committing in a relationship are also indicated.

Pulling the Threads Together

The inward focus necessary for healing is symbolized by a journey into the center of the pupil. All of the patterns in the iris point toward the pupil, which represents inner centeredness. If the consciousness is unfocused ("off center" or out of the pupil), then the individual's unconscious urge to heal will create a series of environmental interactions (experiences with family members and others) in an attempt to bring his attention back to an inner focus. These experiences in turn create emotional and mental tendencies, communication issues and other challenges, all of which encourage the centering of consciousness.

The particular form that these interactions takes is predictable and is written in the iris as characteristic traits of the personality. It then becomes clear that the apparent "personality" of the individual is there merely to encourage that person to get closer to their core essence. The "personality" is a set of lessons.

Once the centering of consciousness is achieved and maintained, the characteristics (traits) in the iris become the means by which the individual shares his gifts with the world – they are no longer "difficult issues" but rather represent the gifts of individuality in communication and bonding, etc. Each iris position provides information about a variety of aspects related to the lesson or challenge, the gift, the way the trait is expressed, how it affects bonding and the fears associated with it. There are also auditory, visual, kinesthetic, mental and emotional effects associated with every position.

Once you have studied the positions in detail, you can be overwhelmed by the sheer volume of knowledge revealed by them. Although there are many aspects to any position in the iris, this is simply the consequence of that particular position's core information being expressed in different behavioral spheres. Bear in mind that the net result of all these individual effects is a long-term impact on behavior: the alignment of the personality to bring about change.

In Consultation

When doing an interpretation, retain your ability to be flexible;avoid creating firm rules as guidelines for yourself. Become aware of the key feeling, attitude or disposition associated with an interpretive area, and then shift your interpretation of its slightly depending on its precise position and the individual's constitutional type.

One of the interesting paradoxes about the Rayid Method is that its ultimate purpose is to help you forget what structure you are, to help you move beyond what the eye reveals. If you are attached to knowing what structure you are, it becomes more difficult to get free of it. The more precise you get in defining someone's personality, the more likely it is that you'll limit his growth, limit his ability to break free of his personailty patterns. That is the main problem with having a detailed understanding of iris positions. Don't forget to free your clients from the limitations of their structure.

So don't fall into the trap of simply reading one area after another. Try to get an impression of the fabric that these threads are weaving. Remember that every position provides you with information about the individual's need for a particular personality lesson.

When you analyze someone in a consultation, remember that you are defining them;the more you define them, the more you limit them and trap them in

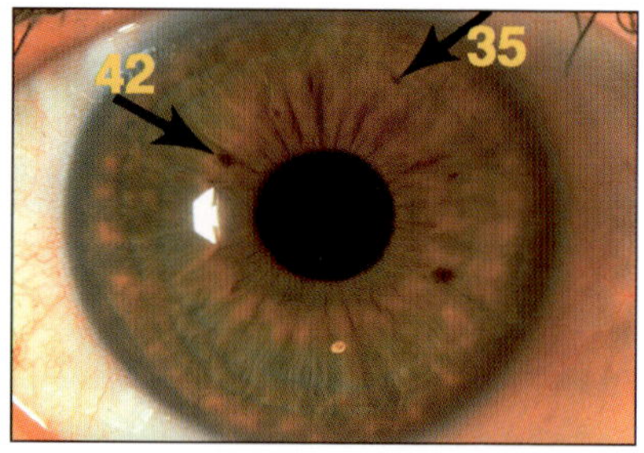

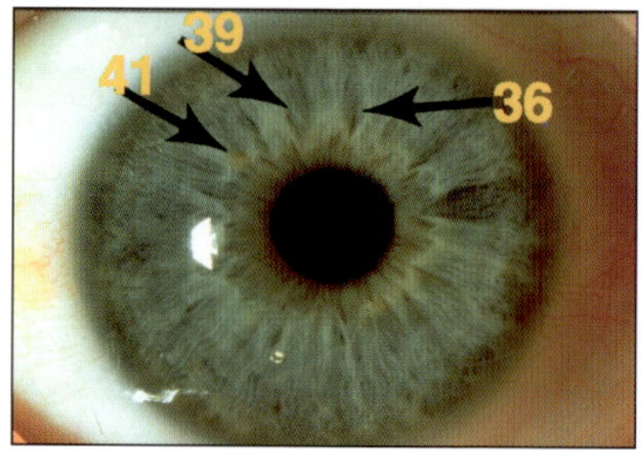

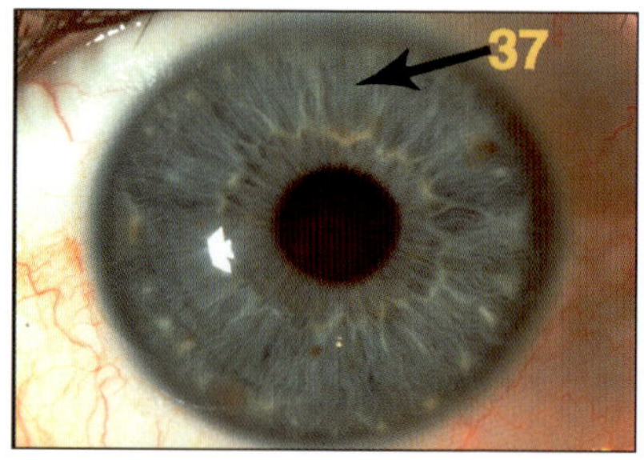

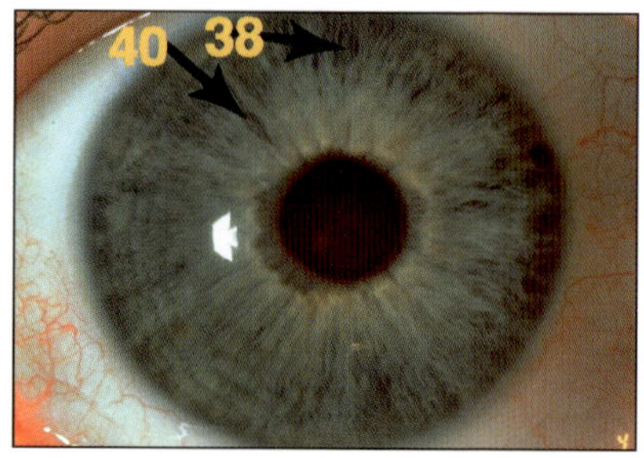

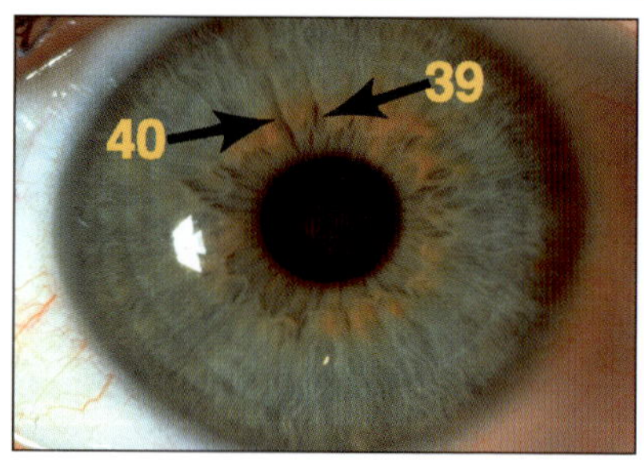

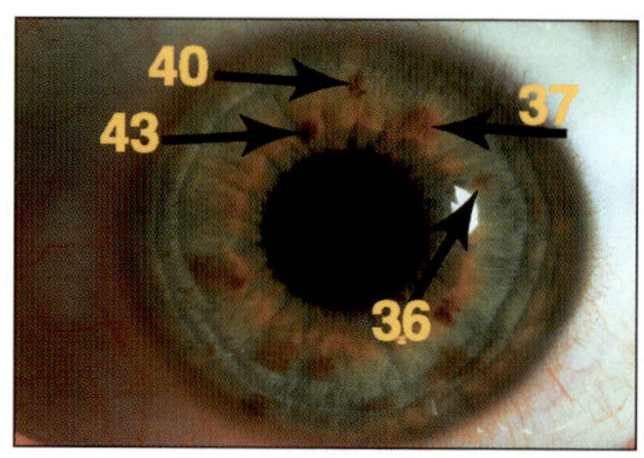

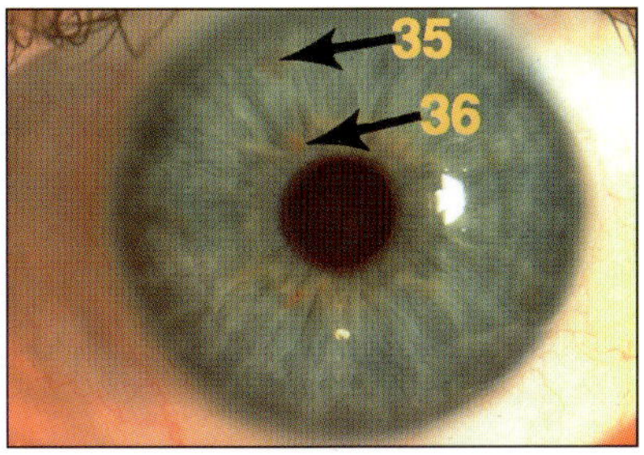

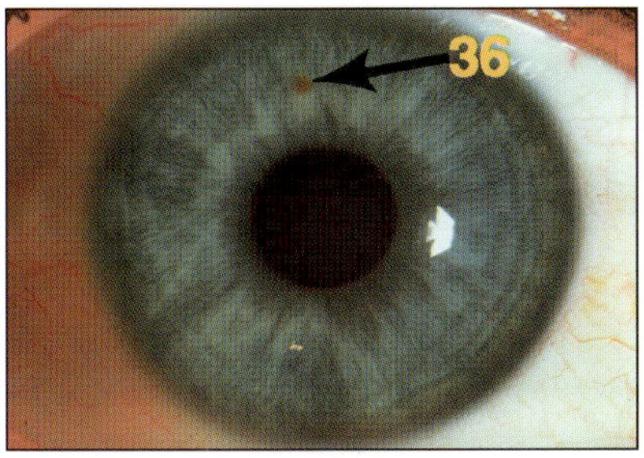

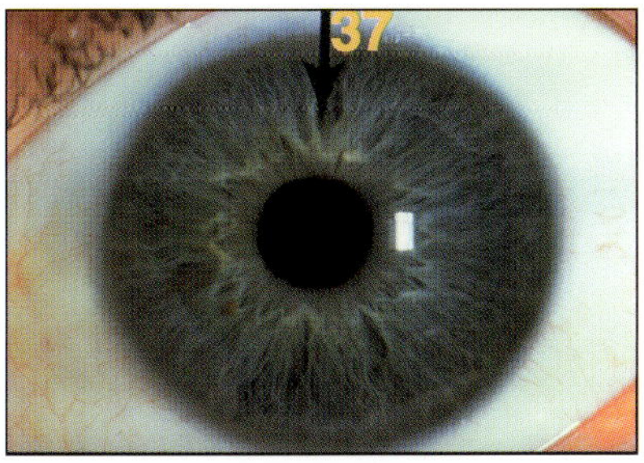

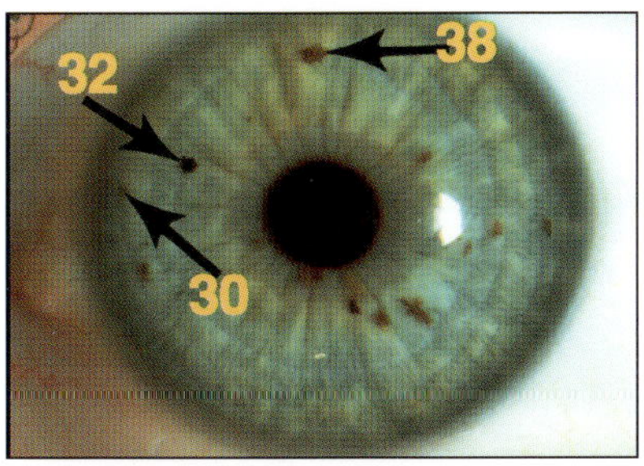

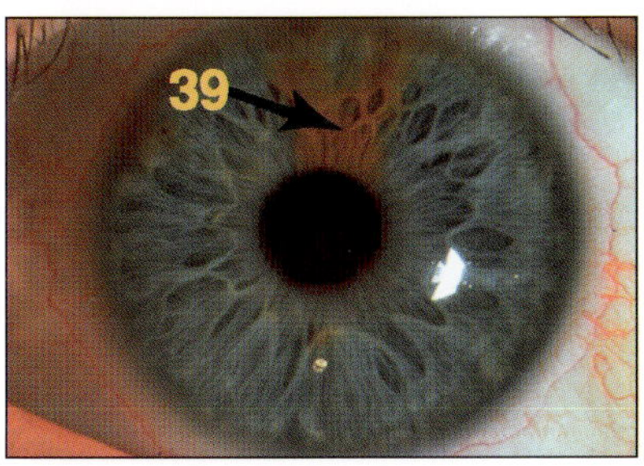

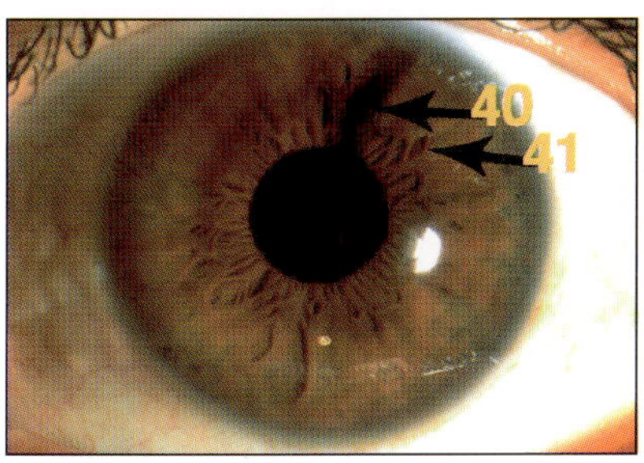

the details. This can get in the way of paying attention to the "macro" lesson: long-term structural balance.

Understanding iris positions is, however, important in helping you to establish a rapport with a client. The kind of interpretive accuracy you get by referring to a couple of very specific aspects of the client's experience will engender confidence in your abilities. So instead of getting lost in the details, try referring to only one or two key positions in the eye, and get confirmation from the client of your interpretation. Use your client's confidence in you to help him. Although you may be referring to particular experiences at certain points in ytour client's development, your primary concern should be with freeing him from those experiences.

The most important thing when interpreting someone's eyes is to ask, "Where is this person's main lesson right now?" So don't fall into the trap of just reading one area after another. Try to find the thread of what they all add up to. There is, of course, a difference between understanding and interpreting. You need to be aware of the implications of the positions to help you in your interpretations as a Rayid practitioner. Understanding the positions helps you to appreciate the life processes each individual has been through as a person, even if you don't necessarily describe everything you see to your client.

In order to prevent a client from becoming attached to the apparent limitations you are presenting to him, it is useful to describe the traits as something that he may have experienced in his past. You can tell the client, "These traits are chapters of the book that describes your life up to this point." What is most important is to give the client some pointers as to how to move on.

The majority of what you see in the eyes is in the past. Help your client to leave it in the past.

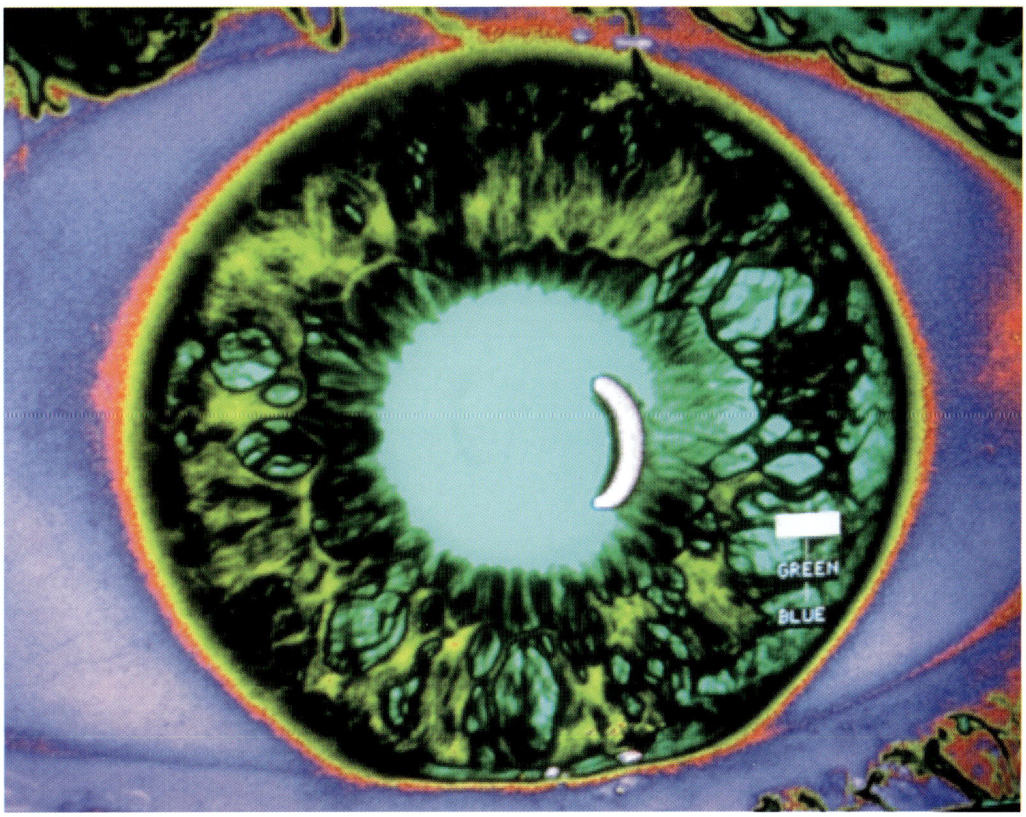

The Effect of a Jewel or Flower in Key Positions

The primary effect of a specific trait in an area is to slightly alter the vibratory pattern of the genetically inherent structure. It does this by increasing (▲) or decreasing (▼) behavioral qualities associated with that area of the iris. This chart describes the impact of jewel and flower traits on eight different qualities of personality:

MENTAL (M): Self-awareness, clarity and control. Thoughts, analysis and the use of words.

EMOTIONAL (E): Expressive feelings and social involvement. Spacial perception and emotions.

KINESTHETIC (K): Grounded awareness and a sense of connection or "belonging." Physical sensitivity.

ACTION/MOTION (A): Vitality and change. Sense of purpose and commitment.

SPACE (S): Openness and receptivity. Similar to "E" but without reactive emotions. The wordless experience of surrender/allowing.

HEMISPHERIC FUNCTION (H): An individual trait will increase or decrease the activity or dominance of the hemisphere in which it is found.

INTROVERSION (I): Inner-directed. Retains structural qualities. Interest in conceptual, future or intangible matters.

EXTROVERSION (X): Outer-directed. Expresses structural characteristics. Interest in actual, past or tangible matters.

The chart looks at the effect on certain key positions only. The positions are listed by number, name and primary energetic quality (mental, emotional or kinesthetic). Personality qualities are listed in order of their observed impact on behavior.

POSITION	JEWEL	FLOWER
1. Nurturing (Kinesthetic)	▼ K	▲ K
	▲ E	▲ M
	▲ A	▼ A
	▲ H	▼ H
	▼ M	▼ E
	▼ I	▲ X
2. Resentment (Mental)	▲ M	▼ K
	▲ E	▼ M
	▼ K	▲ E
	▼ A	▲ A
	▼ H	▼ H
	▲ I	▲ X
3. Anger (Emotional)	▼ H	▼ H
	▲ E	▲ E
	▲ A	▼ M
	▲ K	▼ K
	▼ M	▲ A
	▼ I	▲ X
4. Rivalry (Emotional)	▲ E	▲ E
	▼ H	▼ H
	▲ A	▼ K
	▲ M	▼ M
	▼ K	▲ A
	▲ X	▲ X
6. Independence (Emotional)	▲ E	▼ K
	▲ M	▲ A
	▼ A	▲ M
	▲ K	▲ S
	▲ H	▲ E
	▲ I	▼ X

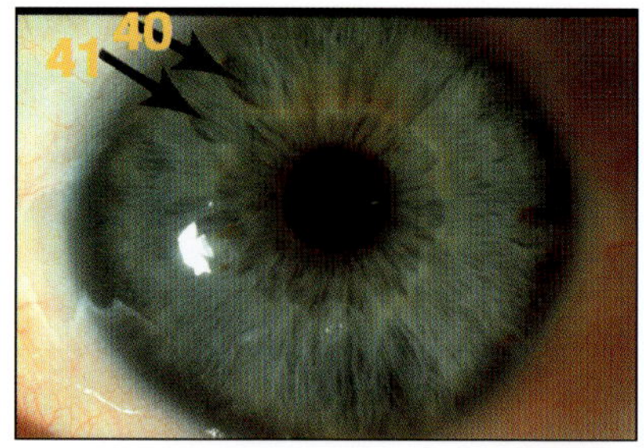

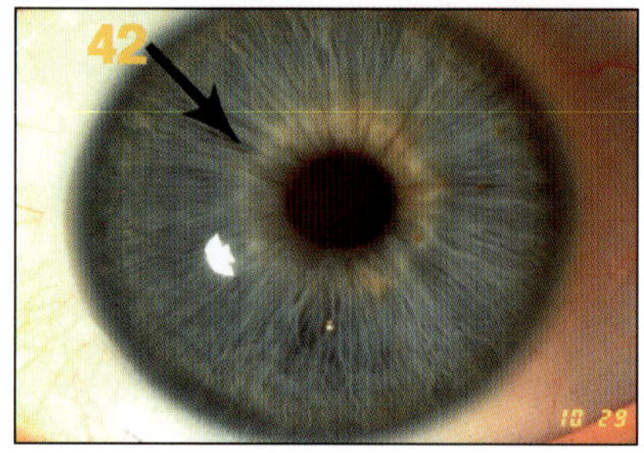

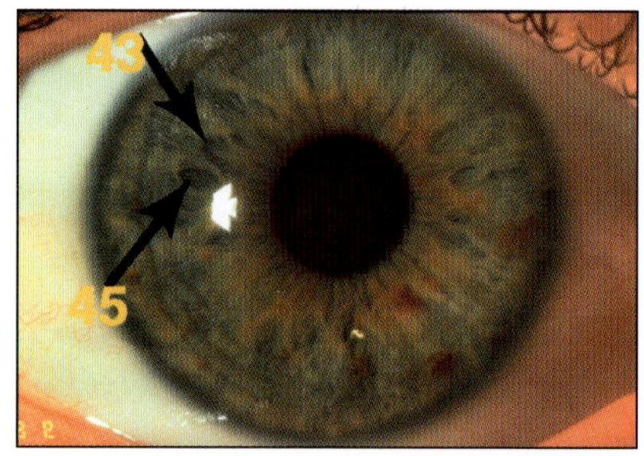

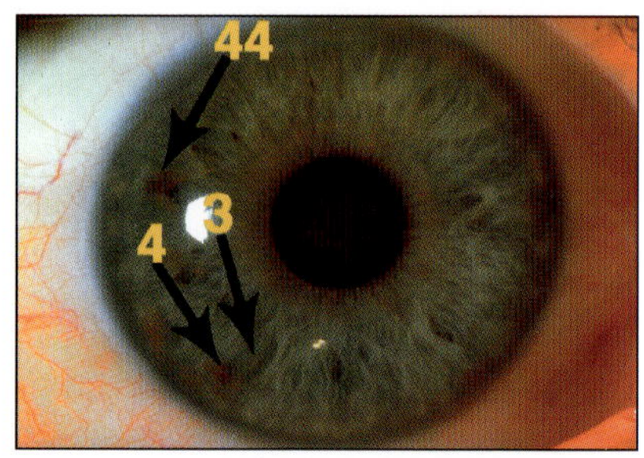

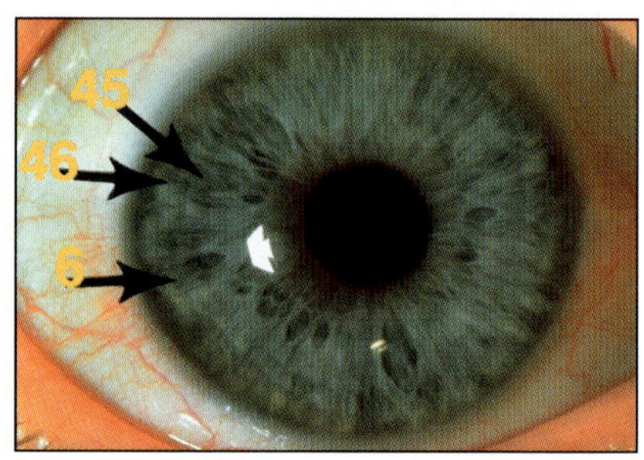

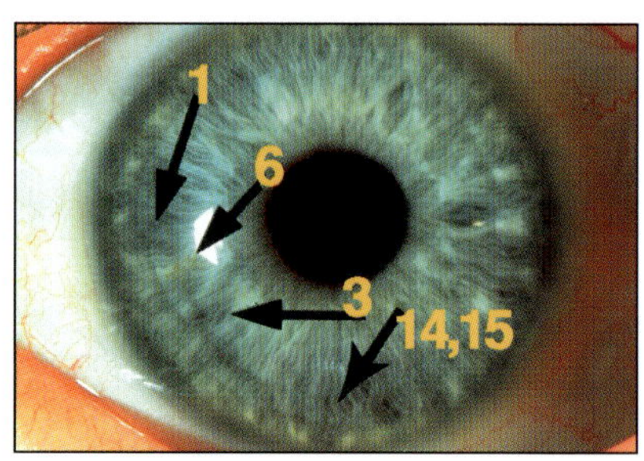

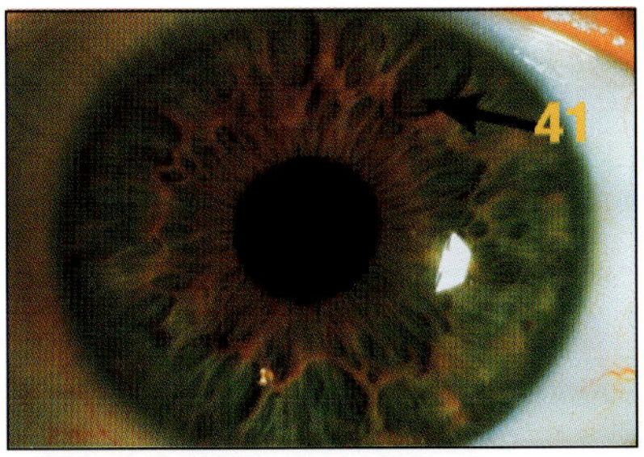

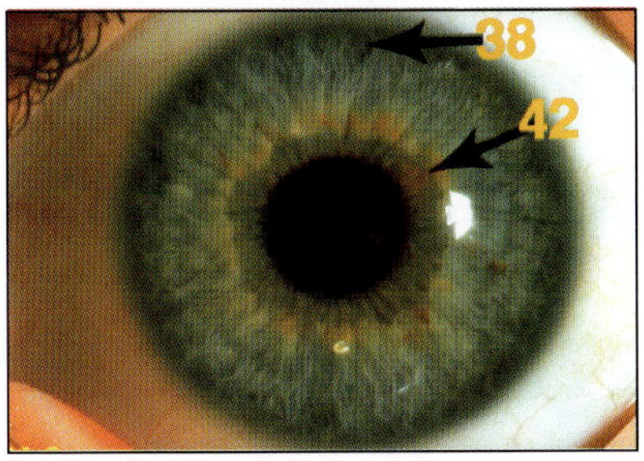

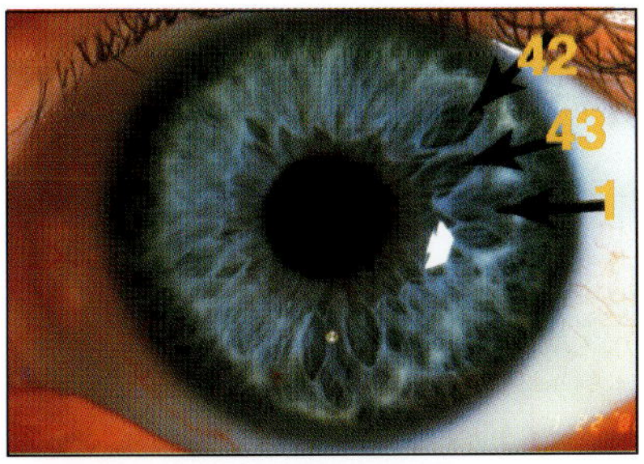

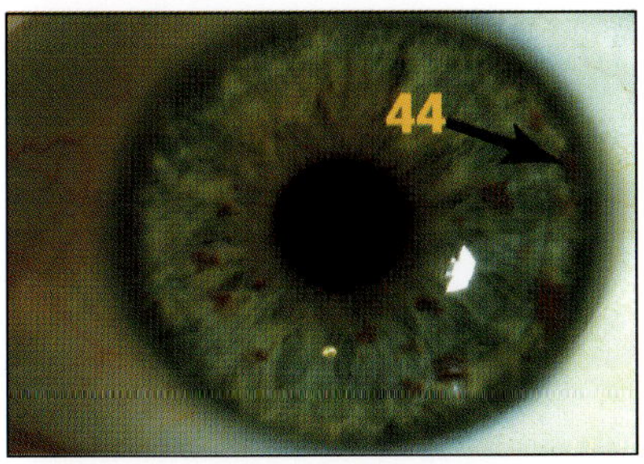

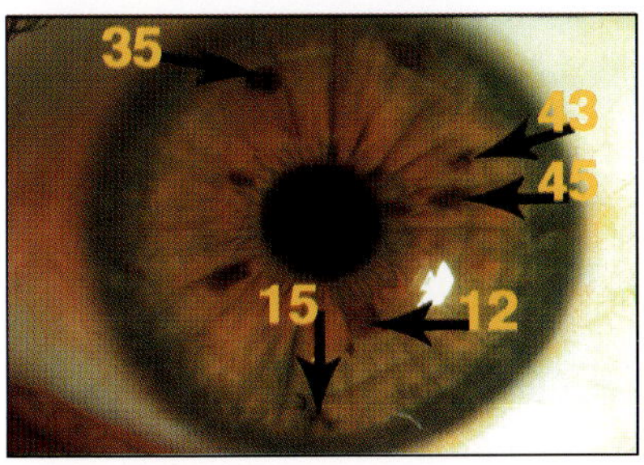

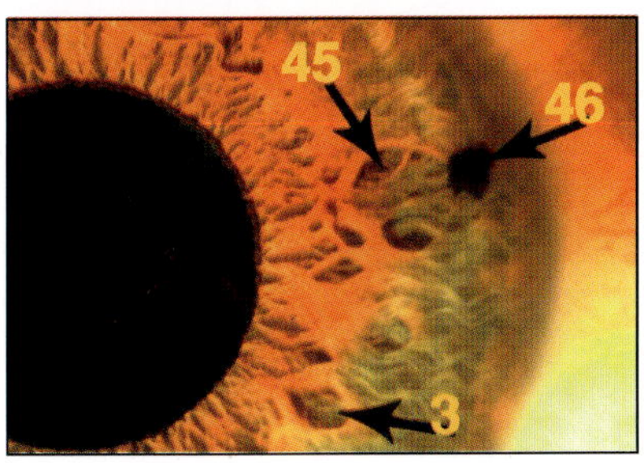

7. Concern (Kinesthetic)

▼ A	▲ E
▲ K	▲ A
▲ H	▼ K
▲ M	▼ H
▲ I	▲ M
▼ E	▲ X

8. Originality (Mental)

▲ S	▼ H
▲ M	▲ E
▼ H	▲ M
▼ A	▲ A
▲ K	▼ K
▲ I	▼ X

14. Patience (Kinesthetic)

▲ M	▲ A
▼ H	▲ E
▼ E	▼ H
▲ K	▼ M
▼ I	▼ K
	▲ X

16. Self-Esteem (Mental)

▼ A	▼ H
▲ M	▼ A
▼ H	▲ K
▲ K	▼ E
▼ E	▲ M
▲ S	▲ S
▼ X	▲ I

20. Gentleness (Kinesthetic)

▼ A	▼ A
▲ M	▼ M
▼ H	▼ H
▼ K	▼ K
▲ S	▲ S
▼ X	▲ I

22. Sexuality (Emotional)

▲ E	▲ A
▲ A	▲ K
▲ S	▲ M
▲ H	▲ H
▲ K	▲ S
▼ M	▲ E
▼ I	▲ X

43. Will (Mental)

▲ M	▲ S
▲ E	▼ A
▼ H	▲ H
▲ A	▲ M
▼ K	▲ K
▲ X	▼ X

45. Heart (Kinesthetic)

▲ E	▲ A
▼ H	▼ E
▼ M	▲ M
▲ S	▼ H
▼ K	▼ K
▼ X	▼ X

46. Compassion (Emotional)

▲ E	▲ E
▼ M	▲ S
▲ H	▲ K
▼ A	▲ H
▲ K	▲ M
▲ S	▼ A
▼ X	▲ I

The Influence of the Family Tree

TRANSGENERATIONAL PATTERNS

Personality is primarily genetically determined. Question any parent of a young child and you will be told that the child definitely came into this world with a distinct personality. Although early environmental factors can have a significant influence on the way in which a child's personality is *expressed,* your childhood experiences were not the *origin* of your personality. The package of behavioral traits that you think of as so uniquely your own is, for the most part, simply a variation on an existing pattern in your family tree.

Genetically, you are a medley of physiological and behavioral programs inherited from your ancestors. Although each individual has the opportunity to exercise free will, most people have difficulty extricating themselves from the invisible influence of preceding generations. Imagine driving in your car with the intention of going where you want to go and doing what you want to do, but riding in the back seat are 30 of your ancestors, each giving you a different set of instructions. One says turn right, another says turn left; one says slow down, another tells you to speed up. This is the nature of the influence of the family tree and how it continues to affect your choices and desires throughout life.

Many of these influences are far from benign; some aspects of our inherited behaviors are decidedly counter-productive in terms of our overall emotional and psychic development. A metaphor that is helpful when exploring the influence of particular ancestors is to think of the family tree as a large river with many tributaries, each of which represents a specific branch of the family. Imagine being at the mouth of the river, where you detect toxic waste in the water and find precious gold deposited in the riverbed. Both the toxins and the gold have their origin somewhere upstream, each coming from a different tributary. The poison of unresolved negativity from a preceding generation influences everyone in the present and needs to be dealt with. It is useful to know from which tributary the poison comes, so that you can travel back to that place and clean it up. Similarly, it is useful to know which specific tributary is responsible for depositing gold along the bed of the river. To find the source of that gold is to access the source of one's true genius. The river must be cleansed and the original source of the gold rediscovered.

As we have outlined in the preceding chapters, the iris is a precise map of the specific toxins and precious metals flowing downstream to that person. The iris structure, specific positions and the individual's hemispheric function are like a highly accurate metal detector or chemical sampling device that can be used to locate the origin of specific behavioral traits.

The Key Influence of Parents

It is commonly accepted that parents are the main influence on a child's biological and psychological makeup. For example, as we saw in the chapter on hemispheric polarity, the parents genetically influence whether a person is predominantly left-brained or right-brained. But parents are really just messengers in the grand scheme of transgenerational influence; the entire genealogy of a person's family tree focuses through the parents, represented in the body by the two halves of the brain.

In a mysterious way, nearly all Jewel patterns emanate primarily from the mother's side of the family. Similarly, nearly all Flower types emanate from the father's side of the family. Jewels "know" that they are from the mother's side, while Flowers will say that they "identify with" the father's side. This innate intuition can be used to help each person enliven his constitutional vehicle and reaccess the genetic source from which he comes. Without dwelling on the past, each person needs to become aware of his origins so that he knows which particular genetic key will open the door to the experience of genius, love and wholeness. Once this happens, the ever-deepening experience of well-being restores the body to perfect function, increasing the person's capacity to feel and raising his vibratory frequency (see standing wave pattern analogy in book introduction).

The path to this experience of wholeness involves the individual in encounters with people who have complementary experiences and personalities. Your parents are the first of the people you meet on your journey through life who have something to teach you, and their impact is profound. They are the primary genetic *and* environmental influences on your personality. Under normal circumstances, they cannot change the *core* personality that you were born with, your parents' behavior toward you can influence the way in which your personality unfolds during your life.

Mothers are the energetic source for all children and, therefore, for all people. A child needs to be loved unconditionally by its mother, to be given of that energy freely without being told how to use it. The most destructive thing a mother can do is to chronically express anger toward her child. This creates a separation of the child from its source.

The ease with which you can go to your father is the ease with which you can be true to yourself. If it is difficult for you to hug your father, to communicate honestly and openly with him, it will be difficult for you to find and/or express your true nature. Your relationship with your father also determines how easy it is for you to attain success. How was it for you to walk up to your father? This is how you will experience approaching your goals. In an ideal situation, a child needs its father to be the one that helps to "direct" its energy, without being critical. The most destructive thing a father can do is to criticize his child or its mother. If your father was critical, your mind and body cannot rest; you will never be able to stop trying to achieve, or else you may give up entirely.

The father becomes increasingly important from the age of two but especially between the ages of four and seven. That is a key period of personality expression. By this time, the mother will ideally have given the child a strong feeling of connection with its source (which in infancy was her), and it is now the father's turn to help complete the process of personality expression into the world.

Parental Disharmony

If the relationship between the parents breaks down, the conscious personality can end up in conflict with the unconscious personality. Neuro-degenerative diseases can result from successive generations of angry, critical fathers and controlling mothers because the child does not feel accepted.

Whenever you see a very slim, nearly emaciated person, you are likely to be looking at someone with a transgenerational criticism pattern. A baby who has a chronic problem with absorbing food probably has a mother and father who are constantly bickering or criticizing each other. The yin and yang elements are not nurturing each other and so the child cannot be sustained.

With such parental difficulties, it is often easier to deal directly with the child than to try to get the adults to change, since their behavior is usually too entrenched. For more information about this topic, see *Parent-Child Relationship Challenges*, in the next chapter.

Ancestral Women

The influence of women on a child's personality seems to be at least eight times stronger than that of men. This correlates with recent scientific discoveries in the field of genetic inheritance. There is a type of DNA, called cytoplasmic DNA, which is inherited only from the cytoplasm of the mother's egg, and which is particularly responsible for energy and respiration, especially through mitochondrial DNA. The Chinese have a system of eight ancestral meridians going back to eight women, the eight great-great-grandmothers. These eight ancestral women are primarily responsible for the personality of any individual today, representing eight ancestral rivers.

Healing the Self and Family

We need to free ourselves from negativity in the past in order to be fully awake in the present. We need to free ourselves from the unconsciousness in us that manipulates the body and mind.

This unconscious is far stronger than we generally acknowledge. In order to achieve a state of physical and emotional well-being, in order to clear up harmful patterns in the personality or the family tree, we must be free of such negative influences. This requires the use of many tools – spiritual, mental and physical – to bring us fully into balance.

You can't heal the personality or relationships of one child without healing the whole family. The influence of the family tree is too strong. If you had the opportunity to explore transgenerational behavior patterns, as family therapists do, you might be surprised at how easy it is to predict that a particular personality trait will repeat itself in a specific child in the family sequence. Most people have "psychic octopuses" that need to be cleared out of their personalities. Tentacles originating several generations back can still jerk you around like a puppet on a string.

Because we are so intertwined with our ancestors, we can't lift ourselves out of our harmful patterns without lifting our entire family tree out with us. It doesn't work to just block off from the influence of the family. If you try, you can end up suffering severe traumas because you are actually trying to cut yourself off from part of the energy matrix that sustains you. It would be like the hand trying to cut itself off from the body. So it is important not to deny the family's influence but to *acknowledge* it so that you can free yourself from it without pretending that you don't have roots.

In order to heal, it is important that you let go of the belief that your childhood created the personality patterns that you were actually *born* with. You came into this world with a vibrational agenda. That vibrational agenda was handed to you genetically and you are now acting it out physiologically and socially. It may appear that your father and mother were the origin of it. They were not. They themselves were only a link in the chain. Even your apparently formative childhood experiences were in themselves primarily a continuation of genetically established patterns.

The influence of the family tree is pervasive and extremely complex. Although it is possible, using Rayid, to determine that certain behavior patterns appear to originate with specific ancestors, remember that you could find the cause of that person's behavior in an earlier ancestor even further back. You can keep going further and further back into time like this, ad infinitum, and gain nothing from your attempts to lay blame. If you do explore the past, content yourself with knowing something about the dominant branches of your family tree, for that can help you to better understand your current motivations. Let go of the need to blame either yourself or your parents, or to blame anyone else in the family tree as being the cause of your pain, because they are not. The influence of your family tree is powerful, and it can be harmful, but it is a web that has no weaver.

Before you can reconnect with your core essence, it is essential to use affirmations and other psychic or spiritual technologies to release the negative influence of transgenerational toxicity. This restores full access to the treasures that are hidden deep within you. You must consciously acknowledge the influence of preceding generations and remind yourself that, with the aid of the true self, you are able to free yourself from that influence before you can expect to effect any real change in your personality. This is one of the reasons why doing affirmations and rituals can be so self-empowering. The body must then be cleansed, nourished, rested, touched and revitalized. With the psychic hooks removed, and with a healthy body, the individual is now prepared to reconnect with his true nature.

The iris is a map that reveals the specific therapies and lifestyle changes that a person can make in order to become fully enlivened. Along the way, the individual will experience changes in current relationship patterns and ever-deepening feelings as all the tributaries of the family river are cleansed and vitalized. This makes it easier to harvest the gold that is also flowing down to you from previous generations. The specific tributary that is the origin of your essence and genius is associated with a single meridian line and a single acupuncture point in the body. From this specific access point in the body all other meridians, and the biological and energetic systems that they represent, can be restored to perfect function and harmony. Your journey toward the experience of enlivened wholeness not only increases the life force in the body, it also intensifies feelings, improves your ability to relate to others and develops certainty and clarity of mind.

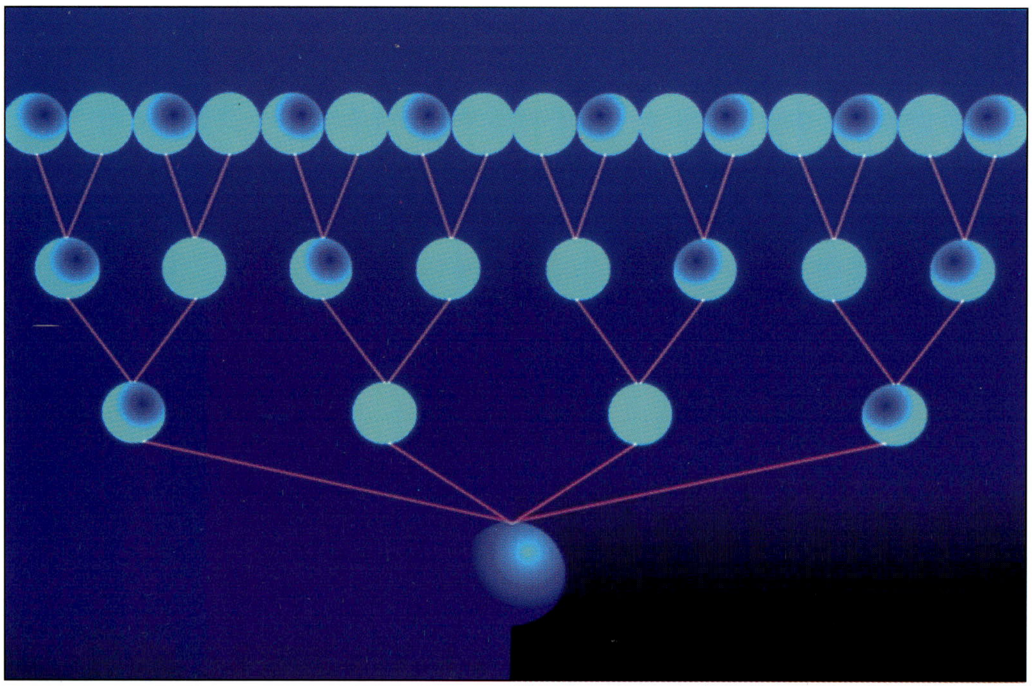

Rayid enables you to determine the Jewel (mental) and Flower (emotional) influences in your family tree for three generations back.

IRIS DEVELOPMENT

The considerable body of photographic evidence accumulated to date indicates that the structure of the iris can be added to but not reduced. In other words, once a trait has developed, it appears to stay. An ongoing project to photograph the same children on a regular basis has given us excellent records of iris development over the years.

We know from individual case studies that all of the flower patterns that will ever appear in the iris are visible at, or shortly after, birth. We have no photographic evidence of a flower trait changing during a person's lifetime. We do, however, have photographic evidence of jewel formation in eyes that had no jewel patterns during the first year of development. Current theory suggests that jewel patterns are latent within the genetic code and are preprogrammed to emerge at specific times.

The photographs of Aaron, top right, are a case in point. Taken six years apart, they clearly show the formation of numerous jewels. An estimated 90% of jewels appear between the ages of three and eight, although we do have photographic evidence of jewels forming in people as old as 40. The photographs of Symon, lower right, show him to be a Flower structure at the age of four months. At 12 months, there is no change in the shape of the individual flowers or iris fibers but there is the beginning of a noticeable shift in coloration toward gold or brown hues. Although a certain amount of this coloration is due to differences in the color tone of the slide film, there is a definite deposition of brown pigment around the Ring of Expression in the more recent photograph.

So far, we have no evidence of the overall iris structure changing in an adult. Although a jewel or ring may occasionally develop later in life, this is never enough to change the fundamental constitutional structure. The group of four photographs of an adult iris (below) were taken four years apart. Consistent, high-magnification photography shows no change in the individual fibers of the eye.

These are just three examples of the detailed research currently being undertaken. Further studies include photographing individual flower structures many years apart.

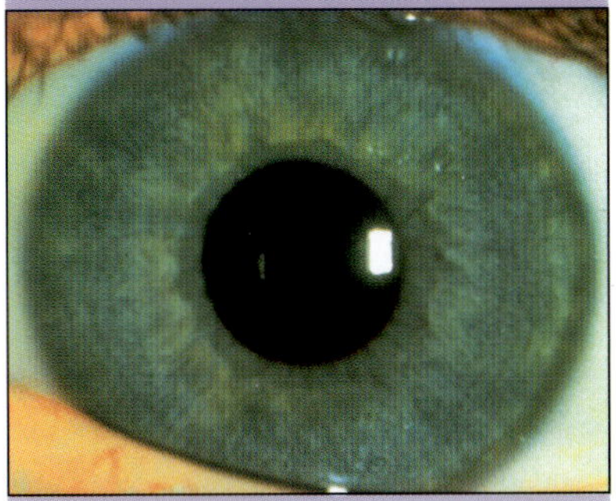

Aaron (age 3), left eye

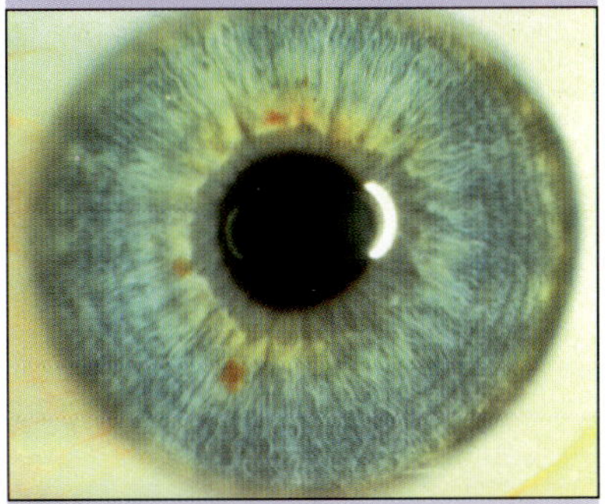

Aaron (age 9), left eye

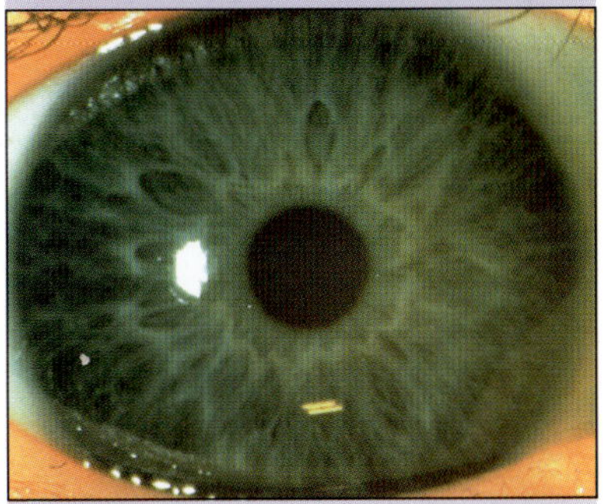

Symon (age 4 months), right

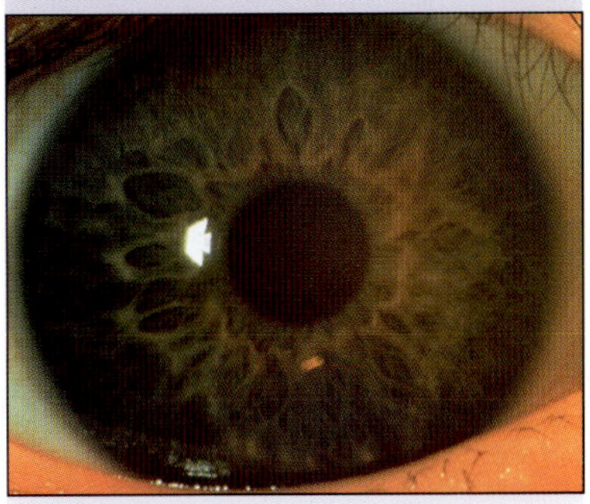

Symon (age 12 months), right

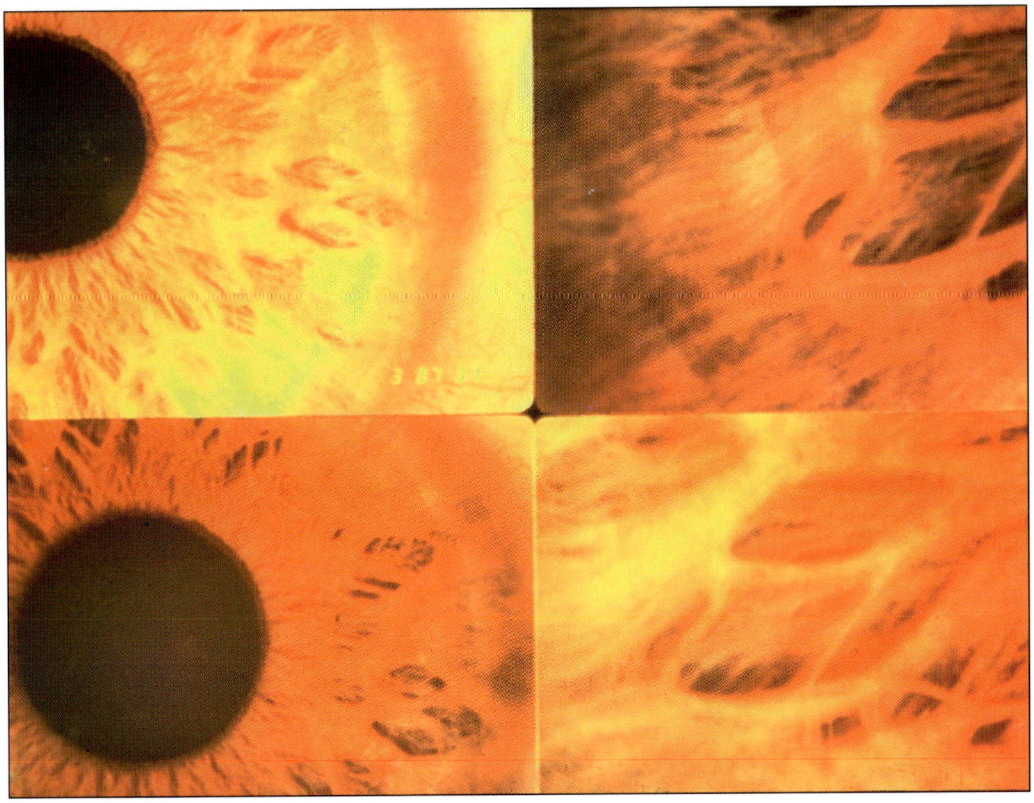

High-magnification photographs of the same iris in an adult, taken four years apart. Even the close-ups of the individual flower trait (on the right) show absolutely no change in fiber structure. The bottom two photographs are the most recent.

THE 16 VIBRATORY CHANNELS

Most people's behavior is predominantly either left-brained or right-brained. Although everybody goes through a daily cycle of oscillations between left- and right-brain dominance, most people oscillate around a habitual degree of deviance to the left or right. In the Rayid system, there are eight degrees of hemispheric dominance on either side of neutrality. These are the 16 vibratory channels, representing relative degrees of mind distraction away from balanced behavior.

Every person occupies one of these channels, or "slots." Each of these vibratory slots represents a specific frequency that modifies the primary structural personality, giving some people behavioral traits that we used to think of as hemispheric adaptation (see *Hemispheric Polarity*). The slots from 1 to 8 describe a left-brained personality; the slots from 9 to 16 indicate a right-brained personality. Slot 1 is the extreme left-brained position; slot 16 is the extreme right-brained position. Someone who isn't noticeably left- or right-brained will occupy slot 8 or 9, the middle ground.

It can actually be quite misleading to use the terms "left-brained" and "right-brained." What we are really identifying is masculine and feminine impulses moving through the entire body, not just the mind, and it is not accurate to think of masculine and feminine attributes as being determined purely by the brain. Unresolved issues in the constitutional personality create tensions and impulses that cause a person's behavior to alternate between either masculine or feminine qualities of expression. This is a binary process in which one mode of behavior automatically excludes the other. In a healthier person, this binary (either-or) process is replaced by the experience of fusion, in which both the masculine and feminine aspects of the personality can be experienced simultaneously. For the sake of easier communication, we simplify our terminology and refer to the expressed personality in terms of left- and right-brain attributes, even though the true nature of this subject is far richer and more complex.

The right brain is associated with feminine attributes, the left brain with masculine attributes. As we discussed in the chapter on hemispheric polarity, the Jewel parent determines the hemispheric orientation of the child. A Jewel father will pull the child into the left (masculine) hemisphere, while a Jewel mother will pull the child into the right (feminine) hemisphere. Jewel energy overrides Flower energy because it is more crystallized. The Flower parent's main influence is in how the child *experiences* his personality, not in how it is expressed.

Each succeeding generation of a particular polarity will amplify the trend set by the Jewel parent. For example, an individual with a Jewel mother most probably will be in one of slots 9 – 16 (right hemisphere). If the grandmother is also a Jewel, then the person will be particularly right-brained, probably occupying one of slots 13 – 16. But if the mother is a Flower and the father is a Jewel, then the person is probably in one of slots 1 – 8 (left hemisphere). And if both the father and the grandfather are Jewels, then the individual will probably be somewhere in the range of slots 1 – 4 (i.e. further left). If the great-grandfather was also a Jewel, the person would be in slot 1 or 2 (very left-brained). Just one Jewel woman in the paternal line would modify this influence. For example, if your father's mother was a Jewel, your father would have been a right-brained Jewel and so, even though you would still be left-brained, you would be less left-brained than if your father had been a left-brained Jewel.

For some as yet unknown reason, this neat pattern appears to break between the third and fourth generation. The extreme left-brained position (No. 1) is when all of the direct male forebears were Jewels, except for an extremely strong Jewel great-great-grandmother. This Jewel woman still exerts incredible influence, even though she is buried somewhere back in the mists of time. Although the 16 vibratory channels represent the 16 lines of inheritance from the great-great-grandparents, it seems as if the most powerful influence on personality formation is usually a woman, one of the eight great-great-grandmothers. It is very unusual to encounter extremely left-brained Jewels, and slot No. 1 is usually occupied only by radical Shaker-Flowers.

The extreme right-brained position (slot 16) is when the direct female ancestors, for four generations back, were all Jewels. The kind of people that occupy slot 16 are typically extreme Shaker-Jewels who have been abused by their fathers. In touch with multiple dimensions, they may see things that are apparently real but are not normally visible to the eye, or may see things that are not there in any dimension, that are simply a projection of their own fears.

As we have shown, the degree of hemispheric dominance can greatly affect a person's behavior, and the concept of vibratory channels gives us the ability to quantify the extent to which someone appears to be more left-brained or right-brained. Jewels are naturally constricted, as are left-brained personalities, and a slot 2 (very left-brained) Jewel would be extremely controlled and tight. A mildly left-brained (e.g. slot 7) Jewel would be less constricted, and a right-brained (slots 9 – 16) Jewel would have some degree of expansion to balance his innate constriction.

Accessing the Core Personality

Each one of the 16 vibratory channels represents a distinct element of personality, one aspect of a whole person. When fully awake and enlivened, an individual can experience the qualities associated with all of these channels simultaneously. Such a person has managed to clear away the emotional and psychological debris that accumulates during life, and which obscures the original genetic blueprint that was present immediately after conception. That blueprint represents the core personality, the true constitutional structure that each person must return to before he can move beyond the iris (see *Therapies* chapter introduction).

Any one of the vibratory channels can represent the slot that a particular individual must center on in order to get to *his* core personality. It isn't the case that any one slot is objectively preferable to another. In order to get to core, however, a person really needs to be operating on all 16 channels at once. This process can perhaps best be understood by imagining the tail of a trout which, moving rapidly back and forth, occupies a wide range of space at nearly the same time. Using this full range of mobility creates a compelling movement that allows the trout to swim upstream and leads the individual person to his true constitutional nature.

The further the tail can move from side to side, the stronger the propulsion and the more headway the trout makes upstream. The greater an individual's range of expression, the more vibratory channels he can occupy and the closer he comes to his core personality. The vibratory slot that a person is said to occupy is like the center of the stroke of the trout's tail. It is the point around which all other expression revolves. If a person has a limited range of motion/expression, and the tail is locked to one side, then the great currents of life will tend to move that person around in circles of great helplessness.

A person who is already at core is therefore able to fully occupy all of the vibratory channels at once. Such a person isn't limited to any particular degree of hemispheric function and so doesn't appear to be particularly right-brained or left-brained. This is very different than the case of someone who occupies the middle ground of slots 8 or 9. Such a person (usually a Stream) has a more neutral expression, and so doesn't appear to be particularly right-brained or left-brained either, but his range of expression is still limited. In our trout analogy, this person's tail is centered close to the head-on position but it isn't moving much from side to side; he may not be swimming around in circles quite as much but nor is he making much progress upstream. The tail has to be able to beat fully from side to side in order to make headway.

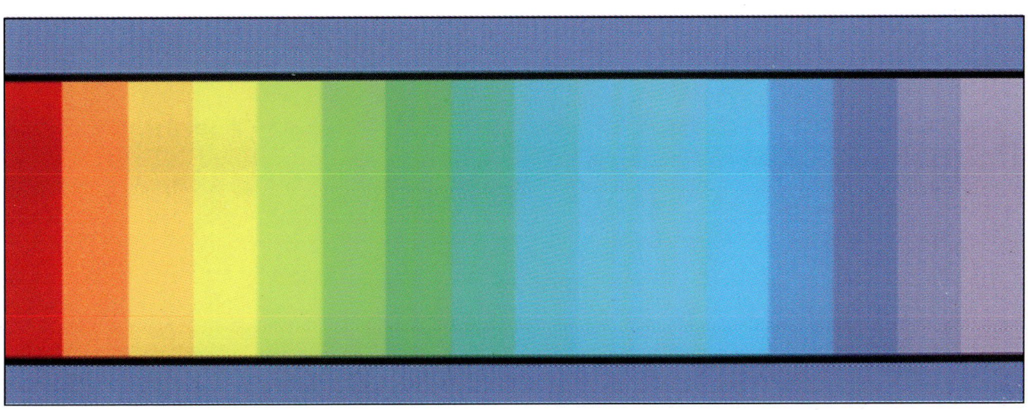

Like the colors in a rainbow, each of the 16 vibratory channels is a different frequency of expression on the personality continuum.

SIBLING SEQUENCES

In addition to being modified by the Jewel parent, a person's overall constitutional structure is also influenced by his position in the sibling sequence and the gender of the firstborn child.

The gender of the first child in a family has a powerful effect on subsequent children. For example, a firstborn girl will strengthen the feminine attributes in subsequent siblings, including making them more right-brained. This means that, amongst other things, subsequent Flowers will be more emotional and subsequent Jewels will be more flowing.

Although we have not yet found an explanation for this phenomenon, we have noticed that the sibling sequence is determined by the father's genealogy. For example, if a man remarries after having just one child, a daughter, in his first marriage, that daughter will pull subsequent children toward the right hemisphere even if the firstborn child in the second marriage is a boy.

Knowing the personality profile of some of the children allows you to work backward to determine the personalities and iris structures of the parents. If the children in a family tend to be very emotional, they are probably left-brained and so the father is probably a Jewel. If the children are generally more conservative and controlled, the mother is probably the Jewel, pulling the children toward the right hemisphere.

If the first child is a girl, the mother is usually a Jewel, and the whole family will gradually become more artistic and feelingful, taking on, as a group, the qualities associated with the right brain. If the first child is male, the father is probably a Jewel, and the whole family will move toward a more material focus (associated with the left brain). This is perhaps part of the reason why, in Chinese society, having a first-born son is directly associated with economic success for the family.

The hardest sibling positions are first and last. The first child often matures too quickly, while the youngest child is treated like a baby throughout life.

A Firstborn Son

Tending to be passively aggressive and silently rebellious, a firstborn boy often gets his character traits from the mother's side of the family. Although he can be intermittently cooperative, this child typically has a strongly independent nature. This independence usually isn't expressed verbally, however. Instead, the boy simply won't do what you want him to do. If you command him to do well in school, for example, he will say nothing in response but his grades will simply deteriorate.

Firstborn sons usually mature early and gain success late. Their inward defiance generally leads them to sabotage anything that is deemed important until they are allowed to choose what they want and feel supported in that choice. If the parental support is too focused, however, or tinged with impatience, they will destroy even the things they want in order to rebel and assert their independence. A firstborn son needs encouragement through respect and to be treated as a friend and equal by his parents. Generally quite comfortable when engaged in adult activities, a good way for the parents to acknowledge his maturity is to spend time with him alone.

Often mechanically dexterous, with inventive, design-oriented minds, firstborn sons are capable of great novelty when left alone. They often have a serious, slightly overbearing nature in their interactions with their siblings and people in general. A stereotype from the animal kingdom that encapsulates the independence and quiet defiance of this child is that of the wolf.

As an only child, his personality profile isn't much different, except that he is more likely to attain success earlier on, especially when his mother allows it and his father encourages it. He needs his mother to love him exactly as he is and his father to love him for what he is becoming. As an only child, this male is particularly capable of using his power in a positive expression, being both inventive yet practical, strong-spoken yet soft.

Child No. 2 After a Boy

Typically almost a diametric opposite to the older brother, this child usually is from the father's side of the family and exhibits a determined nature. More physically and emotionally aggressive than the older brother, this child is competitive, reactive, intense and tends to feel anger toward women. Symbolized by the badger, this person succeeds through intense determination and aggression. Often quietly engaged in one-upmanship and performance comparisons, child No. 2 can become restless through being occupied in too many projects.

Unlike the older brother, this child is

generally most successful when directly engaged by a father who helps provide focus, concentration and discipline. Capable of fine motor coordination and physical prowess, this is the athlete that responds well to the authoritarian coach (dad) and generally likes team sports. While the older brother prefers to go it alone, accepting no criticism, this child is often openly rebellious while secretly needing to be led.

Child No. 3 After a Boy

Like a fox, this child uses cleverness of mind or quickness of foot to attain success. Often secretive, and capable of being insidious, he likes to be in control of the details of the situation. This child typically achieves his goals without being openly aggressive, preferring to work behind the scenes. Diplomatic, and with an air of quiet passivity, he can talk his way into and out of almost any situation. A slippery, amiable achiever, child No. 3 derives his chess master's mind from the deeper strength of the father's side of the family. Comfortable with intense mental activity, this child is often engaged in professions such as accounting or traditional philosophy. In addition to diplomacy and cunning, child No. 3 can draw on his superior networking skills to get ahead in life. He can be quite socially gregarious, even playful, strengths which are sometimes used to his advantage by putting on a socially pleasing facade. He may also be mildly lazy and is often thinner in body than the two older children.

Child No. 4 After a Boy

Usually from the mother's side of the family, this child often has a dual personality: the joker/entertainer and the wise man or woman. Theatrical and service-oriented, with a soft outward personality and a sharp mind, child No. 4 is often aloof yet sociable, playful yet distant, filled with wisdom and yet lacking the practicality that is required to actually achieve results. Despite this lack of practical understanding, this person is generally popular and makes a good leader, typically with the rare ability to delegate.

Physically capable but maturing later in life, child No. 4 tends to experience great success as an integrator and synthesizer. Although readily attracting members of the opposite sex, this sibling none the less tends to avoid true intimacy, and lives in a state of quiet conflict with men. This person has many of the characteristics of the coyote, which is regarded as a wise, creative trickster in Native American mythology.

Child No. 5 After a Boy

This child usually marks a turning point in the family matrix. In some ways reminiscent of a deer, child No. 5 typically has the qualities of innocence, gentleness and kindness. He is deeply inspired by, and learns from, the simplicities of nature. Blessed, and with a joyful heart, this person generally retains a childlike simplicity well into adulthood, tending to mature late in life. Inherently fair, and with a deep desire to earn recognition by pleasing or serving others, child No. 5 typically is drawn to some form of service to family and community, such as the healing arts.

Generally an easy child for everyone in the family to deal with, this ease typically disguises a deep need to enhance self-expression and develop self-esteem. This child often refuses to take a definite position in debates, wanting to avoid conflict or disharmony. Yet when confronted, No. 5 after a boy is also capable of being very honest. This child is most probably from the father's side of the family, although this does vary, since this child marks the switch-over point after which the sibling sequence starts repeating itself.

A Firstborn Daughter

As an only child, this girl can be difficult or selfish, needing to be the center of attention. She is usually at her best when allowed to assume the role of the queen. When in a position of acknowledged strength, she is a potentially powerful administrator and leader. She is often seductively flamboyant, creatively or artistically driven, and likes to do things for herself. Her primary lesson is the right use of power.

A firstborn daughter with siblings, however, gains maturity through being a second mother to the younger children. There is a risk that she can lose her childhood innocence too quickly, becoming serious and burdened too fast. When this happens, she typically spends the rest of her life constantly seeking to recapture the joys of her early childhood innocence. She generally doesn't laugh enough, stays close to home and is drawn to public service, teaching or the arts.

Often the recipient of excessive discipline or abuse as a child, she is usually most happy if she leaves home and gains a sense of freshness and freedom. Even as an adult, the firstborn daughter still needs to be honored and appreciated as a little girl. She is usually from the father's side of the family.

Child No. 2 After a Girl

Expressive and rebellious, this child tends to be independent, determined and often distant from mother. No. 2 after a girl is usually dealing with an underlying feeling of aloneness and a desire for personal security. This often manifests in the form of a compelling drive to prove himself as successful, either mentally or materially. This child also has a detached, conceptual quality that can make him quite artistic or even physically inventive.

Child No. 3 After a Girl

This child is usually the amiable, wise one. Softly controlling yet fair, he is typically sensitive to others and makes a good facilitator. He may also be engaged in the nurturing arts. This child is often religiously devoted, physically strong and gentle in character. Sensitive to criticism or conflict, No. 3 after a girl strives to preserve the peace and hold things together. This child is usually from the mother's side of the family. Wise, philosophical and responsive to the needs of others, No. 3 is usually quite comfortable working in the hierarchy of established organizations.

Child No. 4 After a Girl

This child is usually an extreme example of either success or failure. Shocking and chaotic, both attacking and defensive, yet concerned with the greater good, this person has a revolutionary flavor. A teacher, philosopher and romantic idealist, No. 4 after a girl generally has a sense of bitterness about not being recognized by father. He is is most probably from the mother's side of the family. Potentially addictive, introverted, yet driven to express, this sibling's self-doubt is balanced by an exceptional capacity for farsightedness. No. 4's greatest need is the experience of emotional intimacy.

Child No. 5 After a Girl

As with No. 5 after a boy, this child has the mark of innocence and an air of simplicity. He can be utterly kind or totally neurotic. Usually pleasant, caring and nurturing, working for the approval of others, this sibling is often engaged in taking care of the individuals in a community. His childlike quality makes him good with children. He is also close to nature. No. 5 will not thrive in an atmosphere of conflict, and is very sensitive to any overt differences between the parents or the siblings.

Humble, sensitive and delicate, this sibling also has the propensity to be joyful, robust and creative when raised in an environment in which the mother and father verbally and kinesthetically demonstrate a desire for harmony. As an adult, No. 5 after a girl is typically involved in public relations, seeking to facilitate a sense of community between people. This sibling is the peacemaker, bringing this quality to the world through a variety of means, including words, art and touch.

As this position in the sequence represents a switch-over point in genetic influence, the child's character patterns can be from either side of the family. No. 5 is a fulcrum, a point of balance, making peace between the generations.

Subsequent Children After a Boy or Girl

Beginning with child No. 6, the sibling sequence starts mirroring the pattern of the first five siblings. No. 6 usually has similar qualities to the firstborn child, and No. 7 is similar to No. 2, etc.

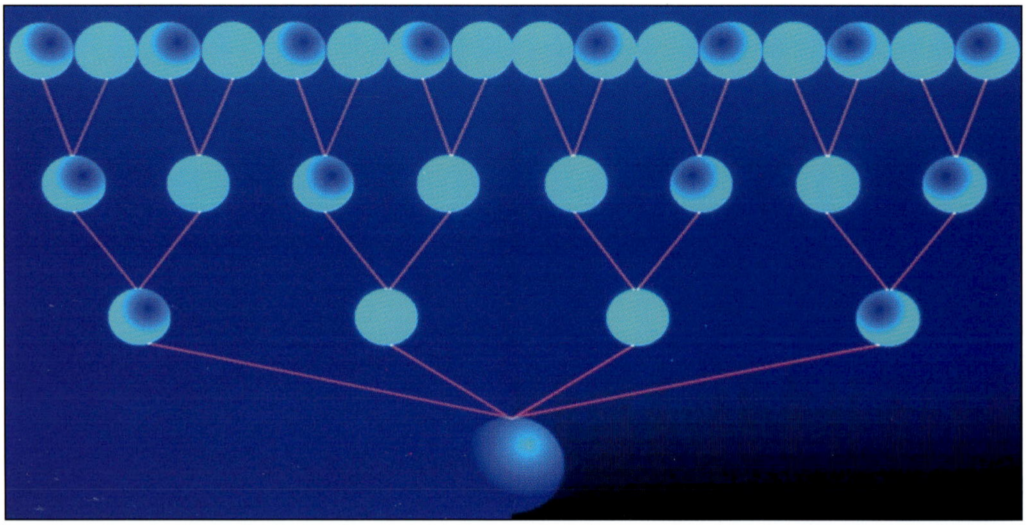

FAMILY CASE STUDY

This family case study covers a couple (Glenn and Mary) and their four children. Mary is a left-brained Jewel female who periodically moves to the right hemisphere and then back again; Glenn is a right-brained Shaker-Flower male who has the opposite hemispheric switching pattern, moving to the left and later returning to the right brain. They are perfectly matched, with a fiery and volatile love-hate relationship.

Mary is in complete control of herself, the house and her husband. She is organized, tidy and thoroughly skeptical. Glenn, on the other hand, is an easy-going sloppy, fun-loving, agreeable person. Although an excellent salesman, Glenn is not at all comfortable in a business suit. He would rather be at the beach chasing women. It is Mary's demanding, goal-oriented nature that keeps Glenn at work and the family together. It is Glenn's easy-going social personality that provides Mary with an atmosphere in which she can learn to relax. Though they drive each other crazy, they are mysteriously in love.

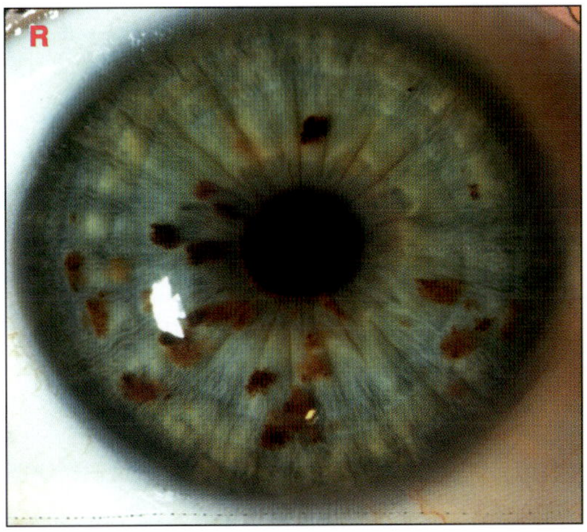

Mary (mother), right eye

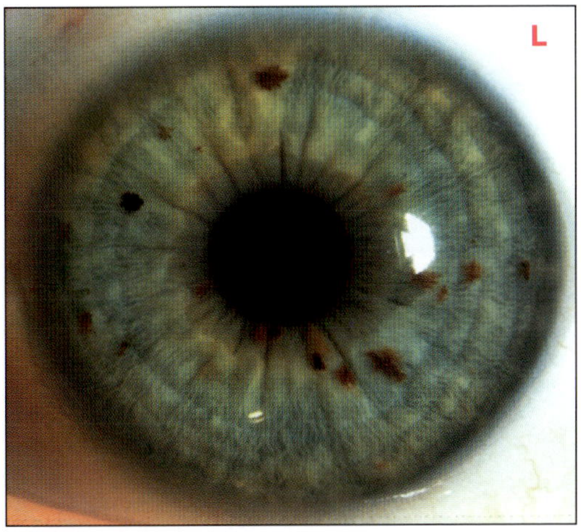

Mary (mother), left eye

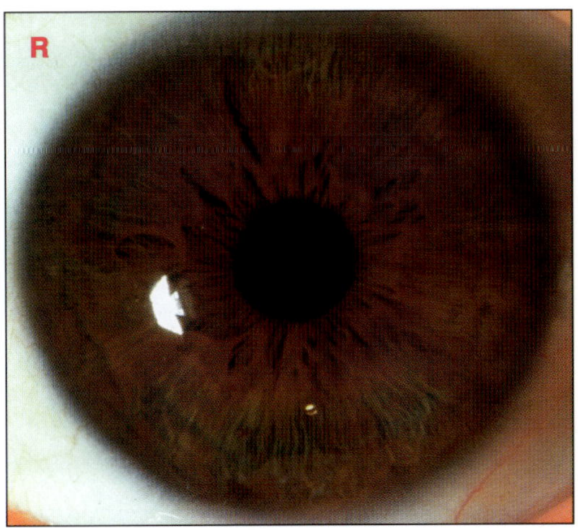

Glenn (father), right eye

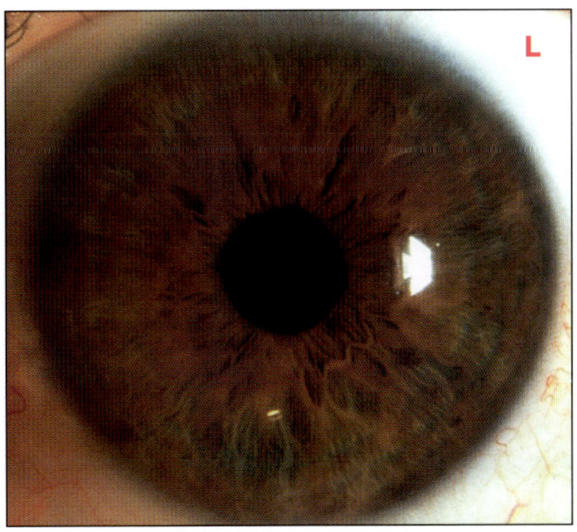

Glenn (father), left eye

For a detailed exploration of Glenn and Mary's relationship as partners, see the description of *The Love-Hate Pattern* in the next chapter. Glenn and Mary are the same couple used for that in-depth investigation. The interplay between these two strong individuals, both of whom have patterns of reaction and expression with the opposite sex, has a noticeable effect on the development and expression of their children (see the following two pages).

David (age 10)

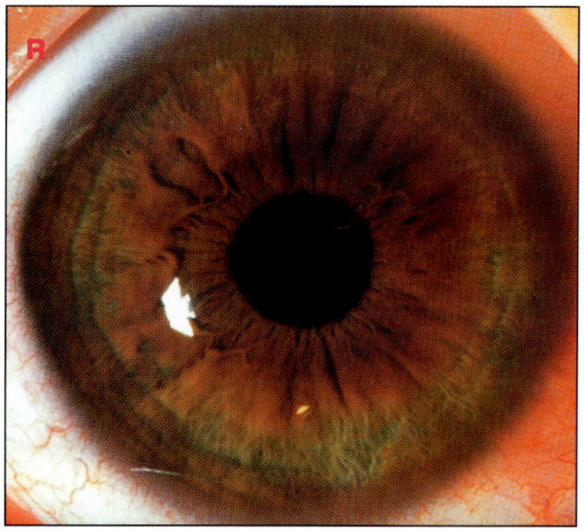

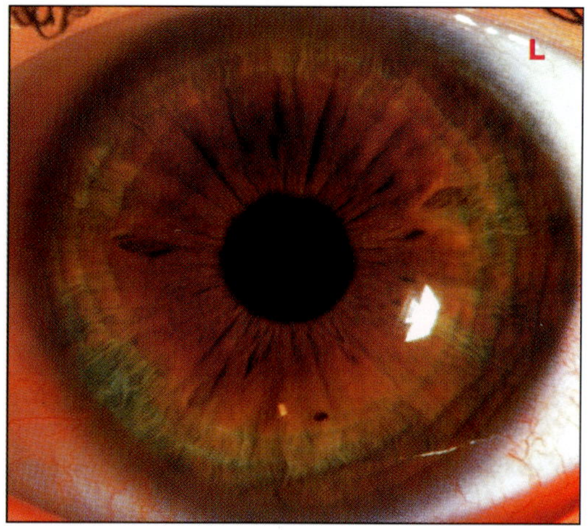

The eldest child, David, is a boy whose constitutional pattern is similar to that of his father but with more of a Stream quality. He has a number of small flower patterns throughout his eyes, a large Anger flower (position No. 3) in the masculine (right) eye, and also a large flower in position No. 42, which is associated with rebellion against authority. This emotionally intense young man also shows a higher concentration of color at the top of the feminine (left) eye. This indicates that he is moving to the right brain, often a consequence of having a Jewel mother. This makes David a right-brained Flower introvert, feelingful, with heightened spatial perception, artistic abilities and perhaps even musical talent. The inner imagery of his emotional nature and his introverted tendencies are filtered through the right brain when he does express himself. This indicates that he is a futuristic, artistic, conceptual boy who may have difficulty actualizing his visions through the left brain. While quite emotionally expressive, he currently keeps his inner feelings to himself, and will probably begin to demonstrate his rebelliousness in his middle and later teenage years.

Kristen (age 8)

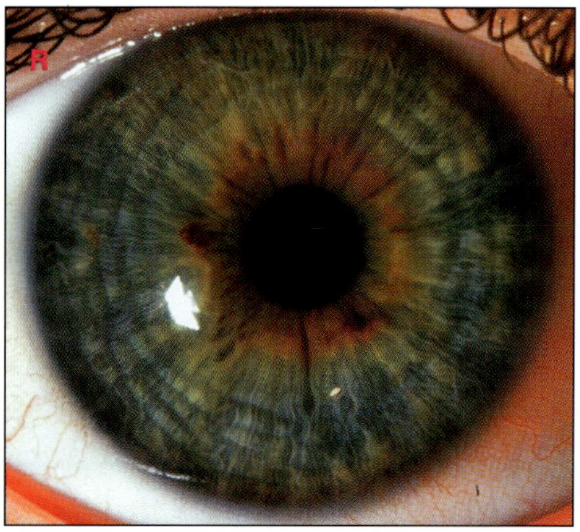

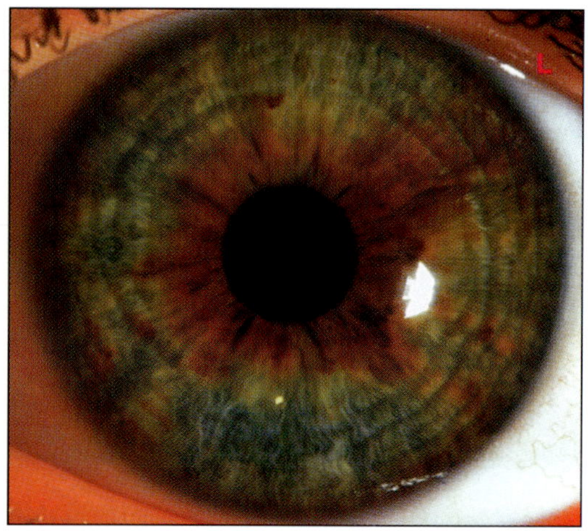

The second child, Kristen, has a noticeable patch of brown through the feminine (left) eye, again indicating that her mother is a Jewel. She has an underlying Harmony pattern and a small flower in the position associated with anger toward the father and brother (position No. 3). This kinesthetic, Stream-Jewel, right-brained girl with strong Freedom rings is likely to be very intense. Having an older brother with a strong temper who is more emotionally and physically aggressive increases the likelihood of her moving to the right brain. It also means that she will have learned how to turn her powerful, sharp mind into a verbal cutting edge that she uses against men. Like her mother, she has strong verbal ability, but her expression will be much more right-brained, abstract or theoretical in nature. Mentally aggressive, the intensity of her reactions in relationships is increased by the Love-Hate pattern of her parents. All Jewels have a tendency to go right; this little girl, pulled by a Jewel mother, repelled by an older brother who is a Flower with an Anger pattern and a father who has an Anger pattern toward females, is likely to be extremely right-brained. In the long term, she will have a tendency for limited emotional expression due to her mental control and may take that repressed feeling and express it as antagonism or sarcasm. Around her mid-40s, she has the opportunity to break through to a high state of innate wisdom.

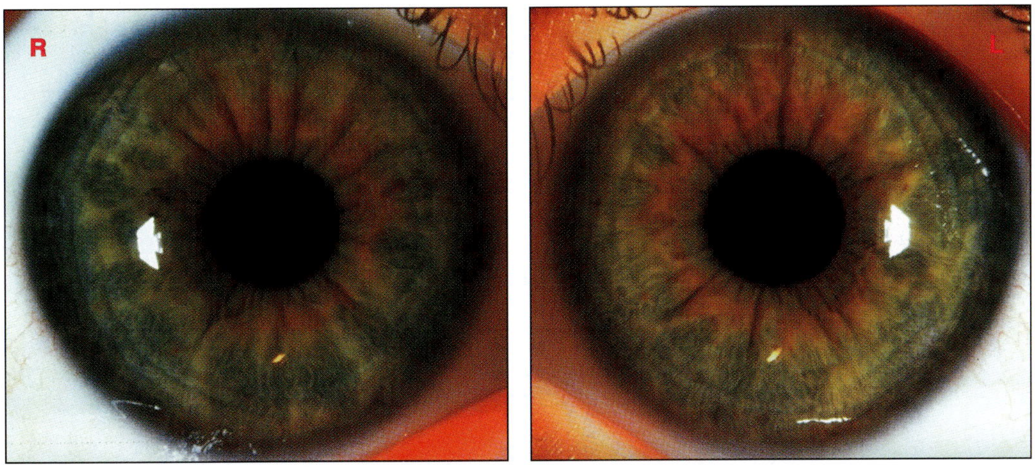

Danielle (age 7)

Child No. 3, Danielle, is primarily a Stream-Flower. The presence of just a few jewels means that she could more accurately be described as a Stream-Shaker-Flower. This is one of the combinations that was not described in the *Essence of the Structures* chapter. It is easy to interpret, however. Simply think of it as a composite of the three distinct personality types of the Stream, Shaker and Flower, giving more emphasis to the elements that are most obvious – the Stream and the Flower. Being the third child, behind a firstborn boy, she will be diplomatic and a natural mediator. With Anger, Heart and Will issues in the right eye, she will be a *determined* child, with great mental clarity, capable of taking care of herself. Her smooth iris structure, with an overall softness of appearance and a density of fiber, means that she also can be quite slippery. *Softly* clever and manipulative, she is good at getting others to do what she wants. Unlike Kristen, with whom everything is up front, Danielle is the sort of person who can smile at you while stabbing you in the back. It is easy enough to get confirmation of your interpretations of children – just ask the parents!

It can be nearly impossible to get a two-year-old to sit still long enough to have both of his eyes photographed. But if you know the iris structures of the parents and siblings, and if you know the child's position in the sibling sequence, you can still draw an accurate picture of his personality.

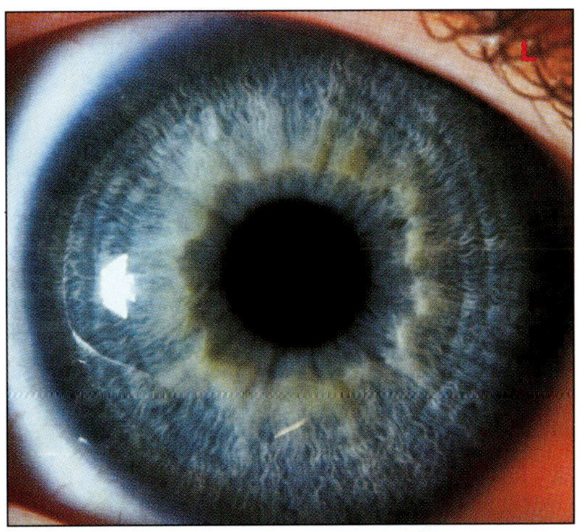

Jack (age 2), left eye

The fourth and youngest child, Jack, is a pure Stream extrovert, with tight, dense iris fibers and a distinct Ring of Expression. He is very different than anyone else in the family. As child No. 4 behind a boy, Jack can be entertaining, charismatic and powerful. People come to him. He is probably left-brained because he is a boy behind a firstborn son (see *Sibling Sequences*). As the second boy behind another boy, he will also exhibit some of the characteristics of child No. 2 behind a boy. (Similarly, Danielle will exhibit some of the personality traits of child No. 2 behind a firstborn girl.) To some extent, each child's personality is a composite of its overall position in the sibling sequence and its position relative to older children of the same sex. (This is an aspect to sibling sequences that was not covered earlier in this chapter.) Jack will therefore be quite physically powerful. The personality traits of the youngest child in the family always seem to be more exaggerated. Another child dissolves some of the characterization, softening up the youngest child's expression. Because he is still the youngest, Jack is particularly masculine in his expression.

Relationship Patterns

Relationships create or destroy life. Essential to our continuing social development and yet continually challenging, they are the most compelling mystery in human experience.

Who we are today is largely a product of the relationships between our genetic predecessors. This is true physiologically and psychologically. At a biological level, we would not exist if it were not for the fact that our parents (and their parents in turn) had interacted in an intimate way. Our preference for specific patterns of communication, the manner in which we express and receive thoughts and feelings, is also genetically predetermined. Our behavioral style is heavily dictated by the constitutional structure of the personality which, as was demonstrated in the previous chapter, is a function of the transgenerational influence from parents and grandparents as well as one's position in the sibling sequence.

While we do most of our intense personal growth through family relationships (with our partners, parents and children), friendships are generally an opportunity to have a respite from difficult change, and workgroup relationships are a combination of social interaction and getting the job done. Each type of relationship makes its own unique contribution to the quality of our lives and also has its own stresses.

Every relationship we have is an opportunity to grow. Interactions with others stimulate a person's constitutional structure and activate life issues connected to specific positional traits in the iris. This is what enables us to get back to our core natures, the way we were when we were born. If the constitutional structure is not stimulated through relationships, it will instead harden. Relationships keep the personality constantly vibrating with feelings and experiences so that the constitutional structure can deepen and change. A long-term, committed relationship with a partner is particularly effective at stimulating our own issues. This is because strong attraction is the consequence of an unfulfilled, separate polarity moving toward union with its opposite. The greater the differences between you and your partner, the greater the force of attraction, the greater the stimulation of your own issues and the greater the opportunity for growth. This opposition also creates a sexually compelling attraction.

As every relationship is a reflection of the personalities involved, and because those personalities are essentially a reflection of patterns in the family tree, every relationship we have today is a reflection of relationships acted out in a previous generations. That is why we can sometimes seem to be repeating age-old family patterns, reliving the lives of our grandparents, parents or other family members.

Every relationship contains shadows from the past and gives subtle pointers to the way forward in the future. Present relationships are a subconscious attempt to free us from the negative influences of the past and to deliver to us the beautiful treasures that are also hidden within the transgenerational toxicity.

The purpose of all of our interactions is ultimately the same: to help us learn how to be who we are and to allow others to be as they are, to enliven our bodyminds so that we can avoid suppressing others or denying ourselves. Relationships are a means of increasing our vibration (see *Therapies)* and ultimately teach us how to be sensitive to the truth in everyone.

Workgroup Patterns

Rayid provides insights into the relative strengths and weaknesses of the constitutional types and the way they relate to each other and society. Although this chapter focuses on relationships between couples; and between parents and their children, it is interesting to catch a glimpse of how Rayid can be used to optimize the efficiency and productivity of a workgroup. As each of the four structures has a different way of interacting socially, it therefore has something different to contribute to society.

Each one of the four primary personality types also represents a quadrant or sector that exists within each person. It is important to understand that each individual has all of the attributes of the different structures within him, and can have them operating simultaneously.

Just as an individual can benefit from being able to call upon the strengths represented by each of the four primary personality types, so can an organization. In large organizations, Stream qualities are represented by the service department and other internal functions that maintain the integrity of the business. The Shaker represents the decision-making authority and motivation. Jewel characteristics are essential to groups involved in planning and control, such as the financial department.

The Flower represents vision and sociability, as well as the public relations group that is responsible for presenting a positive image of the company to its customers. When a business group incorporates all of these complementary patterns of expression, there is a greater potential for professional success.

For example, a visionary Flower may have an exciting image of a bridge he wants to build. But actually building that bridge requires the accuracy and attention to detail of the Jewel mind in order to ensure that every single nut, bolt and cable is put in the proper place. It is the competitive, task-oriented Shaker type that gets the work done by driving the group toward the goal of manifesting the image. But in order for this to occur, it needs the the physical conformity of the group (aided by the Stream) to physically achieve the building of the bridge.

Every business, or department within a business, needs to understand the differing social needs and strengths of its employees. After all, the success of any organization depends on the best use of its human resources.

Just as individuals have a left hemisphere (representing the father, male relationships and authority) and a right hemisphere (representing the mother, female relationships and creativity), so does any social or business enterprise. In some ways, the inner relationship of the enterprise to its own creativity and to its own authority does more to determine its success or failure than anything else.

Companies that have difficulties with authority often are extremely creative, roguish or unmanageable. Companies with difficulties on the feminine side become excessively controlling, show to change and very traditional. The IBM corporation is definitely left-brained whereas Apple Computers, in its early stages, was very right-brained. Like one's relationship to the mother, if the feminine side is too controlling, the child's maturity is often slowed. Like one's relationship to the father, when the father is too controlling, the creative feeling is stifled. Every organization needs a father and a mother, needs to fully occupy both the left and the right brain.

Complementarity: Why Opposites Attract

It is not uncommon to find yourself drawn to someone on the basis of looks or circumstance and then to discover that you really aren't particularly attracted to that person. When incompatible people become intimate, the relationship usually fizzles out quite quickly. The information in this chapter deals with the kind of sustained attraction that can lead to *long-term* partnering relationships.

As we mentioned in the introduction to the last chapter, the path to the experience of wholeness involves the individual in encounters with people who have complementary patterns and experiences. The mechanism is actually quite simple. Our thoughts, feelings and attitudes attract us to certain social and physical experiences in life. Those experiences teach us lessons. These lessons give purpose and meaning to life. Your parents are just two of the people with experiences complementary to your own that you encounter on your path through life. The law of attraction draws together families, friends and loved ones for this common purpose.

The primary source of all stored pain within the human psyche is from relationships in the family tree. That which restores the ultimate perfection of each person is also the experience of relationships. The law of attraction brings together the opposite halves of the same lesson. These opposite halves are the complementary patterns found in most intimate relationships. The people we attract in relationships are the ones that most closely complement our own subconscious processes, for it is from this that we have the most to learn.

There are some general rules that apply to long-term, intimate relationships:

1. Physical opposites attract.
2. Mental opposites attract.
3. *Similar lessons* attract.

The goal of relationships is to create balance, to straighten the crooked parts of ourselves and to round out the rough edges. Stated simply, it is to bring our lives closer to an ideal image through the experience of lessons.

The habits of our self-expression cause us either to attract or repel other people. When these habits mirror the habits of the person to whom we are communicating, it directly increases the level of feeling within the body. If these habits are unmirrored, the feeling in the body is neutral. The reason for this feeling of excitement in the body when experiencing the attraction of mirrored opposites is that it is a sign of the movement toward completion.

The law of opposites does not apply to friendships. We can have friendships with people of the same structure because of an appreciation of that similar structure within ourselves, or because we have interests in common. The more "awake" one becomes, the more likely it is that one can have friendships with someone of any eye structure.

There are only two archetypal patterns in intimate relationships. Any variation from either of these basic patterns is only a variation on a theme. Although other relationship patterns do exist, they are statistically rare. The common patterns are:

1. A Jewel male with a Flower female. He (right-brained) suffers from the Freedom Mirage and she (left-brained) suffers from the Eureka Illusion (see later).

2. A Jewel female with a Flower male. She (right-brained) experiences pain with men and he (left-brained) feels anger toward women.

Either of these relationship patterns can be at any degree of health. As Shakers and Streams tend to be either more Jewel-like or more Flower-like in addition to their primary structure, they almost always fall into one of these categories too.

The attraction of complementary opposites is mirrored at every level of investigation. A Jewel and a Flower in a relationship will, for example, often be dealing with symmetrical positions, of the opposite polarity, in opposite eyes. If the man has a jewel in a certain position in the father eye, it is common for the woman to have a flower in that same (or a similar) position in the mother eye. For example, if the male has a *jewel* in the area of Resentment (position No. 2), the female is likely to have a *flower* in the same area.

JEWEL MALE, FLOWER FEMALE

The Eureka Illusion and the Freedom Mirage

This is the allegorical description we use for a relationship between a right-brained Jewel male and a left-brained Flower female. Approximately 85% of Jewel male, Flower female relationships have this pattern.

She: the Eureka Illusion

Flower women are like a small boat that is constantly searching for a harbor, without ever finding it. The harbor represents security, father, a trustworthy lover. For such a woman, her unfulfilled mind is like a cyclone that creates impossibly strong headwinds, always driving her back out to sea, preventing her from joining with her true love (the harbor).

Some Flower women try to be a bigger boat, hoping that might improve their chances of finding a way through the storm. They may work hard, improving the home, making themselves more attractive, becoming involved in grand schemes or a whole host of different activities that enhance their sense of self-esteem. But the inner cyclone still deceives them.

Most Flower structures try to go left (i.e. operate from the left hemisphere of the brain). A Flower woman going left is doing so to create a sense of security, and is automatically attracted to men. Typically, she has also lost the comfort of her relationships with women or even of social situations generally, so she may tend to isolate herself.

A Flower female with an Anger pattern and sexuality issue (position No. 3, see *Positions in the Iris*) in the right eye can use her sexuality as a weapon. An Anger pattern generally increases the sexual passion (unless it is very extreme, in which case it could suppress it). She likes to build her body – its strength or its beauty – and is commonly involved in sports, dance or gymnastics when she's a teenager, or has a desire to learn to ride horses.

A Flower woman going left is always trying to attain a particular goal, which changes as she gets older. In her teenage years it may be sports-related or material, like acquiring a car. Then it may be an education, a relationship and, later, a home. She effectively sets a series of goals for herself throughout her life. But each time she attains one of her goals, she feels empty. None of her goals provides any real satisfaction. Between the ages of 34 to 38, she usually reacts to this disappointment by wanting to be alone, away from the house, kids and husband. Then, around the ages of 40 to 42, she re-emerges with a new set of goals, wanting a second career, a second house, etc.

All Flowers have a profound sense of aloneness due to a feeling of being "cut off from the source." It is a form of grief. Flower women going left seldom feel complete, and create external goals to cover up that inner emptiness. They are searching for something to fill that inner void. Each time they reach a goal they think they've found it: "Eureka! I've found it. *This* is it." ("Eureka" is a Greek word meaning "I've found it.") But then they realize that they haven't, so they cover up their disappointment by setting another new goal. This is the Eureka Illusion, to keep thinking that, each time they attain a goal, they've found the answer to their inner pain.

She also tries to have the deep hole inside her filled through touch and external security, by her partner. She wants him to make the feeling of emptiness go away. But this compulsive need for security cannot be filled from an external source; it can only be filled from inside, by a deep sense of fullness coming from within. So even if her partner is in the room with her all the time, she still feels alone and abandoned by him. She complains because he's always reading or always working on his computer – he's "not there" for her.

For a Flower female going from right to left, material security is of paramount importance. But for her usual partner, a Jewel male going from left to right, material "security" represents a prison – he would rather play "St. Francis of Assisi" and give up all his possessions.

He: the Freedom Mirage

A male Jewel going right has a relatively easy time being in a relationship with a woman because he has some "yin-ness," some femininity to draw upon. This helps him to relate to women. He readily attracts, and is attracted to, the opposite sex. Because of this ease, he is quite likely to be drawn to having relationships with several women.

A male Jewel going right is seeking a mystical understanding of the infinite. He

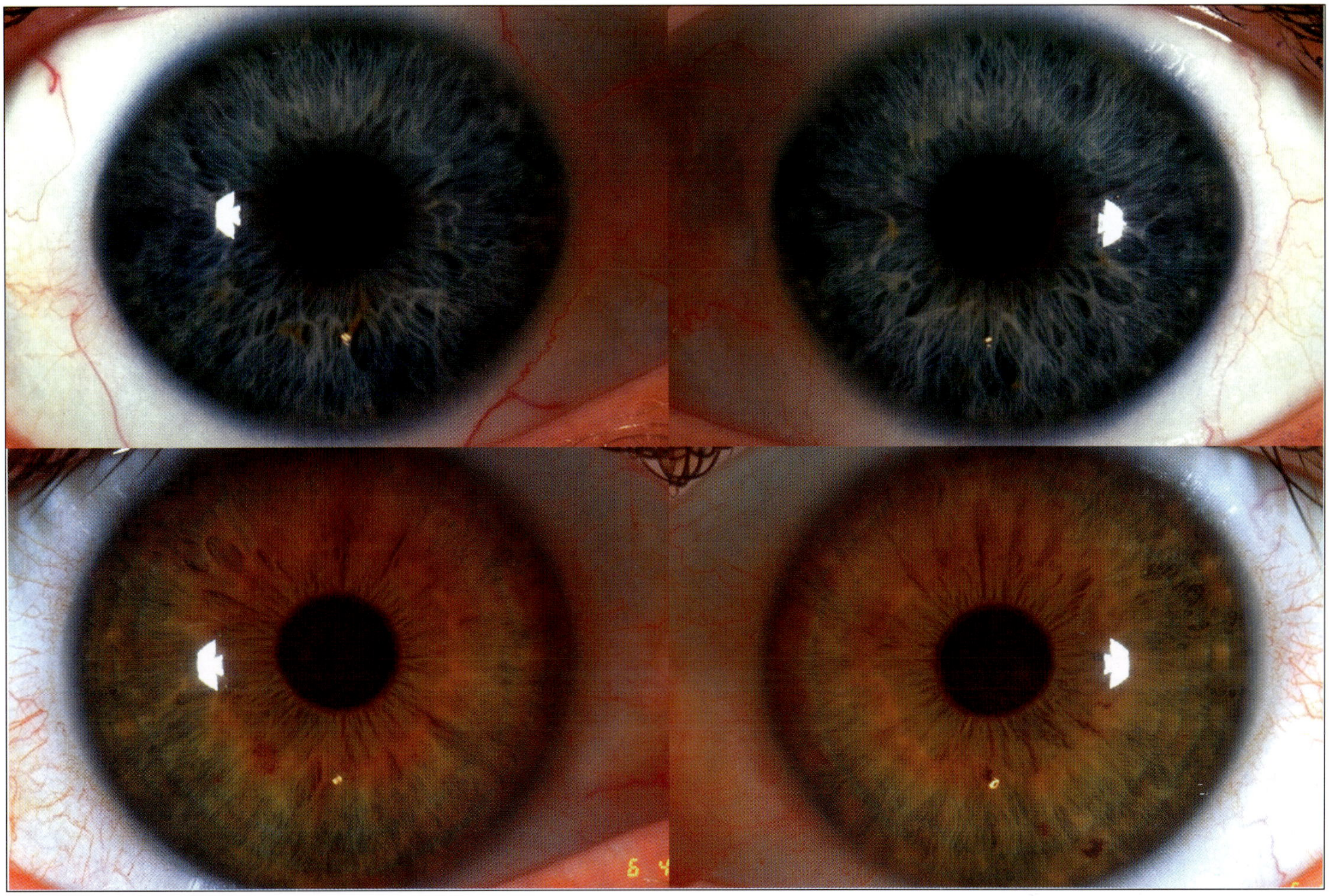

A left-brained Flower female (top) is attracted to a right-brained Jewel male for a long-term relationship.

is using his mind in an attempt to experience the spiritual source that he knows exists, and is prepared to work diligently in order to find it. He is like a mystical, ragged priest crawling on hands and knees through an arid desert, searching through philosophy, art, beauty, and nature for that place where God exists. He longs for emotional release.

Then, in the middle of this agonizing search, he find a cool, restful oasis called a Flower female. She has a castle full of intimacy, which he so desperately craves.

"Eureka!" she thinks to herself. At last she has found the attention she was craving. The very thing she has wanted all along was for someone to be there with her, to heal her aloneness. He notices everything about her, engages her mind and body, and she then begins to try to cloister him, to keep him in her luxurious castle.

But Jewels seek freedom and resent being controlled. They don't like the feeling of constriction. He connects physically with her but doesn't want to be entangled in her web. This may show itself in a tendency to fall asleep after love-making, or to get up for a drink or to go to the bathroom. Thus he experiences release but no real fulfillment.

This man is like a Franciscan monk who is trying to dematerialize his existence, who craves the freedom to be who he is, to find God, to explore. He responds by resenting the material comfortableness that the Flower woman has created, and resenting her attempts to contain him. He looks out of the window and there, on the horizon, is the shimmering light that he seeks. Or is it really there? This is the Freedom Mirage. He takes off in search of "it" again, thinking it is just over the next rise, or somewhere only just out of reach at the extreme limits of his mind, if only he can get far enough out of his body. And so this wandering Jewel never attains his goal, simply resting for a while in the Flower female's oasis before setting off into the desert of the mind again.

He is addicted to mind phenomena, but the true freedom he seeks is inside himself, just as it is for his partner, manifested through relationship. But he cannot experience true intimacy because he is in love with his mind, and she is a jealous lover; it is very difficult to usurp her power over his body. His only hope for happiness is to see that this relationship is the freedom that he has been searching for. In order to see this, however, he must free himself from the restricting effects of his own mental illusions.

His partner so desperately craves just a few seconds of flattery now and then and, if he wants their relationship to work, he will learn to pay her some attention. What the male Jewel wants is an emotional cheerleader to support him in the pursuit of his dreams, and his mate must learn not to get in his way.

Their Interaction

As both partners in this dynamic relate quite easily to members of the opposite sex, their relationship can superficially look a lot closer than that of a Flower male with a Jewel woman. Actually, the conflict is just deeper, more internal and usually emerges further into the relationship. In many ways, this makes it more tragic when the disappointment finally comes, especially because their idealization of the opposite sex is so strong. With her need for a father figure and his fascination with visual beauty, it is not uncommon for her to be younger than he.

Because they mesh so well, the partners in this relationship combination generally become dependent upon each other: she doesn't need a women's group and he doesn't need so much outside stimulation. So when they finally do split up, they typically don't have external support systems, which makes the parting even more difficult.

What a Flower woman likes about a Jewel man initially is his ability to be alert. This makes her feel good because he pays her a lot of attention. But after a while, she begins to perceive and experience that alertness as a constant inspection, as criticism.

As their relationship progresses, the Jewel male is likely to become deeply involved in some project, and his partner is equally likely to try to find some way to divert his interest back to her. She might say, "You're not paying me any attention," or she might even have a small accident. Unconsciously, she is trying to find some way to get his attention, the thing that attracted her to him in the first place. The consequence of this is that he feels restricted by her, and so is even more likely to withdraw.

Once their relationship is well-established, the most common complaint by Flower women about Jewel males is that they're just not there. "You're just not listening," she often says to him. Even when he is with her, it is as if he isn't fully present.

Unlike her partner, a Flower woman likes to be held closely. But until the unconscious issue is dealt with, she can never be held closely enough, because her internal sense of aloneness is so strong. It can feel good to her for a while, but her partner is only placating symptoms that arise regularly. Her sense of aloneness is so profound that she will almost make sure that he leaves her, or else she will leave him first (before he gets a chance to leave her, as she sees it), creating the very thing she is afraid of: abandonment.

Variation: Left-brained Male, Right-brained Female

Relationships between left-brained Jewel males and right-brained Flower females are uncommon because those structures are themselves unusual. Only about 15% of Jewel male, Flower female relationships have this pattern.

She: Creative and Romantic

Soft, feminine and expressive, this graceful Flower welcomes you like the sunrise over a mountain meadow. Highly creative, with musical or artistic talent, she typically has difficulty following through with her creative expression. Although she is primarily a quiet person, her stormy side reveals itself when she snaps into anger or depression. Generally noncompetitive, she usually has several female friends and is quite close to her own family. She has a tendency to have problems with her spine or hips.

A right-brained Flower woman likes being taken care of, and is attracted to a powerful, left-brained Jewel man for long-term relationships. This couple embodies a popular archetype of masculinity and femininity: the strong, silent type (him) in partnership with a devoted, romantic woman. There is as much contrast in their personalities as there can be, creating a strong attraction. They usually enjoy each other's company tremendously, although she can find his "matter of fact" attitude hurtful. When they do disagree, they are prone to bickering, and she can resort to emotional, nonverbal manipulation when she feels slighted. Romantic and strictly monogamous, she is usually devoted to her man, even to her own detriment. She is very motherly and service-oriented, and tends to put the welfare of others before her own well-being. She generally feels inadequate around her mate, working hard for his approval and attention, and she usually defers to his choice on external matters. He treats her better than he treats other people, however, and she is committed to making him more overtly loving. He likes being with her because she slows down the pace of his life.

He: "John Wayne"

Straight out of the movies, this seemingly cold, aloof and mysterious man often closely resembles the characters played by John Wayne in the old Hollywood movies. Usually very physically active, and verbally quieter than right-brained Jewel men, this mountain of strength is equally suited to being a loner or a great leader. Just as intense

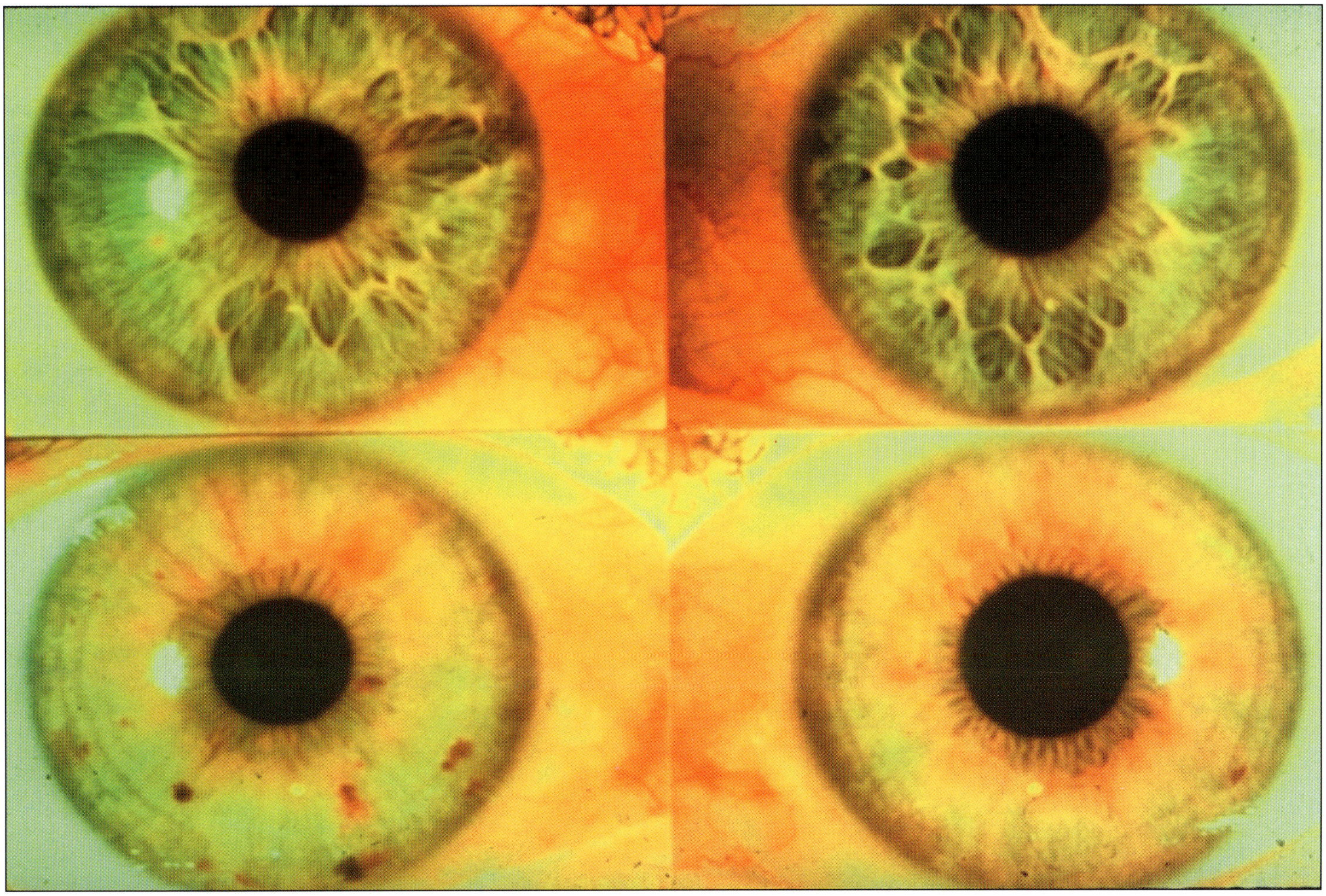

A right-brained Flower female (top) is attracted to a left-brained Jewel male for a long-term relationship.

but less reactive than his right-brained counterpart, he embodies the essence of wisdom and stability.

Preferring traditional ways, and often religious, the left-brained Jewel male demands privacy and commands respect. He likes to be served by women, and tends to place himself in a superior position to his partner. He usually attracts an adoring, soft, right-brained Flower female, whom he may have difficulty accepting because he consciously seeks a strong woman as a mate. Having gone left because of an Anger pattern with women, he often takes out his frustration on his partner by projecting controlled criticism at her. A strict disciplinarian, he none the less enjoys his role as a father and a husband, and just needs to learn how to deliver his message more tenderly. When he lets her in, she can be sustained by the great gentleness and love hidden just below the surface of that cool exterior.

The epitome of the controlling Jewel, his desire for control extends beyond his relationships and into the material realm. He likes to control the finances and can easily find his life's vocation as an accountant. He is often devoted to his work above all else and this, together with his preference for controlling every situation, makes him particularly suited to being self-employed. He is subject to emotional breakdowns under stress and has a propensity for digestive disorders. He often enjoys financial games, such as playing the stock market, and gets pleasure from being close to things with a sense of solidity to them: trucks, rock-climbing or mountain-biking are typical interests.

Often characterized by an absence of trust in other people, or by uncertainty about the future, he can turn this potential limitation to good use by being an excellent planner or organizer, and can make a truly great politician.

JEWEL FEMALE - FLOWER MALE

Right-brained Jewel Female, Left-brained Flower Male

This relationship pattern accounts for 55 – 60% of all relationships.

She: Determined and Sharp

A female Jewel going right is bright, intelligent and a good communicator. She usually knows what she wants, where she's going and how she's going to get there. Most things in her life are in her control and she is willing to work hard for success.

She is usually right-brained because of anger issues with her father that drive her away from the left (masculine) hemisphere. This usually has its conscious root in some fear of criticism or a loss of recognition with her father (or another major male figure, such as an older brother). She typically sublimates her anger with males and authority figures into an aggressiveness towards bureaucracies and large institutions, or into saving the world.

Constantly engaged in improving society or herself, she is often drawn to the professions of teaching, public relations or the social services. She is independent and usually has strong spiritual views, which may fall outside of organized religion. She has a need to analyze things constantly, to understand them and to communicate her perspectives to others. She likes to be asked about her opinions and likes to be listened to. She also needs to be right, especially in her interactions with her partner. She is a gatherer of information and a seeker of truth and of intimacy. Of all of these, it is intimacy that eludes her the most.

The Jewel pattern is primarily masculine and represents a striving for control. It can therefore be hard for a woman to be a Jewel and still retain her femininity. If she has a mesomorphic body, it exacerbates the difficulty. In her interactions with people in general, she can create the impression that she has a knife in her pocket which she is ready to use. Her sharp mind combined with her overt, natural aggressiveness can make her come across as being part rhino and part wolf. This can get in the way of intimacy.

She most often attracts an emotional (Flower) male who is dealing with a complementary Anger pattern with women (left eye). Internally, however, she is sensitive to any form of emotional attack, especially one which questions her credibility and her need to be right. Her Flower partner is a nonverbal communicator, typically uncertain about what to do with his life. Yet what she really wants is a man who can take charge of his life and *do* something.

Not surprisingly, her most common experience with men is friction. Her most common complaint toward her partner is "Why can't you get your act together? Why can't you demonstrate some control in your life and figure out where you are going?" Exasperated by her partner's indecisiveness, she typically ends up telling him how to live his life.

She is quite likely to have a women's group for support, which she needs because her husband probably treats her like a piece of property. The more right-brained and Jewel-like this woman is, the more likely it is that she will reach the point where she (energetically) gives up on men and seeks the sisterhood of other women for intimacy.

He: Soft and Tenacious

A male Flower going left gathers systems, information, types of physical exercise, etc. in an unending progression, and doesn't understand why he never feels like he's getting to what he wants out of life. So he puts his hope into his long-term objectives, and tends to plan far ahead. He is likely to set quite distant goals for himself, such as aiming to get to the top of the corporation in 30 years. Because it takes him longer to achieve his goal(s), it takes him a long time to realize that meeting these goals won't satisfy him. This is in marked contrast to the typical Flower female, who sets shorter-term goals, generally no more than a year or two away each time. She moves on more quickly, having realized that this last goal wasn't actually enough.

The perfect complement to the right-brained Jewel female, the left-brained Flower male typically comes across as being quite distant, not quite there. He is attracted to her presence and her great certainty about who she is. He has a sense of being abandoned and so enjoys the attention her sharp mind focuses on him. He likes the sound of her voice. He will listen to her, be guided by her and at times may even allow her to teach him, although nonverbally.

He longs for a feeling of security, which he believes he can have with his mate if only she would let him in past her mental barriers, if only she would trust him enough

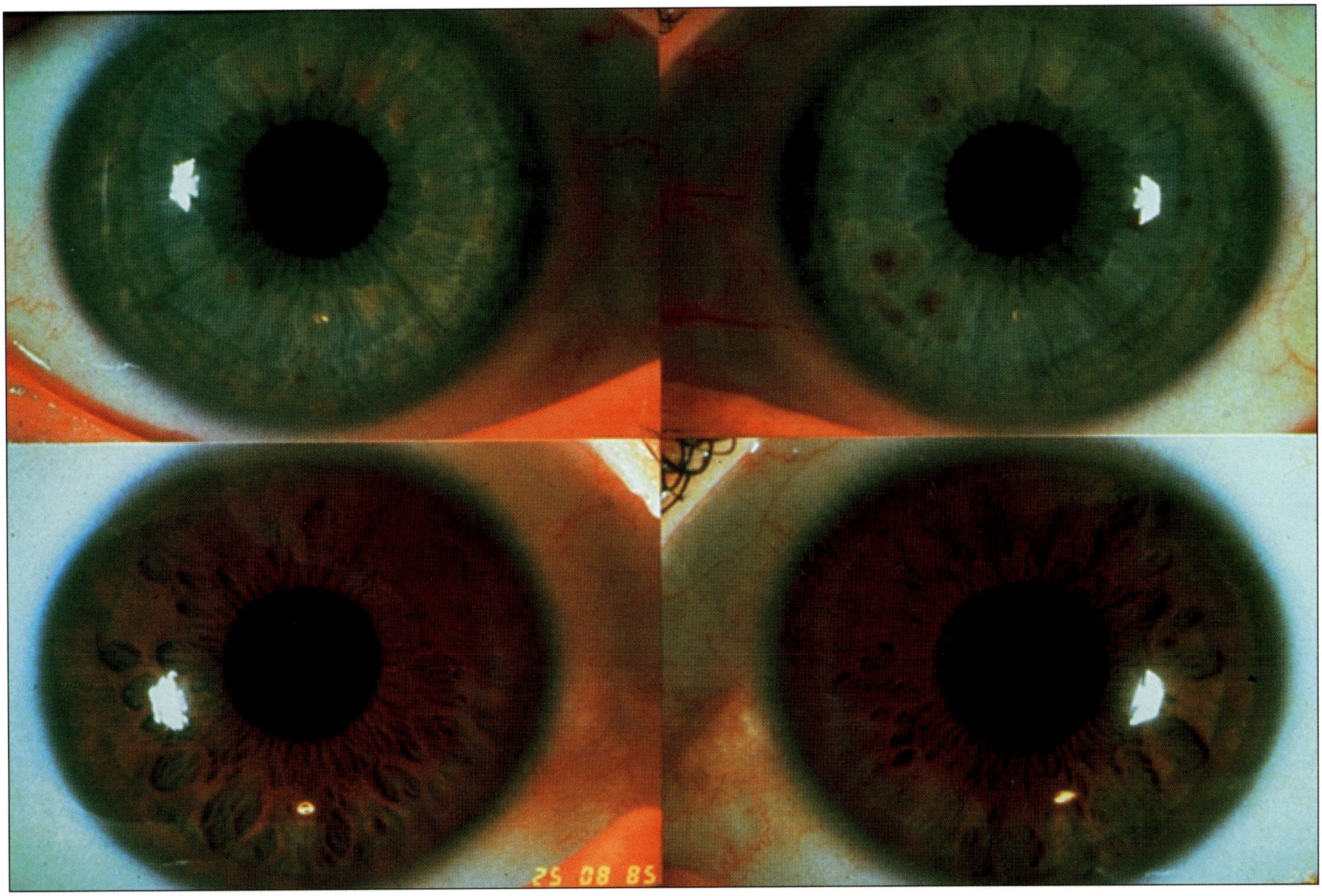

A right-brained Jewel female (top) is attracted to a left-brained Flower male for a long-term relationship.

to let him past her need to protect herself and to control other people, including him.

Although he may not be aware of it, he typically feels angry with his mother for not nurturing him adequately when he was young. But even if he is conscious of having anger issues with a sister or his mother, his wife still restimulates those feelings, and he still responds. When pushed, this cuddly bunny rabbit can be transformed into a roaring lion, or an obstinate water buffalo with his feet planted firmly in the mud. If he is chronically angry, then he is not likely to attract women at all: in nature, the water buffalo and the rhino do not share the same pasture.

Most Flower men create an adaptation to the left brain, which makes them likely to be engaged in very masculine activities. This is a natural way for them to control their feelings. For a male, a movement to the left brain is supported by society, which encourages men to be strong. Although he may express himself as a dominant male for many years, he inwardly misses his true nature, which is soft and receptive. His masculine outer nature shelters an inner femininity.

He typically doesn't question who he is until the middle of his life. Then, suddenly, he realizes that he has been living someone else's life. Nothing around him has deep meaning anymore. He either withdraws, gets depressed, gets angry or may even become suicidal.

If he chooses to allow it, his strong, thinking, mystical mate can help point him in a new direction at this difficult time of his life. He can feel like a small boy learning to grow all over again, and would do well to surrender himself to feeling childlike.

Their Interaction

This couple is like a snow-capped mountain rising from the shores of a large, high-country lake. From the top of the mountain, she can see the lay of the land for miles around, which she feels is a good perspective from which to make decisions and plans. He, on the other hand, prefers the quiet, spontaneous peace of being completely open, like the waters of the lake. At a core level, his Flower nature is very feminine and allowing, and he feels a sense of tranquility and expansion deep within. Like the lake, he is usually clear and receptive to the things around him. The lake loves the mountain, loves to quietly receive the streams that flow down from the mountaintop. His peaceful reflection gives her the mirror she needs in order to see herself. Her great certainty is like a rocky shoreline that gives him a sense of border or form. It comforts him.

Their relationship is a delicate but perfect balance between his feminine, feelingful nature and her masculinity. Like a mountain lake, he may have many moods. Her incessant mental jabs and critical words can be like rocks thrown one after the other into the lake. When there are too many of them, coming too fast, they may stir up angry waves that destroy the image of the mountain. When the mountain is excessively dominating, the lake fills up with stones and other avalanche debris and the water flows away. So while he likes his partner's strength, the left-brained Flower male may also be stifled and suffocated by it. On those occasions, her masculine willfulness buries him like an avalanche, and he loses himself.

She yearns for a man to open to her, to allow her to reveal her truth and to go in the direction she sees, for in her heart she is a teacher. She must be wary, however. If she gives him too much guidance she misses her own lesson, which is the realized experience of peace, allowing and silence. When she learns to create a receptive space with her words and gestures, she gives her mate room to expand and feel his own self-worth.

When he is allowed to be who he is, he feels strong. When he begins to take responsibility for his life, his sense of dignity returns. Although he loves the certainty she has about what to do and how to do it, he shouldn't allow himself to be led by his wife too often. If he does, he could end up feeling like he is in a mother-child relationship with her. If he does not follow her at all, however, it creates a constant state of conflict between them. The wise Flower man will allow his brilliant partner to lead him at times.

A Flower man is sensitive to being manipulated and a Jewel woman is sensitive to being criticized. Even if he is particularly soft and nonconfrontational, this couple quickly get to the point of disagreement. At some point, his controlling partner inevitably begins to direct his life, criticizing him, his clothing, his work, his attitudes. She wants to make him be better, wants to improve him. When she asks him, "What are you thinking? Why aren't you alert? Why aren't you there?" this irritates him. It makes him feel attacked, suffocated , controlled and limited.

When he gets angry with her, he says "You're always criticizing me! You're not listening to me! You're not hearing me!" She responds by telling him to put his feelings into words. He tries, struggles a bit with it, and she cuts him off and tells him what he's feeling.

She doesn't understand that, while she thinks that she's right there with him, trying to be alert and concentrating so hard on trying to understand, she's actually manipulating him and preventing him from expressing himself and not allowing him to be who he is.

When he feels overwhelmed, manipulated, not respected or abandoned by her, he will try a variety of nonverbal methods of communication first. His responses might involve quietness, withdrawal, depression or even the use of drugs. When these fail to improve the situation, he may leave before she hurts him any further, or he may react with angry outbursts; in some cases, he may even be physically violent.

She gives up on him, gets involved in her work or other activities, and immerses herself in the outer world. He reacts because his worst fear is abandonment. He's afraid she's going to leave him.

A Flower man (whether left- or right-brained) wants his wife there when he gets home. He needs her to be close by. All Flower structures, but particularly Flower men, have an intense, unconscious fear of abandonment. He needs reassurance that she will stay with him. Flower structures do not like being left alone, although at times they may feel that it is *easier* to be left alone.

She may respond to his overwhelming need for security by giving him reassurance in the way that he craves, by giving up something that she likes doing that makes him feel abandoned. But this won't last. Both left- and right-brained Jewel women will eventually get involved in other activities. If she's right-brained (or is going right) she's likely to get involved in social activities, and he'll try to find some way to keep her home, even if he has to sabotage her attempts to go out into the world.

Once he finds a way to deal with his fear of abandonment, he can allow her to be as active in the world as she wants. When this occurs, he will feel deep pride in her achievements and develop an abiding respect for her insightful wisdom.

Variation: Left-brained Female, Right-brained Male

She

This Jewel female's logical, analytical nature is increased by her linear, left-brain orientation. This concentration of constrictive energy slows down the mind, body, feelings and gestures. A natural gatherer and synthesizer of information, she is a pack rat of consciousness with a compartmentalizing mind. It grinds fine. Anything worth considering is to be reconsidered from every angle, making decision-making often excruciating and unlikely.

She tries to control her environment. With great dexterity and fine motor control, she makes a natural, hand-oriented sculptor. Like a strong dam holding back a large

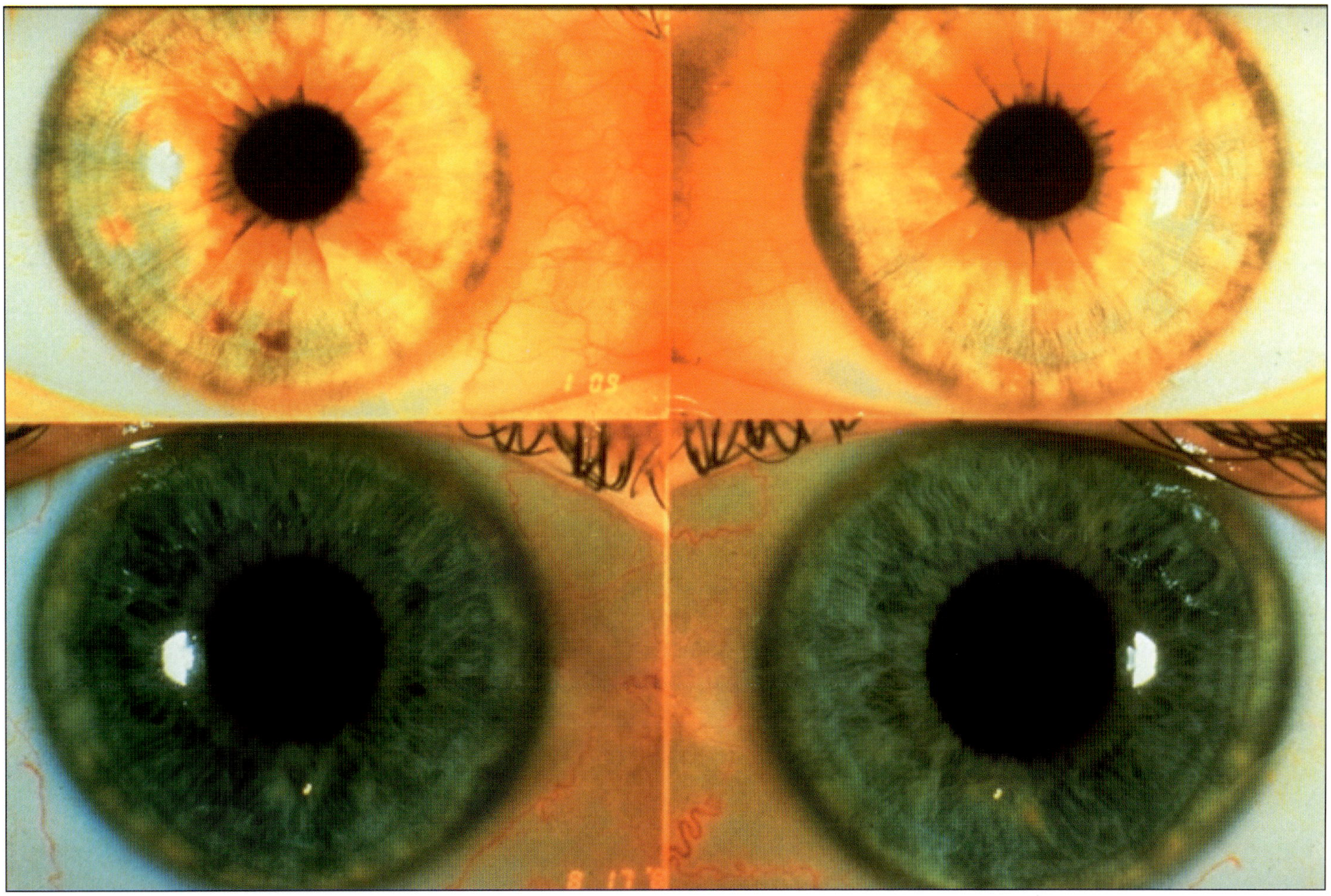

A left-brained Jewel female (top) is attracted to a right-brained Flower male for a long-term relationship.

reservoir of water, she has an extremely powerful inner holding force. A lot flows into the reservoir but little flows out. This inner focus gives her the potential to be a Chi Kung master, and the large reservoir contained within her gives her the capacity to be physically nurturing.

She has an innate fear of criticism, yet still has a tendency to constantly correct and try to control her mate. Desperately needing the experience of feeling, she is attracted to a theatrical Flower male who is as overstretched and overinvolved as she is narrowly focused.

He

Naturally fluid and feelingful, with an abstract, conceptual, right-brain orientation, this Flower male has the potential to be extremely creative. As a musician or actor he is capable of emoting great feeling in his audience. Playful and theatrical on the one hand, he usually has an anger issue with women and also has the capacity to be quietly blaming or vexatious. His father didn't give him a feeling of confidence as a male, partly because he didn't have the ability to flow with his own feelings. If this Flower male wasn't allowed to have his feelings as a child, it could restrict his ability to have the experience of his natural joyfulness as an adult. If he channels his emotional energy into creative exertion and works really hard, he becomes more masculine, gets his act together, and satisfies her deep need for material success.

Their Interaction

Dramatically polarized, the natural level of irritation in this couple's interaction is heightened by the fact that they feel like equals. Feeling more confident and more secure than a right-brained Jewel female, she is prone to tackle her mate head-on, like a mosquito confronting a lion. She keeps on and on at him with little jabs; he tends to be regally patient until he's had enough. And then he roars. When the male Flower finally erupts, she is momentarily shocked into silence, may even break down and start crying.

Their complementary strengths are most evident in the arena of work. This relationship combination is often very materially successful, because what she dwells on, he becomes. When she sets the goals and he follows her guidance, he usually becomes successful. He must be careful not to overexert himself, however, for he can't keep up with her amazing endurance. His energy ebbs and flows in a cyclical pattern and he will tend to exhaust himself before he realizes it. But since she is pushing him, it can be hard for him to avoid depletion.

THE LOVE-HATE PATTERN

As a mate, we inevitably attract a structural opposite with complementary patterns to our own. Sometimes the relationship includes elements of attraction and repulsion that can produce quite a stormy interaction. Such love-hate relationships are often very passionate and at the same time very uncomfortable. They are usually short-lived because the two individuals are too different to really relax and be comfortable with each other. They may learn a lot from each other, but eventually most relationships of this type end through sheer frustration.

In most love-hate relationships, the act of breaking dishes, throwing lamps or slamming doors is "standard operating procedure." Acts of violence only seem to strengthen the passion of reconciliation. It is truly an incredible process to behold.

In some cases, the couple stays together. While most people might find the endless ritual of attraction-repulsion to be an agonizing way to live, others seem to enjoy the excitement that comes from a violent outburst followed by the passion of making up. This process is usually repeated endlessly until the real root issue is uncovered. That issue is buried deep in the relationship patterns of the dominant parent.

The strongest example of this pattern is seen when left-brained females meet right-brained males and *both* have either Anger or Resentment in the dominant eye. The left-brain dominance of the female means she has a closer relationship with her father, hence a closer relationship with males in general. The right-brained male has a correspondingly strong attraction to females. This is the pattern which binds them together and keeps them coming back for more. The pattern which keeps them at war with each other is the resentment that the left-brained female has toward males, and the resentment that the right-brained male has toward females. The attraction pulls them together and the pain of anger or resentment in the same hemisphere tears them apart.

Illustrative Example

The Love-Hate relationship depicted in the iris photographs (right) is between a couple called Glenn and Mary. See the *Family Case Study* in the preceding chapter for an interpretation of their children's eyes.

Mary is a left-brained Jewel-Stream female. This is essentially quite similar to a Stream-Jewel iris structure, but in her case the Jewel pattern clearly dominates the underlying Stream pattern. Glenn is a right-brained Shaker-Flower male.

Their iris structures are unusual. Most Jewels go right and most Flowers go left, but here we have a left-brained Jewel female with more jewels in her masculine (right) eye and a Flower with more traits in his feminine eye. They are mirror opposites.

Mary is a Jewel pulled to the left brain by her father and older brothers. In her right eye, she has a jewel in Nurturing (see *Positions in the Iris*), but also a series of jewels around the position of Anger from Jealousy out to Resentment. This means that she has a tendency to be nurturing but also has rivalry, competition and resentment issues with males (right eye). She is actually attracted to the hemisphere where there is pain with the opposite sex. When she tries to get away from her pain with men, an invisible rubber band pulls her back to them again. Some Jewel females have so much pain in the masculine hemisphere that they stop having relationships with men altogether. Mary also has a jewel in the area of Impatience, indicating a sharp tongue in her communications with men. There is a jewel in the Heart position, indicating a sense of betrayal or hurt with men. So the thing she is attracted to hurts her. She hates what she loves.

Typically, a person goes to the left brain because of difficult issues in the right brain or because the father's side of the family is keeping the individual in the left brain. This means that there is probably a series of Jewels behind the father that are the source of the jewel structures in Mary's masculine eye. She will be attracted in relationship to someone who is emotional because she is mental, seeking her opposite in order to find balance.

Whatever issues she had with older brothers, he had with sisters. He fought well. He is attracted to the right brain probably because his mother (right hemisphere, left iris) was a Jewel. This would keep him in the right brain. So he marries another Jewel woman. He acts out his issues with women in his relationships just as his wife acts out her issues with men. She acts more masculine on a mental level, he acts more feminine. The two are attracted to each other but on some level they also dislike each other intensely. That is the nature of the Love-Hate relationship.

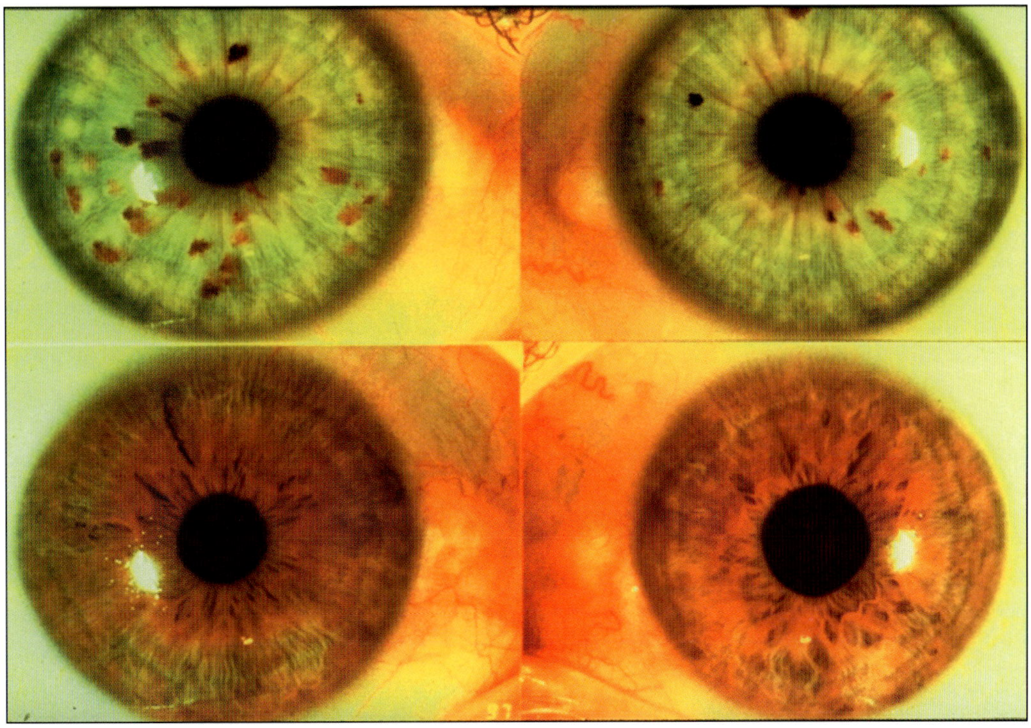

Mary (top) and Glenn, a classic Love-Hate relationship.

The man who can't quite get it together with women but always does. The woman who can't quite get it together with men but always does. They oscillate back and forth in a duality of extremes: admiration, control, laughter, volatility, joy, sex and anger. A passionate roller-coaster.

One of the challenges in the relationship is that, not only does her Jewelness make her act masculine and controlling, her left-brain orientation *also* makes her act masculine and controlling. She has turned off the right brain, which is rare for a Jewel, and he has turned off the left brain, or is only *partially* accessing both hemispheres. His allowing, emotional, Shaker-Flower disposition can handle her harsh, masculine ways for just so long before triggering his emotional issues with women. He explodes; the lion roars at the wolf and the wolf becomes a little puppy. (Sometimes when you yell at Jewels they actually feel better, as long as the outburst is brief.)

When things are going well, their opposite strengths and weaknesses enable one to empower the other. If they were to work at their relationship at a deeper level, more consciously, they could help each other considerably.

SIMILARS RELATIONSHIPS

Opposites attract. This is one of the fundamental laws of relationship. In 95% of all couples, it is a relatively straightforward matter to determine the opposite and complementary patterns by looking at the irises. But there are some apparent exceptions and these we call similars relationships.

Simply put, a similars relationship is when it is difficult to tell the difference between the iris structure of two mates. They may both look like they are Streams, Flowers or Shakers and you can't really tell why these two people are together.

Relationships in which both partners have similar eye structures are rare. They are most likely to occur when both people want to experience some comfortableness for a period of time, for example after a traumatic opposites relationship with someone else. These relationships are, in many ways, more like a friendship. The partners typically enjoy being together and sharing their lives but the relationship often lacks passion. Such relationships usually don't last because they don't contribute much to the work of transformation that we are all subconsciously engaged in. They are an opportunity to rest and recuperate from the stress of relationships; they are not so much about personal growth.

All relationships have *some* degree of opposite attraction. There are many polarity systems dealt with in the Rayid Method (Jewel/Flower, left/right brain, introvert/extrovert, etc.) and all of them need to be considered when examining the eyes of a couple. In extremely polarized relationships, there are very strong similarities and differences and the couple experiences a strong attraction/repulsion dynamic. At the other end of the spectrum, with similars relationships, we have found that the law of opposites attracting still holds true, but to a lesser degree than normal, and it may be hard for the practitioner to observe.

Case Study

The eyes (opposite) show a couple in a long-term relationship who are both apparently Stream-Flowers. In the case of the female (top), this is certainly true. She has an openness of structure, an absence of fiber, and shows a hemispheric movement from right to left which is characteristic of most Stream-Flower patterns. In addition to the fact that she has more traits in her right (masculine) eye, there are also a number of active trigger positions in her left (feminine) eye which support the notion that she has moved toward the right eye (left brain). In particular, she has a loss of heart and ideals (position No. 45) as well as a sense of rebellion (position No. 42) in the left eye.

Her mate is also a Stream, with a number of flowers in both eyes, particularly the left eye. Your initial impression might be that he is a Stream-Flower. But with a practiced eye, you will notice that his irises have a much greater density of fiber than hers, enough to mean that he will act more like a Jewel than a Flower. It is true that there are cases when it is very difficult to determine someone's iris structure. Being able to see the mate's eyes can be very helpful.

So the couple is similar in the sense that they are both Streams, but they are different in their fundamental expression. Her relative openness and extreme feeling orientation, further amplified by a Harmony pattern, gives her a very emotional, empathetic nature. He is more mental. He had a difficult relationship with his father, she had a difficult relationship with her mother. He is right-brained, she is left.

In most relationships, the partners are like two opposite pulses that come together only periodically. Couples in a similars relationship are different. They like to do the same things. Like two fish swimming along side by side, they explore the world together. They usually find it very easy to be around each other and have little conflict. Theirs is a comfortable relationship, based on companionship. But they also have very little passion because there is no underlying tension to create the necessary attraction. A couple like this might live together for years as friends, waiting for something to change, always on the verge of expecting something better.

The couple in this case study have had two children in nine years, but never got married. In similars relationships, not getting married but living together is quite common. People who have been in difficult opposites relationships sometimes seek out a similars relationship because they are, on the surface, so much easier. When a clearly opposite right-brained Jewel and left-brained Flower get together, there is lots of emotion, lots of passion and a physically magnetic attraction but they typically have few interests in common. It can be very stressful.

The absence of strong emotional and

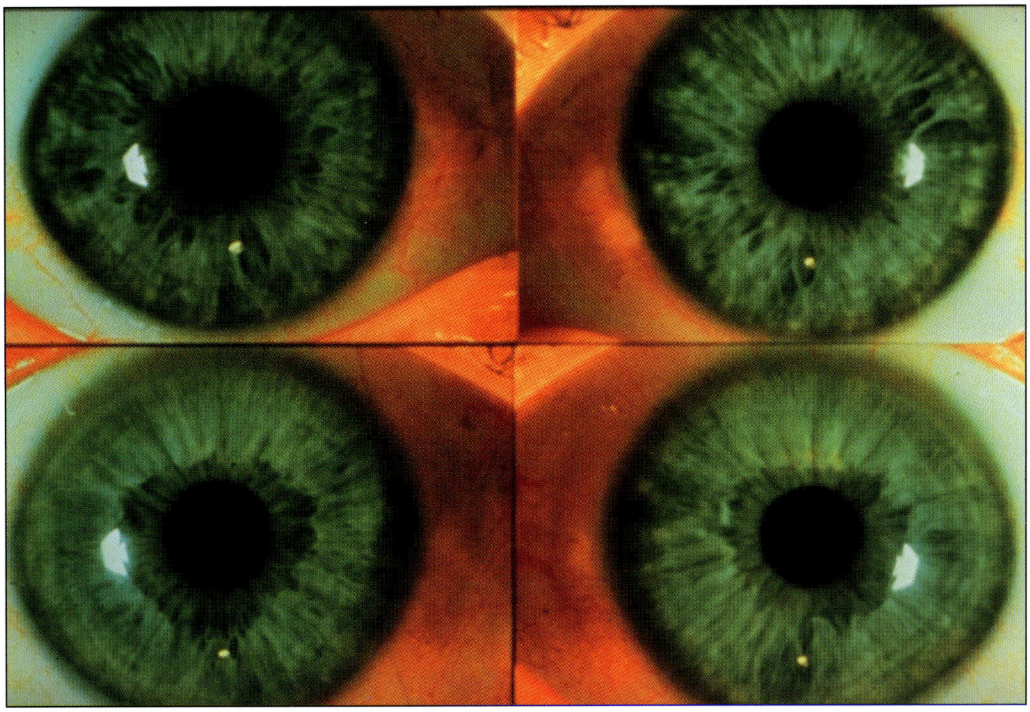

A female Stream-Flower (top) in a long-term relationship with a man who, at first glance, may also appear to be a Stream-Flower.

physical attraction in similars relationships creates a silent, unfulfilled yearning for more, yet there is also a sense of peace with the relationship that makes it difficult for the couple to part. It is like hurting a friend when you leave. It usually takes one of the partners being overwhelmingly attracted to someone else in order to make that jump outside the relationship. If this doesn't happen, the couple tends to stay in the relationship indefinitely. The quiet state of peace makes them act very much like brother and sister. They can be quite nurturing and good to each other.

The woman in this case study has a flower in the Nurturing position (No. 1) in her masculine eye, indicating an absence of nurturing. Her mate also shows an absence of nurturing but in his feminine eye. This is a typical similars pattern. In a similars relationship, you often find the *same pattern* in the *opposite eye*.

In a polarized relationship, you find the *opposite pattern* in the *opposite eye*. In other words, if one partner has a jewel in the area of Nurturing, the other partner is likely to have a flower in Nurturing in the opposite eye.

It is probably only one relationship in a hundred that is a genuine similars relationship. Usually the opposites are there even when the practitioner can't see them. When you can, use other body signs to supplement your iris interpretation. In this study, for example, the man has a higher half moon on his left thumb. This indicates a movement to the right, implying that he is from his mother's side of the family and hence that his primary structure is that of a Jewel. So when you reduce this couple's iris structures to the fundamental level of a Jewel or Flower, he is the Jewel and she is the Flower.

Variations

Of all the structures, two Flowers or two Streams are the most likely to be engaged in a similars relationship. For reasons not fully understood, two Jewels are the least likely combination to form a similars relationship. Of the Shakers, the Shaker-Flower is the most likely structure to be involved in some type of a similars relationship.

Again, it is important to stress that the similars relationship is a rare exception to the overall picture of complementary structure, hemispherically opposed, male/female relationships. Nearly all similars relationships still adhere to the law of opposites in order to attain their ultimate outcome. In what we call a similars relationship, only one facet, the *structural* component of polarity, is lessened. In many cases this is overcompensated for by greater polarization in the areas of introversion and extroversion or left- and right-brain orientation.

Homosexual Relationships

Nearly all homosexual (gay) relationships are similars relationships. About 90% of homosexual men vividly demonstrate some form of Flower iris structure. About 10% are some form of Jewel structure, usually Stream-Jewel.

There appears to be a specific pattern of iris structures in the family tree that makes homosexuality in men more likely. Research has revealed that nearly all gay men have at least one deeply controlling Jewel grandmother who still influences the family, usually the father's mother. Often the mother is a Jewel and there is also an older sister who is a Jewel. This means that the homosexual man typically has experienced the women in his family as being more masculine in their expression than the men, with a tendency to control the family either quietly or overtly. Where it is possible to delve further into the past, this same predominance of Jewel females is also evident in the third and fourth generations back, with a corresponding and complementary accumulation of Flower influence in the male line.

With most of the men for two or three generations back being Flowers – generally passive and emotional – there is a strong, underlying current of femininity that inevitably expresses itself in the present generation.

This research implies that a homosexual orientation is not directly determined by the present environment, that it is genetically preprogrammed. Another way of looking at this type of genetic influence is that it is an accumulation of environmental forces for several generations. The imbalanced accumulation of unconscious, controlling, feminine energy in his family tree has a tendency to open up creative, feminine attributes in the male, while at the same time limiting the expression of his masculine nature, often nullifying his relationship with his father. It also creates a need in the man to compensate for this excessive feminine influence by having intimate relationships with men rather than with women.

Their shared struggle gives gay men a strong bond. By being sexually involved with another man, they increase the masculine presence in their lives. When people are engaged in love-making, they are in a very suggestible state. A gay man thus absorbs a masculine influence through his sexuality. This mechanism is usually unconscious, an automatic compensation for an excessively feminine influence in the family tree.

The dynamics of attraction in lesbian relationships are often less obvious than those between gay men. There are usually two generations of extremely controlling Jewel males on the father's side of the family tree, with a powerful Jewel woman three generations back. This transgenerational influence has the effect of pulling the woman dramatically to the left brain, increasing the likelihood that she will be attracted to another woman for intimate relationships. All of this left-brained, masculine energy in her family increases her innate need for femininity.

Unlike male homosexuals, lesbians sometimes form Jewel-Flower opposites relationships. Most lesbians, however, are some form of Stream or Stream-Jewel, with an accumulation of mother-daughter difficulties that have persisted for several generations in a row. These family dynamics are generally more consciously recognized by lesbians than by gay men.

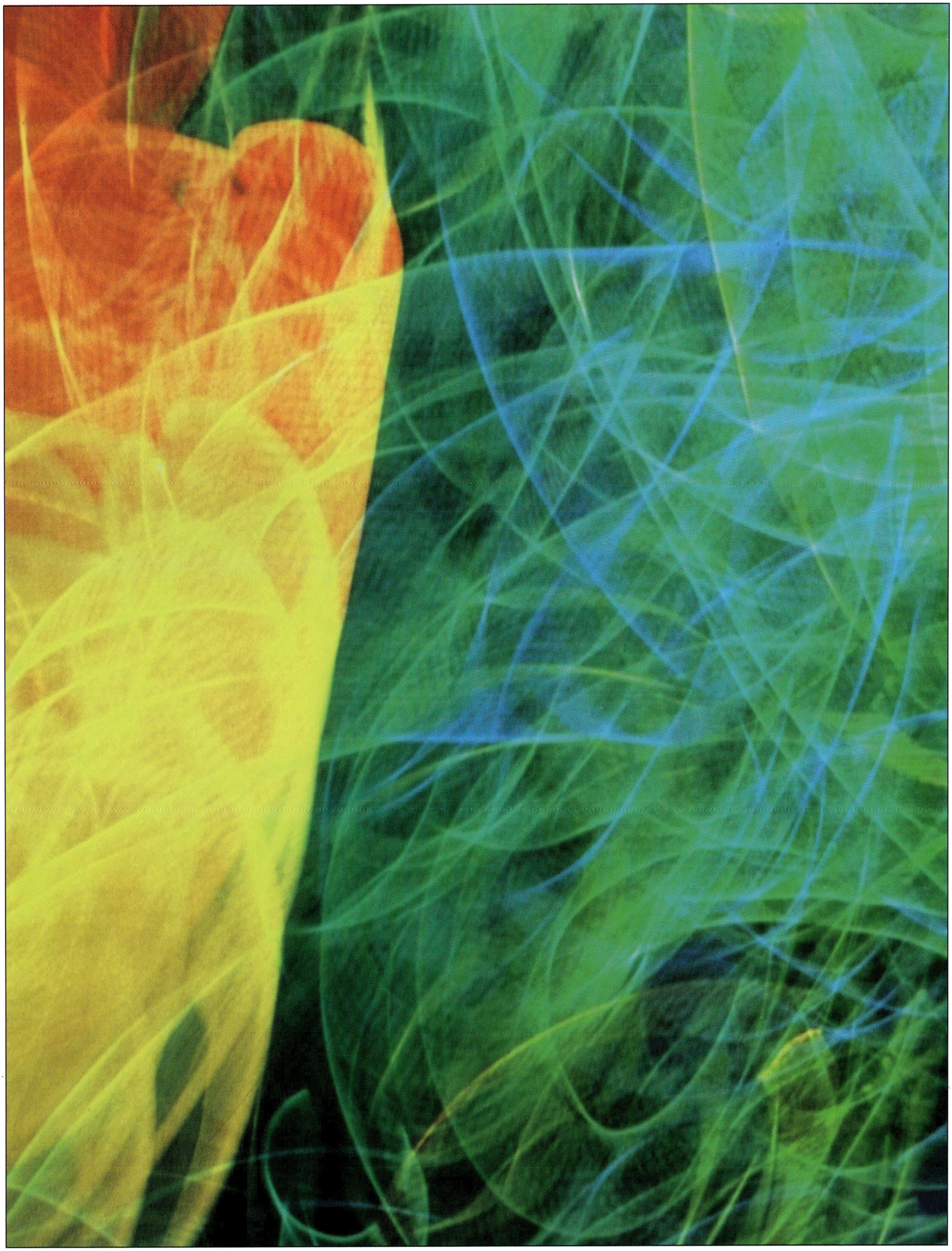

Parenting is simultaneously a joyful experience and also an intensely challenging one. This section briefly describes some of the potential pitfalls. All of the issues outlined here can be successfully dealt with by conscious, loving parents. Before we examine specific challenges, let's consider a couple of general recommendations for parents who seek healthy relationships with their children.

Parents must not put their relationship with their child before their relationship with their partner. Not only does this put up a barrier between one partner and the other, it also damages the child's ability to form healthy relationships later in life.

Don't take it personally if you feel your child is avoiding being intimate with you. Be aware that it is probably developmentally necessary in order for the child to find internal balance. For example, a Jewel child needs to move away from the father toward the mother in order to experience the right-brained (feminine) qualities of the unconscious, becoming more philosophical and emotional to balance the Jewel's innately analytical disposition.

Parent-child relationships are strongly influenced by the existence or absence of complementary patterns in the iris. The greater the degree of complementarity between a parent and a child, the greater the attraction of the child for that particular parent. This increases the activity of the hemisphere associated with that parent. If this complementary energy is extreme and unbalanced, it can disrupt the relationship between the parents and can in turn interfere with the child's ability to bond with a mate.

Following are a few examples of challenging parent-child dynamics. Some are blatantly obvious to the outside observer, others are so subtle that the individuals involved are often unaware that they are engaged in potentially harmful behavior.

Jewel Mother, Jewel Son

By being too controlling, a Jewel mother can keep her son trapped in an infantile state until he dies, especially if he was the last-born. He will always be "her baby." This is particularly likely if he is a Jewel. Although he can attract women quite easily when he grows up, he will tend to attract a woman who grew up too fast, who typically ends up feeling like he is still a baby. When she starts feeling this about him, her sexual energy drops off and, if his wife treats him in the way his mother did, he has no sexual attraction for her either. His intimate relationship with his mother unconsciously blocks his sexual energy with other women.

If the couple then has a child, the wife typically shifts her focus to her infant, trying to get from the child what she isn't getting from her husband. If that child is a male, she doesn't just destroy her relationship with her husband, she also destroys the boy's future relationships with women through her unconscious manipulation. It is important for mothers to fully understand this. If a woman uses the love of her son to replace the affection she should be receiving from her husband, she is establishing a pattern of interfering with her son's successful bonding with other women, whether that is her intention or not.

Flower Mother, Flower Daughter

One of the most difficult situations in a family is when a Flower daughter has a very similar iris structure to her mother. The daughter will feel like she is more from her father's side of the family, and will be more attracted to it. She can develop a very intimate bond with her father, even more so than his bond with his wife. This is especially true if she is the first-born child. If this happens, the Flower mother can become extremely jealous; she probably married her husband for security, and is now unconsciously afraid that her daughter is taking her husband away from her.

When the mother and the daughter are competing for the affections of the male, a terrible, undeclared war ensues. If the mother feels rejected as her daughter gains favor with her husband, she has the means to nullify the daughter's attraction for her father. The mother has the ability, not only to prevent the daughter from successfully bonding with the father, but also to interfere with her capacity to relate and be sexually intimate with other men, even after she has left home. This can potentially make it very difficult for the daughter to successfully bond with a future mate.

To cope with this kind of situation, it is important that the father makes it clear to his daughter that her mother is still "Number One" for him. *Do not honor the daughter above the mother.* Otherwise the mother may well try to pay her husband back by destroying the daughter's ability to relate to all men. When you have two Flower women in the house, they cannot *both* be the queen.

A hopeful aspect to this relationship is that there is also the potential for the mother and daughter to relate as friends once the daughter has left home.

Incest

Feelings are like a river; they flow continually. They cannot be destroyed, they can only be denied. Feelings can, however, be dammed or interrupted by the mind. When this occurs, the feelings create a deepening reservoir behind the dam, gradually building pressure against the retaining wall. Eventually, this pressure causes the body to animate the feelings that have been suppressed by the mind. In families where there is an emphasis on intellectual or verbal communication, but very little space for the expression of feelings, the emotional pressure builds. Like a large body of water pressing against an inadequate dam, this pressure can overflow into the meridians of the body, where it can create compelling and irrational desires.

Cases of parent-child incest usually involve unresolved feelings that have been mentally dammed for more than two generations. This creates an unconscious desire within the body to express intimacy on a physical level, compensating for the absence of feeling on a mental level. This physical pressure is often stronger than the capacity of the will to control it. The mind may not choose to act inappropriately, and may even be against inappropriate action, but a body that is filled with the pressure of unresolved feelings is stronger than the moral or ethical choices of the mind that pretends to controls it.

With any Jewel child, there is a strong chance that the relationship with the father will be difficult. Incest patterns occur most commonly with a Flower father and a Jewel daughter.

Types of Parental Influence

Children are, of course, deeply affected by the degree and type of interaction they have with their parents. And they need different things from the mother and the father. See *Transgenerational Patterns* in the preceding chapter for more about this.

A child needs the mother to be constantly close and yet continually freeing. He needs the father to show the way forward without blocking it, to engage in periodic instruction that assists the child to fully realize his innate purpose and dignity without criticizing the free will of the child.

Inappropriate or nonexistent action by the father or excessive intervention by the mother or the mother's mother can have a greatly detrimental impact on the development of the child. If there is an absence of masculine encouragement, it reduces the child's potential to be materially successful. The child's mother, and her mother in turn, typically influence a child in subtle or hidden ways. Their mechanism of control may not always be overtly obvious, but it is none the less powerful for that. Whenever the controlling influence from these two female sources becomes excessive, it can drastically inhibit the child's ability to fully express himself.

All power and creativity rises through the invisible before it becomes visible, through the feminine before it becomes masculine, through the unconscious before it becomes conscious. If the invisible (i.e. the mother) is too controlling, it limits the conscious expressions of the child.

Potentially the most damaging of these negative influences occurs when the father's mother has not fully released control over her son. When this occurs, her lingering influence interferes with the wife's natural need to engage the positive involvement of the father in raising the child. A father held back by his own mother fails to fully assume his role as a wise and guiding parent of his offspring. The grandmother's controlling influence also interferes with the connection between her son and his chosen mate. This distortion in parental bonding in turn interferes with the full creativity and success of the child. In such cases, the grandmother's influence typically continues even after she dies.

It *is* possible to eliminate such invisible and unconscious negativity. The conscious application of natural law, especially by the father, increases the spiritual, mental and physical success of the entire family. Most cultures and religious groups acknowledge this truth and have developed rituals, invocations and other processes which are intended to apply natural law to the development of a healthy family. See *Universal Therapies* in the next chapter for more information on rituals.

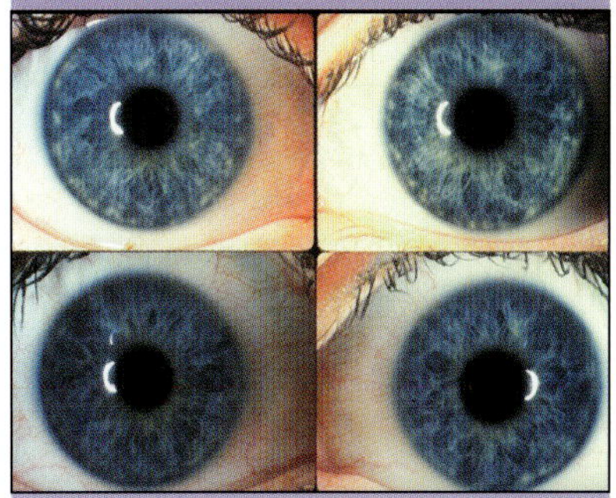

Flower mother (top) and Flower daughter irises

"Serve God, love me, and mend."
- Benedick to Beatrice, in William Shakespeare's *Much Ado About Nothing*

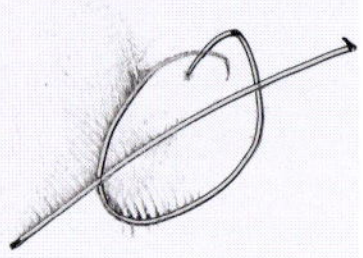

LIFTING THE VEILS

Most couples, whether consciously or unconsciously, come together in order to grow and change. This is the generally unseen force driving most long-term, intimate relationships, something that Shakespeare recognized in his light-hearted look at Elizabethan love. There is no faster way to heal and grow than in the context of a committed relationship in which both partners are focused on a higher purpose.

As described earlier in *Complementarity: Why Opposites Attract*, partners in long-term relationships have chosen one another because each represents the other's unembraced self. The differences between them are not just an unfortunate source of irritation and misunderstanding; they are the very reason the couple have joined together. They are an opportunity for increasing love.

If this otherwise hidden agenda is consciously accepted and openly acknowledged by both parties, then many of the difficulties that inevitably come up during the relationship can be embraced with compassion and understanding instead of being experienced through the mechanisms of resistance and pain.

There are many veils of illusion between a man and woman that must be lifted with consciousness in order for either to realize his or her full potential. The starting point for mutual growth and healing is for a couple to become aware of the behaviors that can harm their relationship and those that can help it.

Factors That Harm Relationships

Some of the behaviors listed are quite common in relationships, but that does not make them healthy. The list concentrates on the subtler forms of sabotage that are often overlooked; physically violent or criminal behavior is obviously harmful too.

1. CONTRADICTION. By far the most damaging to intimacy and extremely common. This includes any action that interrupts your partner's expression. Couples interrupt each other in many ways. One will do it auditorily, with verbal contradictions or disapproving noises; the other will do it with posture or body movements, or maybe by mentally "switching off," developing a blank stare. Usually both partners do it. Such movements or noises; are interruptions of intimacy. You may not think they are, but that is because these movements are inspired by the unconscious. Grimacing, tapping your foot irritatedly or wringing your hands is, at the level of the subconscious, just as much of a contradiction as are verbal interruptions and other "noises of protest." Any kind of neurological interruption of what someone else is saying gets in the way of direct communication and intimacy.

When you contradict your partner by cutting him off or by trying to give a different perspective on his experience, you are effectively denying his experience of reality. This is extraordinarily undermining to the possibility of intimacy between you. Just because you are in a relationship together doesn't mean that you have to agree about any particular issue.

Other behaviors are much less powerfully destructive than contradiction, but in order of importance:

2. Keeping secrets from each other. Like the first small crack in a windshield that eventually grows to destroy the whole windshield, keeping important secrets from your partner ensures that you can never fully "let go" and relax with him, and so you are forever divided.

3. Criticism or impatience directed at your partner make it difficult for your partner to trust you.

4. Noncommunication. By not communicating important things that you feel, you are making it difficult for your partner to know you and so intimacy is kept at bay.

5. Attempts by one partner to control the behavior of the other is perhaps just a particularly overt form of contradiction. It denies the freedom of each person to be who he is and makes intimacy impossible.

6. Mistrust or the absence of support for your partner's actions gives the subconscious signal that you don't really like who he is. How can your partner then be intimate with you?

7. Covert interference by other family members in the functioning of the relationship can drive a wedge between a couple without them even realizing it.

Factors That Help Relationships

1. AGREEMENT. Even when there is disagreement, agree to allow disagreement. This means stifling the various forms of neurological contradiction previously described. It is not just the verbal responses of the Jewel that indicate disagreement; every

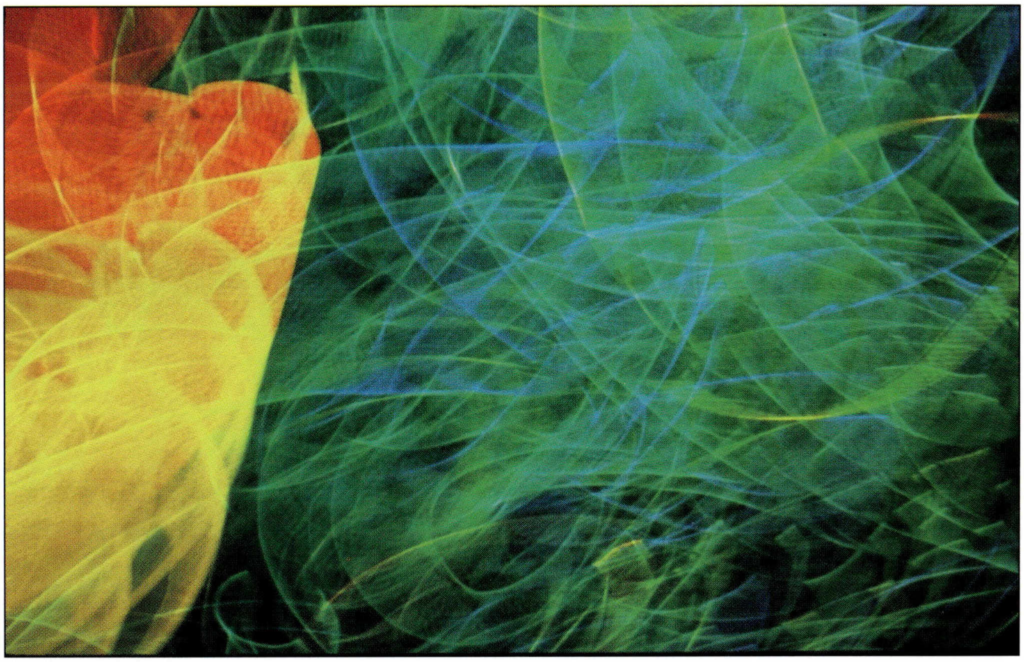

Masculine energy, represented by the yellow and red patterns in this image, has a hotter, more yang, but less long-lasting quality. Feminine energy, represented by the green and blue swirling light, is many times more powerful but it is cooler energy and so has less short-term influence.

structure has its own way of interrupting.

Try being still. It can seem uncomfortable to be still while someone is communicating to you, but just do it. Don't nod your head, twitch, "blank out" or make any other internal or external movement. Even if your unconscious disagrees with what your partner is saying, allow his message to sink in for a few seconds after he has finished before you respond. This can be particularly difficult for a Jewel who is so used to seeing interruption as affirmation.

2. Conscious acknowledgement of your partner and the validity of his choices.

3. Taking personal responsibility for what happens to you in your life. Don't blame your partner or anyone else for your misfortunes.

4. Achieving something together. It is important for couples to set aside time to engage in teamwork. By going through the motions of cooperation, they are actually setting a neurological precedent for intimacy. Try to accomplish and finish a specific (nonsexual) goal together within 20 minutes. That acknowledges your bond. Or create an affirmation that you agree on, and say it out loud to each other, at the same time, as you go to sleep.

There are many other factors that influence the potential success of a relationship. In some cultures, for example, it would not be acceptable for a right-brained Jewel woman to express her natural assertiveness toward her mate. Cultural norms that conflict with the relationship pattern of a couple will not change the pattern; rather they will simply add more tension to the relationship.

No matter the context of your relationship, the loving use of conscious will can enable you to lift the veils that separate you from true, intimate union with your partner. Remember: *Any* relationship can work. You are not in bondage to your structure.

Introduction to Rayid Therapies

"If we do not change our direction, we are likely to end up where we are heading."
- Chinese proverb

Healing is not just the eradication of symptoms; it involves removing the *causes* of the symptoms of distress. Whatever it is that you're suffering from, it won't help matters to accuse someone else of causing your troubles. Blaming your parents, your boss or your partner for your plight is no more likely to create good health than taking medication to dry up your runny nose is likely to get rid of a chronic sinus infection. Tackling the symptom can provide much-needed short-term relief from suffering but it doesn't change the inevitability of the pain returning. Good health and a sense of well-being is everybody's birthright. But we are each responsible for changing our own direction in life. No one else is going to do it for us.

One of the less obvious causes of distress can be an inherited or acquired constitutional predisposition to particular ailments or self-limiting patterns of behavior. These unconscious causative factors must be addressed and appropriately compensated for until you can be free of them altogether. You don't have to live with internalized pain if you can acknowledge who you are and find a way to learn what you need to learn in order to fully realize your potential. There is a whole, perfect being contained within each of us. Shine a light into your own darkest shadows, the parts of yourself that you have hidden away, and you will find him there.

The goal of Rayid is to help the individual to integrate and balance the internal energy systems responsible for creating health, vitality and well-being, so that major life lessons can be experienced joyfully. Not only is it an accurate tool for understanding an individual's personality and relationship style, Rayid also incorporates the use of many different types of therapy. It is not intended to replace other systems but is, rather, designed to be used in conjunction with a practitioner's existing repertoire. Rayid is highly compatible with existing therapeutic systems including nutrition, energetic therapies such as acupuncture, bodywork, physiological therapies, psychological counseling and spiritual practices.

Rayid therapies address every level of a person's being – from correcting vitamin and mineral imbalances in the body through dietary changes and homeopathic treatment, to explaining the individual's relationship patterns and optimal career choices. Every person can benefit from appropriate nutrition, bodywork and mental training. The goal of these therapies is to enable people to free themselves of the unconscious patterns of control in their family tree, allowing them to live in a way which is more vibrant, open and balanced.

Some of the Rayid therapies are universally applicable to all of the constitutional structures, others are highly specific and should be recommended only to people with a particular iris structure. For this reason, it is important that you are reliably able to identify someone's constitutional structure before you begin recommending structure-specific therapies. You must clearly understand the basic iris structures and their associated behavior patterns. Once you have grasped these fundamentals, you can begin to make use of the program of natural therapies that has already been developed for each constitutional type.

This chapter provides an introduction to the principles of Rayid therapeutic theory, focusing on therapies that are applicable to all of the constitutional structures. A comprehensive therapeutic program should also include elements that are specific to each individual iris structure. For a detailed description of structure-specific therapies, contact Rayid International at the address on the last page of this book.

The Body as a Vibrational Pyramid

Your temporal vehicle, the body that you inhabit, actually is made up of several different elements or "selves" which have differing needs and different motivations. At times these selves even seem to behave like noncooperating, independent entities.

Think of yourself as a pyramid (see diagram on page 108). Your being has a physical aspect, which forms the base of the pyramid, an emotional aspect and a mental aspect. The needs of each level of your being must be addressed in any therapeutic program that aims to do more than just relieve the symptoms of suffering.

In addition to these selves, you also have a spiritual nature. Instead of thinking of it as another level to your being, it can perhaps best be regarded as the glue that holds everything together. The appearance of your body, and your mental and emotional responses, are genetically programmed. Your spiritual essence does not have the same programming. This aspect of your self contains the blueprint of perfection that can be released and expressed through the other levels of your being – your body, your heart and your mind.

At the subatomic level, all matter is a vibration in an energy field. The body, then, can be regarded as a vibrational pyramid. Each part of your being must resonate in harmony with the other aspects, or the pyramid will be weak and cannot tolerate many stresses or cope with much additional vibrational energy.

Feelings, too, are vibrations. The body must be cleaned up in order to be sensitive to the feelings that flow through it. You must also train your mind to let go of its control over the body in order to experience those feelings instead of just thinking about them. As you work through your therapeutic program, you will become increasingly aware of the transgenerational lines, hooks and tethers that bind you down. If painful emotions arise from this work, be aware that they are actually part of the healing process. They are not something to be avoided. If we are to be free of our fears, if we are to be capable of feeling limitless joy, vibrant aliveness and embodied bliss, we must also open up to experiencing more of our (previously suppressed) emotional reality.

Many people believe that the way to attain a transcendent state of consciousness is to get out of the body. Although some form of altered consciousness is possible this way, the higher states of consciousness are accessible only by being fully *in* your body. This doesn't mean that *you* should be limited by *its* present limitations; instead, concentrate on opening your body up, *freeing* it from limitation, allowing the blueprint of perfection to come forth. Remember: You cannot move past the limitations of the body simply by denying the needs of the body. You must address those needs, strengthening the body from within.

There is a great difference between changing the issues and making someone more comfortable with the issues they have. With powerful therapeutic work, don't confuse *feeling* better with lasting change. The correct application of targeted therapies can create apparent change by overlaying a destructive vibration or pattern with a dominant, healthier vibration. Such therapeutic "band-aids" may help to correct the imbalance without correcting that which is causing the imbalance. This change may last for several years but, unless you address the deeper molecular, mental and unconscious imbalances that are maintaining the symptomology, the underlying structural imbalance will eventually come through again.

Your body is there to serve you in your life purpose, not to limit you. Think of it as a biological computer that can be reprogrammed by using the right type of input to access and change the core program code. That is the purpose of the complete Rayid therapeutic program, available from Rayid International. It works at every level of your being, dealing with the symptoms of disease as well as changing your core program.

The Process of Change: The Three Rs

The *willingness* to change is the first step toward building the new you. It is the foundation of the pyramid that you must build in order to ascend to a state of spiritual, emotional, mental and physical integration. Your willingness to change involves accepting that you cannot realize your full potential by denying any aspect of yourself, including your "shadow" (or opposite) self. You must seek out your opposite and fully integrate it so that you can be free of the need to live at one polarized extreme or the other. This allows you to connect with your core, the essence of your personality. You must accomplish these steps before you can be genuinely free of your self-limiting psychological programming.

Following Rayid therapies takes a person through three transformations:

1. Reverse the constitutional structure – by using therapies that encourage you to fully experience your opposite structure, i.e. that which is hidden in your unconscious.

2. Return to the core – return to the constitutional expression you had as a child, before you started shutting it down in order to experience its opposite.

3. Reach beyond the iris – meaning, go beyond the constitutional structure, beyond the limitations of personality itself. This element is discussed in the final chapter.

A Jewel, for example, should use therapies that give him the experience of Flowerness. Doing so will facilitate his return to the constitutional structure that he was born with, without all the fragmented maladjustments and adaptations made during life. This original state of immaculate, untrammeled Jewelness is very different than the sometimes harsh, coldly analytical Jewel most of us know. A Jewel who is *at core* will be as alert as an eagle, without the need to analyze what he perceives. He lives in a state of *absolute knowing*. He experiences anticipation, alertness and connection to a universal presence without the anxiety or need to analyze all of the details or ask lots of questions (all of which are signs of imbalance).

A Flower at core experiences feeling without anger or other forms of reactivity. He is constantly connected to his spiritual source at a feeling level.

A Stream's primary means of communicating is through body posture, and secondarily through touch. The Stream structure thus represents therapies associated with stillness, such as "received" bodywork or Chi Kung. You would therefore prescribe an opposite therapy to encourage a Stream to move toward his core structure, for example using a movement-based exercise such as Aikido (which is associated with the dynamic, Shaker personality).

Actually experiencing our creative potential means utilizing what we have to the fullest extent without being restricted by the source from which it was derived. This means that, in order to heal, we don't have to figure out everything that "went wrong" in order to fix it. We do, however, have to go through a sequence of steps to become more conscious, to free ourselves from the genetic hooks that jerk us around, to enliven our bodies and open our hearts. This is the value of the therapeutic techniques outlined in the following pages.

Your temporal vehicle has different levels, each of which needs to be addressed in a comprehensive therapeutic program.

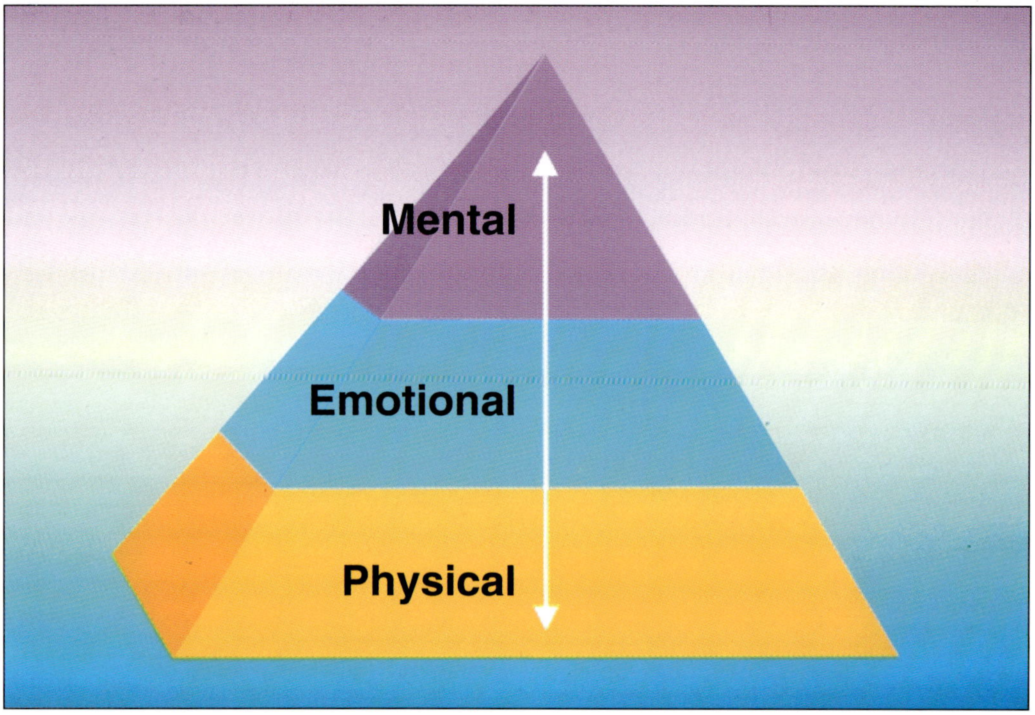

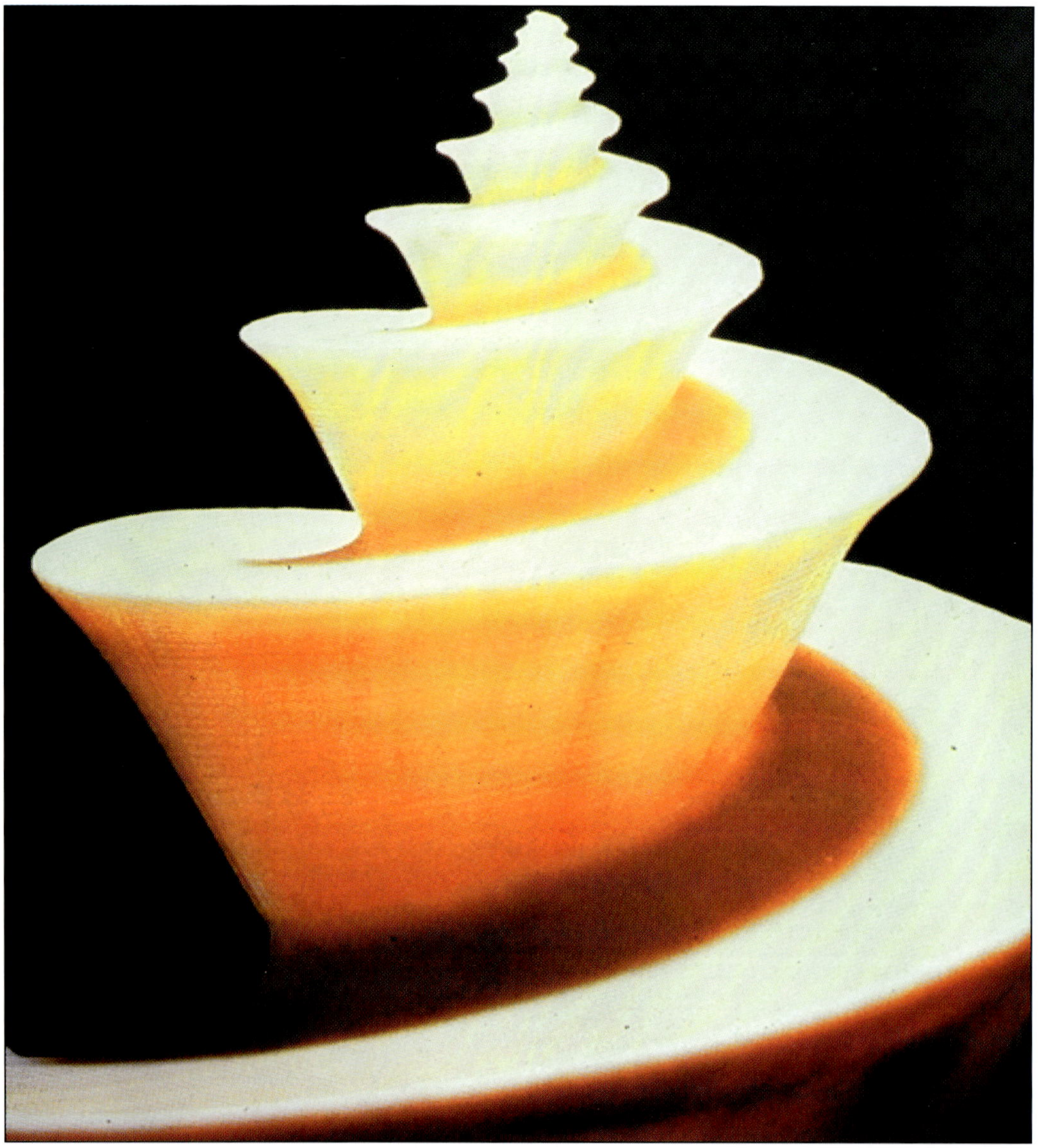

THE STAGES OF HEALING

Healing is a continuous process, in which change in one aspect of life can profoundly affect every other area. For the sake of clarity and simplicity, this section breaks the continuum of transformation into four stages, and briefly describes some of the attitudinal shifts and tools that can be applied at each of four different levels of experience: physical, relationship (to the self as well as to others), mental and spiritual. The spiritual aspect of transformation is included because it is as critical to the process as the others. We need to open ourselves up to a higher power in order to heal. The process of change is not necessarily under our control. Because we are moving into unfamiliar territory for ourselves, we cannot really "lead" ourselves through it. By definition, we don't know where we are going; otherwise it wouldn't be fundamental change. A therapist or Rayid practitioner can help smooth the road for us but has no more idea of where it's leading than do we.

Stage One

This first stage of healing is the most critical and often the most challenging. It involves cleansing, letting go of all self-limiting feelings and surrendering the mind's need to understand. As you progress through the chart, you move from the feminine to the masculine realm. All of the elements in stage one deal with unconscious (feminine) or hidden issues.

Physical: Cleanse. Jewels and Flowers must follow different different cleansing programs (see *Structure-Specific Variations in Therapies*, overleaf). To support this cleansing, it is important to pay attention to the biochemical system of the body, to make up for any vitamin, enzyme or mineral deficiencies and to balance the body's pH. Use the *Harmony of Health* homeopathic remedies and eat more alkaline-ash-forming foods. Rest is essential in order to integrate all of these changes. It also helps the body to cleanse and rebuild, decreasing the incidence of unpleasant physical or psychological reactions to the cleansing process. In this context, rest means much more than relaxing or getting more sleep; it means experiencing regular periods of complete physiological stillness during the day (see *Alpha-Meditation* under *Universal Therapies*, later in this chapter). Most people are chronically deficient in quality rest.

Relationship: Nurture yourself. Let go of the notion that someone else should take care of you. Let go of your need to blame others for what you have gone through. Whatever happened to you in the past, hanging on to these old emotions won't help you to deal with your life *now.* Don't dwell on past pain. You need to go beyond your childhood experiences to the source of who you are, and that is contained in the patterns of your family tree.

Mental: Surrender the mind's need to control. Let go of your need to understand everything. You don't know where you are going, so you can't figure it out. Trust the process of healing and surrender to your spiritual source, whatever or whomever you perceive it to be. Make of your mind an empty cup, create an opening for change.

Spiritual: Find meaning in your life. This process can take a variety of different forms, depending on your spiritual background. If you are not spiritually inclined, it may involve a deeper reflection on the purpose of your life; if you are part of an established religion, you might suddenly rediscover your faith; for some people, their new purpose in life comes in the form of a dramatic revelation. Ask, pray, plead or beg; do whatever you have to do to find direction. If it is not actively chosen, this stage may be accomplished unconsciously (and even unwillingly) when you experience a great tragedy in your life, such as a long illness, a divorce, a loss of self or a near-death experience. Sometimes called the dark night of the soul, such events can force people to take a long, hard look at their lives, to go inward and reflect on the meaning of it all. If you are finding the process of change difficult, try doing clearing rituals (see *Universal Therapies*, later).

Stage Two

Physical: After cleansing, the body must be rebuilt through nutrition and appropriate bodywork.

Relationship: Begin the process of self-acceptance, of improving your self-image, of taking responsibility for who you are. Who *are* you? Don't just recreate the old you; build a new self.

Mental: Start making choices for yourself. If you want to change, you must first determine *how* to change. Evaluate the options open to you, then choose the path that will bring results.

Spiritual: The process of reconstruction will bring with it a

"View your body as an extension of your soul, the spoken word of your being."
- Emmanuel

newfound sense of optimism and a longing to do something more with your life than what you've experienced in the past. Typically, this involves contemplation, actively seeking a way to "live in the mystery."

Stage Three

Physical: Vitalize the body. Now that your body is stronger, animate it. Express yourself through movement, a Shaker quality.

Relationships: Take your new self and put it in social situations. Play, interact with groups of people. Taste the fruits of your self-development work. If the body is integrated, cleansed and healthy, the new self has a greater capacity for success.

Mental: Apply what you have learned. Keep up the program. Be self-observant; watch yourself to see how you waver from your chosen path. This can be very difficult but you must be persistent in moving in your new direction. This is the stage at which many people interrupt their own healing process, when the old habits come knocking at the door. Some part of you still wants the status quo. Say to yourself, "No more will I be ruled by this old, self-limiting pattern." Intensify your affirmations and rituals to help remind yourself to stay on track. Use the *Body Harmony* tape (see *Universal Therapies*). Watch yourself as you interact with others. This is when you return to the core, act out your constitutional creativity.

Spiritual: Appreciate the oneness and the mystery of life. Be thankful for your new discoveries. Open your soul to the connectedness you share with all things.

Stage Four

When you have completed stage three, you have successfully returned to your core constitutional structure. Stage four is when you free yourself from the limitations of your personality. The only way to do this is through relationship; you don't get there alone because it requires the fusion of opposites. Your left and right brain, your internal Jewel and Flower must be in such a state of vibratory aliveness that they can meld without dissolving into each other. Your internal polar opposites actually occupy the same space and retain their integrity. Two must become one, both internally and externally. This stage is an experience of the freedom that can only come through relationship, when two awakened, vibrant beings unite in a mutual, joyous exploration of life.

Structure-Specific Variations in Therapies

Although there are several elements of the healing process that are common to all people, each of the constitutional structures also has several unique therapeutic requirements.

At the physical level in stage one, for example, Jewels and Flowers need different types of cleansing. Jewels usually benefit greatly from strict cleansing diets or fasts using only a single food source, such as carrot juice, rice or a specific fruit. For the Jewel, this type of fasting is a Flower-like experience of allowing or letting go, and it helps with elimination. This is *not* the appropriate way to cleanse a Flower. Flowers need to feel *nourished* at all times. It is best to cleanse their systems using a variety of simple, healthful foods such as steamed and raw vegetables. Their digestive systems need to learn the Jewel-like qualities of assimilation and containment, *not* elimination.

When working with touch in stage two, Flowers will experience the best results from a gentle, peripheral massage technique using soft strokes. For Jewels, it is appropriate to use deeper massage strokes, or techniques such as rolfing that get into the underlying tissues more quickly.

At stage three of the physical level, when movement exercises are introduced, different techniques should be used by Shakers and Streams. As we mentioned earlier, Streams, who are naturally still, would benefit from dynamic movement exercises such as Aikido. This would not be appropriate for Shakers. Chi Kung is one of the most useful therapies for Shakers because it simultaneously creates a sense of stillness while focusing attention on *inner* movement; Shakers are externally active and outwardly directed. Chi Kung teaches them about "holding."

The structure of the iris is, thus, a precise and objective tool for determining exactly which therapies, attitudes and actions will most contribute to an individual's growth at each stage of unfoldment.

	STAGE 1	STAGE 2	STAGE 3	STAGE 4
Spiritual Connection to the Source	Reflection Religion Revelation	Contemplation Longing for more	Thankfulness for the mystery Oneness	Bliss Presence Embodiment
Mental Self-control	Surrender Go inward	Evaluate options Make choices	Self-observation Persistence Creative self-expression	Objectivity Service Genius
Relationship Emotions Connection to others	Nurture *yourself* Release the past	Self-acceptance Taking responsibility	Group interaction Play	Union with a mate True feeling
Physical Stillness Bodywork Biochemistry Movement	Cleanse Rest	Nourish Touch Rebuild	Vitalize Move! Reach out	Experience aliveness, dynamic joy

> *"It is our natures that are the physicians of our diseases."*
> - Hippocrates

UNIVERSAL THERAPIES

Optimum progress through the various stages of transformation and healing requires that all aspects of your being are in alignment and receptive to increasing levels of vibrancy. Every individual, regardless of iris structure, needs aerobic exercise (such as walking) to oxygenate the cells, a clean diet in order to strengthen the body, and quality rest in order to integrate all of the changes. In combination with bodywork, mental training and an active respect for the sacred laws of relationship, this comprehensive approach will create of your disparate inner selves a cooperative community.

This section takes a look at some of the therapeutic techniques that can be applied to all iris structures. There are other, more advanced therapies that are not mentioned here because they require instruction and guidance, especially those involving breathwork.

Releasing Mental Control

After many years of research and experimentation, Denny Johnson has determined that the best techniques for releasing the mind from its controlling influence are those developed by Dorothy Gates, PhD of California, USA. Her work teaches people to release the inner strength necessary for the creation of a well-balanced, talented human being. Her programs include the Spectra Dynamics course, the two relaxation tapes and the *Gifting Your Child* tapes described here. For copies of these materials, contact Rayid International.

Spectra Dynamics

This self-managed therapeutic program is designed to increase your ability to be fully present in, and able to enjoy, your body, mind and relationships. It uses the conscious mind to access the healing power contained within each person.

The mind must be included in any process of growth and change. It controls the feelings in your body, it affects the way you relate and so must be correctly engaged if you seek a lasting transformation. The mind and its controlling mechanisms are regulated by natural laws. What the mind is focused on, it can create as a pattern of behavior. The mind is like a hyperactive child who is overeager to do something to please its parents. It needs to be encouraged yet simultaneously calmed and gently prevented from taking over the whole show. It needs to be given something to *do* rather than something to *stop*. Give the mind something else to do *in place* of the self-limiting behavior.

Words are the natural domain of the mind. Words, in the form of carefully designed affirmations repeated over an extended period of time, can be used to amplify specific mental attributes, thereby achieving changes in self-image and behavior. The Spectra Dynamics course uses the mind's natural need for activity, focusing its strength in such a way that the mind gradually instills into itself a new pattern of expression. The Spectra course is unique in that it uses the language of the mind to ensure that the new program can be received by it. Two other key components are the consistent repetition of the new information, which ensures that the program is retained in memory, and regular relaxation in order to allow the program to be absorbed.

Relaxation Tapes

In addition to the Spectra program, Dorothy Gates has developed two audio tapes that combine relaxation with carefully chosen words to further recondition the mind.

Releasing Self-Sabotage is an instruction to the wounded mind to stop maintaining the patterns of denied feelings that are interrupting the outer expression of your inner perfection. The release of these feelings naturally allows a healthier pattern to emerge. Once the flow of positive feelings has been restored to the body, the next tape can be used.

Building Body Harmony trains the mind to be alert and sensitive to the different body systems, which gradually increases the level of feeling in the whole body. A mind that is fearful blocks the light like a window covered with mud. A mind that is alert, sensitive and open allows health, harmony and vitality to flow though the body, restoring the blueprint of perfection. A clear mind, like a clean window, doesn't just let the light through in one direction. Your relationships and creative expression will also reflect your inner experience of true feeling and harmony.

Gifting Your Child

Parents can help their children to mature into well-balanced, talented and brilliant young adults by using this program developed by Dorothy Gates and offered through Rayid International. It is a remarkable series of audio tapes that use classic fairy tales to stimulate the child's imagination, clarify his emotions and address his anxieties and aspirations.

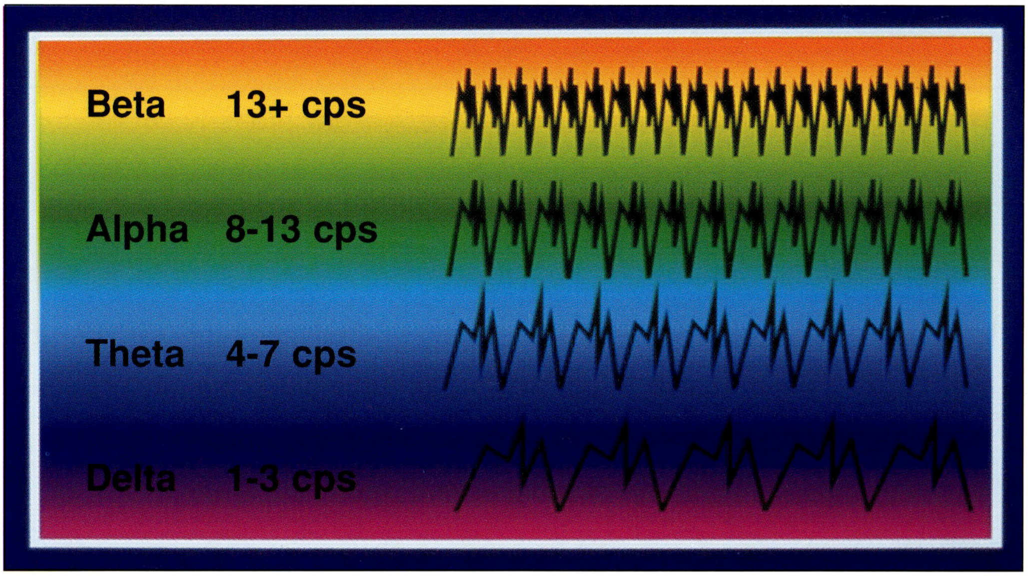

Dominant brain-wave patterns at different states of consciousness. The beta waves (top), at more than 13 cycles per second (cps), are dominant in a state of alert wakefulness. Alpha waves are associated with meditative states; theta and delta waves are emitted primarily when sleeping.

The *Gifting Your Child* program uses the language of the child's mind to influence the child's perceptions and behavior.

At the end of this chapter, there are two examples of original fairy tales created by Denny Johnson (see *Stories for Children*) that have a similar effect.

Stillness (Alpha-Meditation)

Stillness is necessary to ground the various therapies in the body. If you don't keep emptying the cup (your body) of experiences, how can you fill it up with something new? There are many different techniques to keep the body still for a period of time; whichever system you use, do it regularly, for 20 minutes, at least twice a day. The alpha-meditation described below is one of the least complicated.

Sometimes referred to as "conditioning rest," this simple meditation technique is vital in developing and maintaining the functions and integrity of the central nervous system, muscle tissue and the lymphatic system. It is a very easy way to recharge your internal batteries and everyone can benefit from doing alpha-meditation two to three times a day. The purpose of the exercise is to rejuvenate the body and to create a feeling of inner stability – both of which are particularly helpful to anyone who is in the process of creating new life patterns.

Sleep is not rest; it is a different state of consciousness (see the Brain Waves diagram). When the brain is in deep sleep, emitting theta or delta waves, the body is not being renewed; the state in which the brain emits alpha waves constitutes the most physically sustaining rest. Exhausted sleep is therefore not as useful as people generally think. Twenty minutes of focused alpha-meditation gives your body the same amount of rest as several hours of sleep and opens a channel to the unconscious. Alpha-meditation helps you to gather and integrate energy, while creating a feeling of "belonging." You feel more secure in your body and so relate better to other people.

The exercise itself is very simple: Lie down, close your eyes and be still. Breathe slowly and steadily for about 20 minutes. Don't go to sleep. If you find that you simply cannot still your wandering mind, and that your mental activity gets in the way of you relaxing your body, contact Rayid International for a copy of the Spectra program, which includes a more directed alpha-meditation technique.

Transformation Through Ritual

Many people find it difficult to accept that the use of directed consciousness is more powerful than some of the physical remedies that can be offered for an imbalance. The spoken word has a great impact on the mental patterns that hold your present personality, as well as your physical and emotional imbalances, in place. The extent of its power as a healing tool is rarely recognized outside of religious circles. The Kirlian photograph (p. 114), showing the dramatic difference in the quality and level of a person's energy before and after performing a clearing ritual, should give some indication as to its effectiveness.

Designing your own rituals and invocations is easy. Develop an appropriate affirmation and then invoke

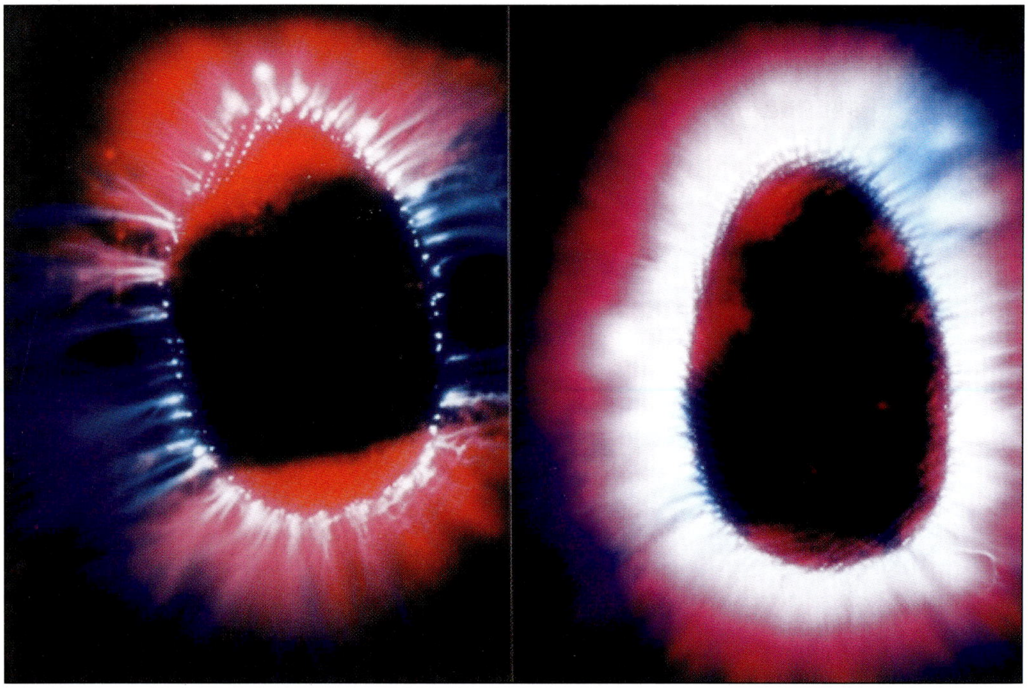

Kirlian photographs of the same fingertip, taken before (left) and after the person performed a clearing ritual. Kirlian photography records the electromagnetic field (sometimes called an "aura") emanating from all living things. These photographs demonstrate the power of ritual to balance and magnify a person's energy.

the spiritual power that fits your own religious background. Do the ritual in the name of Jesus Christ, Allah, Buddha, Love or any other creative and loving force. The important thing is to call on a higher power to help you. Many of the issues we face can seem too weighty to deal with alone.

The following example should give you a starting point from which to develop your own rituals. It is for Jewels, who typically suffer from anger and criticism from the father's side of the family. It is designed to release the accumulated negative mental control from that side of the family. The wording is intended as a guideline only modify it according to your own circumstances:

"I now lovingly release all negative mental control from my father's side of the family, known or unknown to me, including anger and criticism, for four generations back and for four generations into the future. This now allows me to be free and open, to experience my true self, and to experience the vibrations of true feeling. I do all of this in the name of Love."

Write your ritual down before saying it out loud and then burn the piece of paper after reciting it. The last purification is by fire. You have to do your ritual only once, although you may wish to repeat it if other specific forms of transgenerational control become evident.

The more precisely you word the ritual or invocation, the more powerful it is. If you are aware of the ways in which your family controlled you, be specific in naming the forms of control. If you can name all of those people in the preceding four generations, do so. If you can name individual family members in association with each form of control, even better.

If you want to clear out the unconscious control from both sides of the family, wait at least three days before doing a ritual for the mother's side of the family. Substitute the dysfunction associated with that side of the family in place of the phrase "anger and criticism."

Use a ritual or invocation whenever you have cause to believe that some transgenerational issue is creating "dis-ease" in your client or yourself. You could design similar rituals to release any element of the unconscious connective tissue binding you to unhealthy patterns in your family tree. Once you have done this kind of ritual, it is important to stop going into your past; otherwise you are simply recreating, through memory, the very influences you are trying to free yourself from.

If you don't know the origins of the dysfunctional pattern, try this invocation:

"I do not need to understand how or why or when I acquired the specific spirit of this pattern. I ask you, the sprit of Love, to intercede on my behalf in the realm of the unconscious, to free me from this pattern. I will do my best, physically, mentally and in my relationships, to break this pattern in my own domain, the conscious realm, for four generations back and for four generations forward. I need you to release the invisible, hidden influence from whatever part of the family tree this pattern came from."

Angel's Wings

This is a simple therapy that uses the hands to integrate the energy of the four structures in your body. It helps you get a feeling for the different qualities associated with each structure, and actually helps begin to balance the body by getting it to express all four of those primary energies in a sequence. It gives a physical context to the energy pattern and direction noted in the tables accompanying the structural descriptions in *The Essence of the Structures*.

Performing this sequence of hand and arm movements on a regular basis gives the body a physical experience of the energy associated with each structure, and actually helps to retrain the mind. The body and the mind are physiologically "wired" together, and if you train the body to experience dynamic equilibrium, it has a cumulative effect on the mind. In a sense, the Angel's Wings sequence "lubricates" the other therapeutic practices that are being undertaken.

As you perform the sequence, dwell on the feeling associated with each motion and position. The forward postural function is Jewel, the experience of allowing is Flower, the uplifting postural movement is Shaker, and the integrating, physical connection to the whole body through stillness is Stream. This exercise consciously integrates the energy of all four of the primary structures.

Do the exercise three times a day to maximize the experience of integration. Hold each position for as long as feels comfortable to you. You cannot possibly do this exercise too slowly; the slower the better. If you could take 20 minutes to perform one sequence, that would be ideal.

A powerful variation of this exercise is to do it together with your mate while the two of you are standing eye to eye. This amplifies the experience, and is a nonverbal acknowledgement of your partner's energy. By mirroring your partner's energetic expression, you are surrendering to it, agreeing with it, feeling it, rejoicing in it and consequently embodying that sense of union in your relationship.

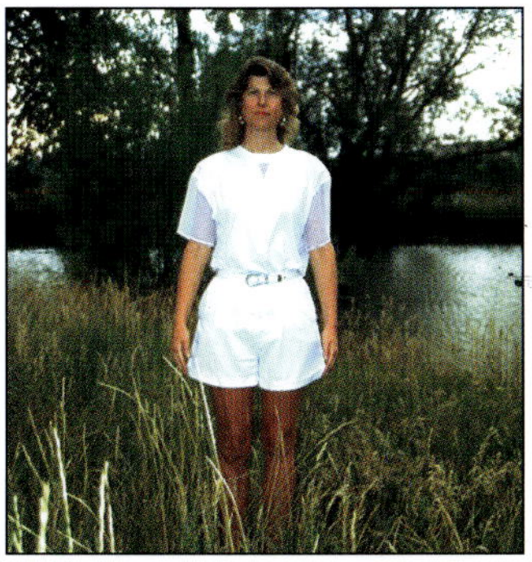

1. Stand with knees slightly bent, feet placed comfortably and arms down by sides. Relax. Slowly lift the hands up, keeping them level with each other, as if they are reflections of each other in a mirror that is placed along the vertical axis of the body. Gradually stiffen the fingers and thumbs so that you have a feeling of sharpness.

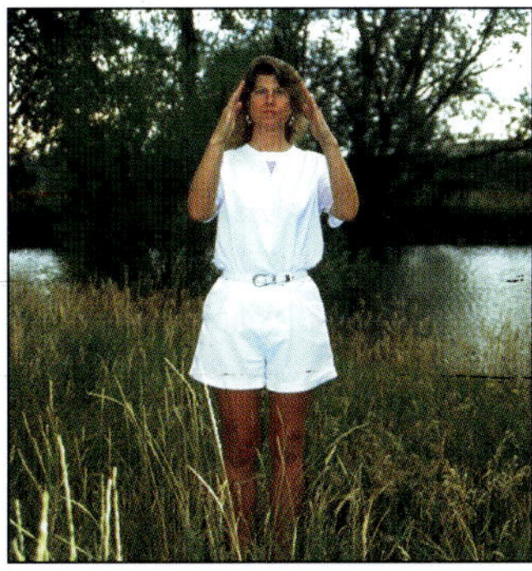

2. Keep raising the hands until the arms form a triangle between the elbows and the fingertips. The fingertips should now be approximately level with the mouth, and the distance between them should be equal to the distance between the eyes. This position embodies the angularity and forward-oriented focus of the Jewel. Feel the precision, the clarity.

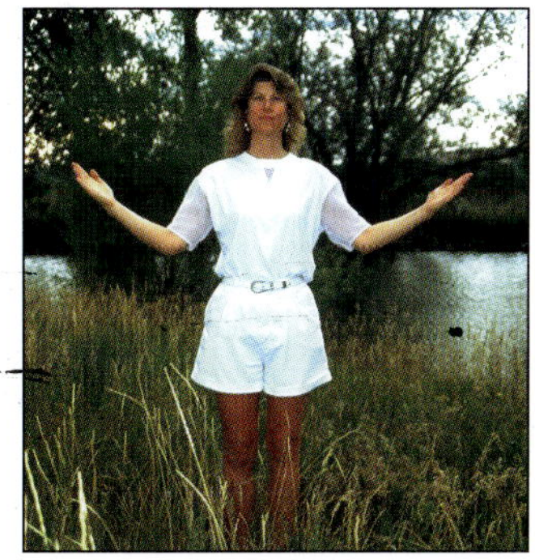

3. Starting from the tips of your fingers, begin moving your hands apart with an open, circular motion, like a blossoming flower unfolding its petals. Gradually bring the hands back until they are almost level with the hips and just out of sight. This motion embodies the receptivity and openness of the Flower.

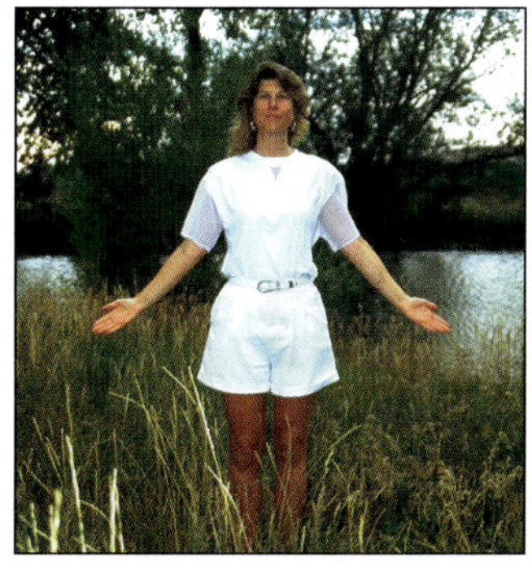

4. When your arms are fully extended but still curved, you are experiencing the opposite polarity of the Jewel, representing a place that you can't see with your peripheral vision. The energy is now behind you and around you, like the all-embracing, allowing surrender of the Flower.

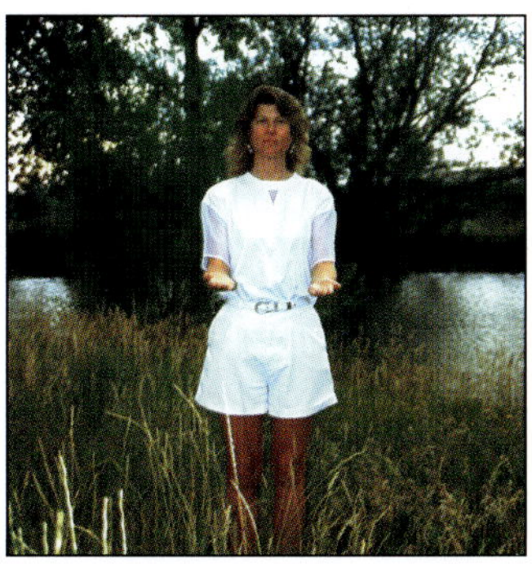

5. Experiencing the Flower and the Jewel in combination creates the energy of attraction. Acknowledging this, bring your hands forward toward each other until they are level with the waist, palms up. As the energy created by the union of the opposites starts to rise, raise your hands, keeping your arms parallel to each other, as if bidding a crowd to rise.

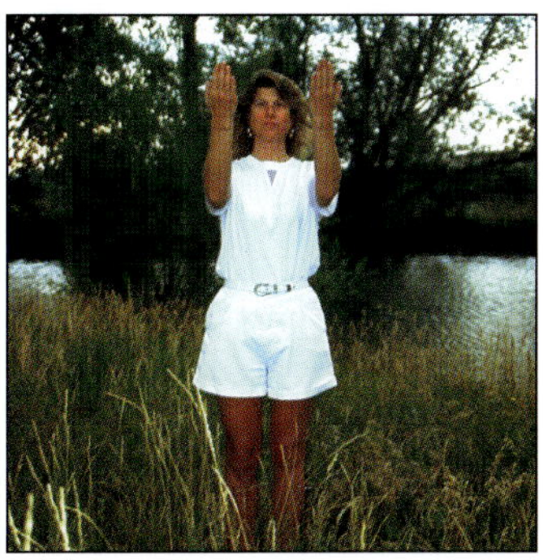

6. Continue the motion, feeling the energy rise up through the middle of your body, until your hands are level with your forehead. This motion embodies the Shaker quality of raising energy and motivating people. It is thankful, alive and awakening.

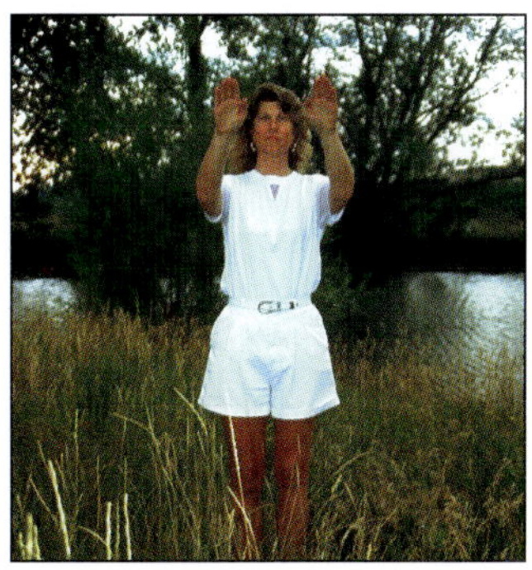

7. Keeping the arms in the same position, turn the palms around to face away from you. The energy you have gathered now spills outward, like sunlit water from a waterfall. Connect with the Shaker energy, which represents that which is up, forward and above. Then begin to lower your arms, as if bidding everyone in front of you to calm down.

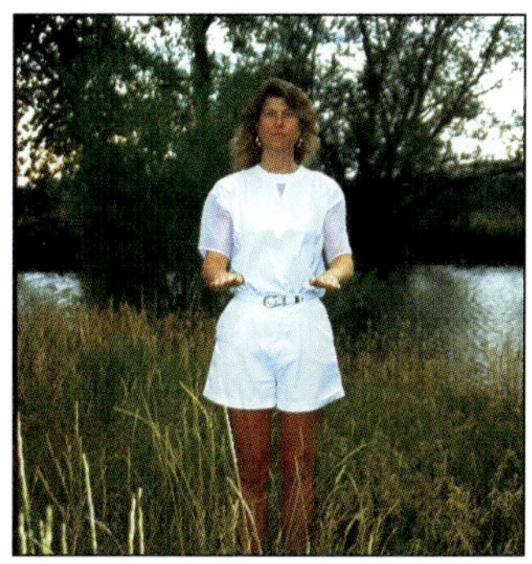

8. Like water flowing down the waterfall into a crystal pool, continue the motion, keeping your arms parallel to each other, until your hands are at waist height. This motion embodies the calming energy of the Stream, bringing all of the other energies back to earth, integrating them. Continue the motion until your arms are back to the starting position.

THE *HARMONY OF HEALTH* HOMEOPATHIC REMEDIES

Everyone with a particular iris structure tends to have similar personality traits and similar physiological weaknesses. The *Harmony of Health* chart lists homeopathic dilutions and other supplements that can correct the underlying constitutional imbalances common to each iris structure.

These remedies have been developed and proven by Margaret Summerville, a Rayid practitioner and multidisciplinary naturopath practicing in Queensland, Australia. Much of the text in this section is paraphrased from the notes Margaret has produced to accompany the *Harmony of Health* chart.

Homeopathy and Rayid

Homeopathy is a system of medicine that has been in use for almost 200 years. It involves prescribing substances to match the energy pattern of a person at a particular time, thus bringing him to the experience of harmony and healing.

One of the principles of homeopathy is that people vary in their response to an illness according to their basic temperament. It follows, therefore, that a homeopath does not automatically prescribe a specific remedy for a specific illness. The patient's temperament and responses need to be taken into consideration, and the prescription determined on an individual basis. Different patients suffering from the same diseases often require different remedies because their basic constitutions are different and therefore their reactions to the stress factor or illness is different.

In homeopathy, then, the classification into a *diagnostic* group is never used for therapeutic purposes. The individual patient is treated as an individual belonging to a constitutional category. Attention is paid to the symptoms that are peculiar to or characteristic of the patient rather than those that are common to the disease.

The need to assign remedies based on a person's temperament has led to homeopaths developing extensive descriptions of particular constitutional types in order to accurately match remedies to people. Until recently, there was no concise or easy way of doing this. With the development of the Rayid Model and its classification of constitutional types based on iris structure, homeopaths can now very precisely assess the person's constitutional "portrait" and accurately choose the remedy which is best able to stimulate that person's individual healing powers.

By combining the Rayid Method of iris classification with a basic naturopathic philosophy of strengthening the constitution in order to stimulate the body's natural recovery mechanisms, we can accurately choose homeopathic remedies in a particular sequence that will bring all aspects of our being into awareness and harmony.

For homeopaths, knowledge of the Rayid Model can give a new understanding of the importance of constitutional prescribing. For other practitioners, this integration of Rayid with homeopathy provides an invaluable link with the therapies of cleansing, nutrition, bodywork, exercise and relaxation, creating a comprehensive and holistic health-care system.

While much of the information on homeopathic remedies in the complete *Harmony of Health* chart is intended for use by trained health care practitioners, the information on the mineral and vitamin requirements of each structure can be applied by anyone.

Mineral and Vitamin Requirements

Minerals have been called the lowest common denominator of any illness. They are essential for building the body and maintaining health. Minerals can also increase an individual's susceptibility to homeopathic remedies which in turn act more effectively, not only resolving ailments, but harmonizing the body's energies as well.

The mineral listed in the chart for each iris structure must be in adequate supply in order that other minerals can be assimilated but it does not mean, for example, that a Jewel automatically is deficient in potassium. Start by taking foods and herbs rich in the indicated mineral as well as foods that are rich in the indicated vitamin.

If a person has digestive problems that include difficulty absorbing certain foods, improved nutritional practices and mineral supplementation may not be enough to correct the deficiency because the body may not be able to absorb or assimilate the dietary minerals. In such cases, it is advisable to use a homeopathic mineral preparation in addition to the dietary supplementation.

Formula 12, developed by BioResearch Pty in Australia, is an excellent combination of 12 homeopathic mineral salts that addresses the needs of all of the constitutional structures in one preparation. Because it is not structure-specific, it can be used by nonspecialists. It is designed to improve the body's ability to absorb minerals taken in as food or supplements. *Formula 12* is available by mail-order from Rayid International.

Tissue Salts

The structure-specific 1M tissue salts listed in the chart should not be used until mineral assimilation is good and chemical residues, food intolerance and miasms are cleared. Homeopathic remedies should really be taken only if symptoms warrant their use, so it is best to work with a homeopath when planning to follow this course of treatment.

The *Harmony of Health* Chart

This is a considerably abridged version of Margaret Summerville's chart. The complete chart, available from Rayid International, includes specific constitutional remedies that take into account iris structure, hemispheric dominance and gender. It also includes remedies for all 12 of the iris structures recognized in the Rayid system.

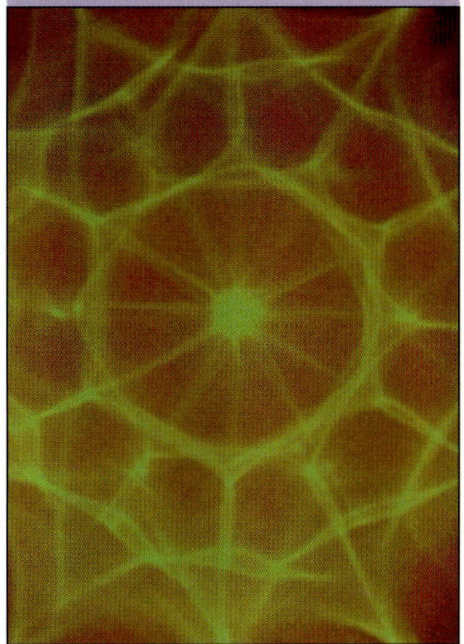

Iris Structure	Mineral	Vitamin	Tissue Salt (1M)
Jewel	Potassium	B Complex	Kali Phos
Flower	Calcium	C	Calc Phos
Shaker	Iodine	Essential Fatty Acids	Nat Mur
Stream	Silicon	E	Kali Mur
Shaker-Jewel	Magnesium	PABA	Nat Sulph
Shaker-Flower	Chromium	Bioflavinoids	Calc Fluor
Stream-Jewel	Selenium	K	Nat Phos
Stream-Flower	Sulfur	A	Kali Sulph

STORIES FOR CHILDREN

It is much easier to develop effective therapies for children than for adults. For one thing, children are much more impressionable. The younger the child, the less separation there is between the conscious self, the unconscious mind and the body. This means that a child's physical behavior can be easily influenced by mental imagery. That is the power of fairy tales.

The two stories that follow are worded using symbols and archetypes that help a child's unconscious to release itself from harmful programming. Read these stories out loud to your child in the evening or record them onto tape so that your child can listen to them each night as he falls asleep.

The Boy Who Goes Fishing for the Sun

A long, long time ago there lived a village of very poor people surrounded by nearly barren rock. There were no trees or bushes, only small blades of grass and almost nothing to eat. The children of the village were hungry most of the time. Every day the children would have to walk to a nearby lake in the hopes of catching a fish so they might have something to put into the night's meager soup. Every day their parents would search the landscape from dawn to dusk just to try to find something to put into the soup to feed their children.

One day, a little boy sitting by the edge of the lake looked into the water and there, just below the surface, he saw a huge fish, the biggest fish he had ever seen. He got really excited because he knew that, if he could catch that fish, his family would have enough food to eat for a long time. He was just about to cast his line into the lake when the clouds parted and the sunlight reflecting off the surface of the water shone directly into his eyes. He looked up at the sky, startled.

"Hmm," he thought, "The sky is blue, just like the lake is blue. I just saw a fish swim by in the lake, like the sun passes by overhead each day. What if the sun is just a very big fish swimming through the sky? If I can catch *that* fish, my family will eat for a *very* long, long time."

The boy was so excited that he dropped his fishing pole and ran home as fast as he could. He ran up to his father and said, "Daddy, Daddy, I want to catch the sun!" His father was silent for a minute. He looked at his son, at the big grin on his little face, and he said, "You know, this sounds like a really big job. For a big job like this, we need to go see your grandfather. He's the wisest man in the whole village, and he'll know exactly what to do. Let's go to him."

The little boy grabbed his father's hand and ran over to his grandfather's house. When he saw him, he shouted, "Grandpa, Grandpa, I want to catch the sun!" And for a long time his grandpa looked at him silently. Then this gentle, wise old man finally said to the little boy, "If you *really* want to catch the sun, I will help you. You are going to need a magic fishing line. I happen to have one right here." He pulled out a beautiful fishing pole and a magical line. He put the line on the reel and, as he handed the pole to the little boy he said, "Remember, hang on to what you want and don't give up. You just have to know what you want, and hang on."

The little boy nodded his head, took the fishing pole and ran out of the house into the field. He started throwing his line up into the sky right toward the sun. It kept falling back down but that didn't matter because, when he threw his line into the lake it would drift back to him anyway, so to him there wasn't really any difference between fishing in the lake and fishing in the sky. But the other kids came by and said, "You idiot, you fool, you stupid little boy. You're so dumb. What makes you think you can throw your line up in the sky and catch anything?" They started laughing at him and ridiculing him. They wanted to throw rocks at him but they were laughing so hard they had to put them down and walk away.

The little boy's body began to tremble and shake so he laid down on the ground. From deep within him there came an avalanche of tears. He cried for all the pain he had ever felt. He cried because these children were his own friends, his neighbors, and they were ridiculing and teasing him for the very thing he wanted most. He cried and cried, and he also cried for his mother. She had died giving birth to him and he had never known her. The only thing that he knew about his mother was that she had loved the fragrance of the rose. As he cried, he remembered his grandfather saying, "Hang on to what you want and don't give up."

The little boy stood up and looked up at the sky. It was no longer blue. He must have been crying for a long time because now the whole sky was filled with dark, thunderous, heavy clouds. A wet rain started falling and he noticed that the sun, almost obscured by the clouds, was about to go down in the distance. So he grabbed his pole and cast the line right up into the sky. And the line just kept on going all the way up past the clouds. It hooked into something but he couldn't see what it was. That something was pulling so hard that it almost ripped the line off the pole. But the little boy hung on, even though he didn't know what he had hooked.

He pulled and he pulled and he pulled, but no matter how hard he pulled, he couldn't pull it down below the clouds so he could see what it was. But he kept pulling anyway until his arms ached and his legs were exhausted and the sun went down below the horizon and darkness filled the land. The air was damp and cold and he felt so terribly alone as he hung on to his fishing pole. But he knew he didn't want to give up.

All through the night he clung to the pole as the sky filled with thunder, lightning struck around him and the earth itself trembled. At one point during the night, a wolf appeared in front of him and growled menacingly. "You can eat me if want," said the boy bravely, "but I won't let go of this pole." And the wolf slipped away into the darkness. Then, right before dawn, he nearly fell asleep and the pole was nearly pulled out of his hands. But the feeling of his grandfather awakened him just in time. The strength surged through his hands and he pulled his fishing pole back. He pulled and he pulled as the sun began to rise and, as the light grew, he got stronger and stronger. After the sun rose, he got so strong that he pulled and he pulled and he pulled all the line in, and he could finally see what he had hooked. There up in the sky was the most magnificent, radiant angel.

The little boy got so excited that he pulled that angel right down to the ground. And there before him stood an angel nine feet tall. The angel looked down at the strong little boy and said, "What is it that you want so badly? All night long I threw lightning at you. I tried thunder, I tried earthquakes, I tried darkness and fear, I even sent a wolf to frighten you and yet you wouldn't let go. What do you want?"

The little boy said, "Angel, you are very beautiful, and that is a very nice sword you have there but I don't really want you. I want to catch the sun. If you help me catch the sun, I'll let you go."

The angel looked at him and said, "Little boy, you've got a deal. Now would you mind taking this fishing line out of my wings?"

The little boy climbed up on the angel, pulled the fishing line out of his wings, climbed back down to the ground and gathered up his line. Then he looked up into the sky and saw that there was not a cloud anywhere to be seen. It was bright and clear and full of sunshine. It was now mid-morning; he had been there all night long, fighting and talking with this angel. He ran home and, just as he arrived, the whole village went into panic. At first he thought it was about him but then he saw them looking up into the sky and screaming, "The darkness is taking the sun! The darkness is taking the sun!" And they ran about in utter terror, for indeed the darkness *was* taking the sun.

The little boy shouted to the villagers, "Don't worry, everybody. I can get the sun back. I can catch the sun." Everybody got very angry with him and came after him with sticks. But his grandfather stepped into their path and he said to the people, "He can do it. I believe him," and so they let him be.

So the little boy took out his fishing line, put it onto his fishing pole and, as he cast the line up into the sky he yelled out, "Angel!" The line kept on going. Up and up and up it went, up past the clouds, over the moon and on to the sun. He hooked the sun and then he pulled and he pulled and he pulled. He pulled so hard that the sun came all the way out of the darkness. This made the villagers very happy and they started saying what a magnificent young man he was. "We should make you a prince. We should make you a king," they shouted, but he didn't even listen to them. He just kept on pulling and they could see that he was pulling the sun all the way down to the earth. Again the villagers became totally terrified. "You must stop this!" they said. "If you pull the sun any closer, surely we will all perish in the flames." They went after him again, this time to kill him for sure. "And if your grandfather gets in the way this time, we'll kill him too," said the crowd.

Then, suddenly, standing in their path, was an angel nine feet tall. The people fell to their knees before him and dropped their weapons. They all started crying because of the utter beauty of this angel of grace. The little boy was joined by his father and his grandfather, and all together they pulled that sun all the way down to the earth. From the north to the south, from the east to the west, the whole sky was filled with the sun. But there was no heat coming from it. All that came out of the sun was a pure, radiant love, as sweet as the purest nectar laced with cream. It had the texture of moon velvet and the essence of the all-pure mother within it. It was so utterly nurturing, it bathed the bones and every mineral in the bodies of those around it.

And the little boy said, "Look, look, look!" For at that moment an opening appeared in the sun. The little boy went up inside the opening and from there he could see another opening. He peered through it and what he saw was an absolute paradise. Beautiful rivers, forests, fruits and animals and birds and an abundance of everything that would sustain and nourish life. Paradise was on the other side of the sun! The little boy came back out to his people and called, "Look, everybody; through here!" One by one, the villagers walked past him to the right and went up and through the sun.

The last one to leave the barren land was the little boy. But he was no longer a little boy. He was a most magnificent, radiant man who stood nine feet tall. As he walked back into the sun, he picked up the fishing line because he knew that, someday, another little boy somewhere would need it. And everywhere there was the fragrance of the rose. His mothers favorite flower.

The Sacred Stone

A long, long time ago, deep in the heart of a vast and endless jungle, there lived a community of people who believed they were the only people in the whole jungle, for they had never seen another human being. They lived in an unusual way: they shared everything. They shared joy, laughter, food and the parenting of all of their children. The birds were always singing, fruit and flowers were always blossoming, and all of the 12 great rivers in the jungle were filled with pure, sparkling water.

One day, while walking in the jungle, some of the people found a crippled little girl. She was dragging herself along by her elbows because she was paralyzed from the waist down. She knew not where she was, where she came from or even her own name. She could remember nothing. Surprised as they were to find her, the kind and loving people took this little girl into their community and raised her as one of their own. For years, they took her out every day and set her in a little chair in the most beautiful part of the village, so that she could watch everyone else go by. But not once did she laugh, for she knew not who she was. Who were her mother and father? How had she come to be there? It was very painful for her not to be able to remember. But it was most painful for her not to be able to dance. Dancing was the one thing she really wanted to do.

One day, quite suddenly, some men no one had ever seen before came charging into the village. They were evil men and they made slaves of everyone. They put up a very high fence around the village and every man, woman and child who was old enough to walk was made to work in deep pits in the earth. They

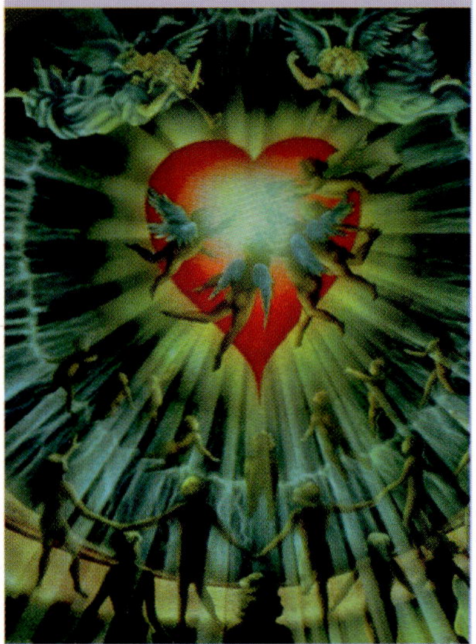

had to carry out big rocks that the evil men broke open to search for precious gems and minerals. Seven days a week, the men, women and children had to crawl on their hands and knees into these deep holes in the earth. There was suffering, sadness and death. The birds stopped singing, the flowers blossomed no more and the great rivers filled with mud and then started to dry up. There was no fruit to eat any more, so the people went hungry.

The little girl saw all the people of the community suffering, and it touched her deeply because she knew what it was like to suffer. She cried for their pain. One night, the people of the community were so burdened that they had forgotten to bring her in at the end of the day. Sitting in her chair, she looked up at the moon and called out, "Please help me to free these people. I'll do anything you ask." Almost instantly, a voice spoke to her right through the middle of her chest. It said, "Throw the white stone into the sun."

And the little girl knew what that was! In the middle of the village, not far away from where she was right now, there was a small hut that had a secret, sacred compartment. And inside that compartment was a white and precious stone. That stone was symbol of all the stored memories of all the people who had ever lived in that community. The little girl dragged herself to the hut, opened the compartment, and took that small, white stone and put it into her pocket. She then began to crawl out to the barbed wire fence that surrounded the community. But before she could get through it, the evil men saw her and captured her.

They had made a law that whoever tried to escape would immediately be killed. They were just about to cut her head off when one of them said, "Wait, this is the crippled girl. I've got a better idea. She certainly can't run away, so let's just throw her into that deep gully. She won't be able to get out and the black leopard will eat her. We'll hear him as he crunches her bones." And they laughed.

The evil men carried the little girl into the night and threw her into the deep gully. Down she rolled, down, down, down into the slippery darkness. When she hit the bottom she was covered in slime and muck and, trembling, she realized that she couldn't see *anything*. She couldn't see the moon or the stars, nothing – it was total, absolute blackness.

Suddenly, she heard the scream of the black leopard. It was not very far away from her. She was terrified. It screamed again, closer this time. It was moving toward her. In a panic she turned and tried to crawl away as fast as she could. But then a voice came to her in the middle of her chest and said, "Turn around. Face your fear." She stopped, took a deep breath and turned around. And there, standing before her in the jungle, was a most magnificent, radiant man. He was filled with such light, her whole body felt love and joy, and in her heart there was peace.

The man looked at her through the soft, radiant blue and white light that shone from him and illuminated the jungle all around. He said to her, "Because you have been willing to sacrifice your life that others might be free, you now have mastery over the entire jungle, and all the creatures therein will serve you. And if you are able to throw the white stone into the sun before the sunrise of the third day from now, you will remember your name, you will know who you are, and all the people of the community will be free." Before he left, he said, "Remember, I am always with you." Then he vanished.

Now, instead of being surrounded by darkness, the little girl could see with ease, because the man had left the light behind. At the edge of the light, she saw a huge black leopard. It was nearly seven feet tall at the shoulder and was staring at her. The leopard had blazing green and yellow eyes and sparkling, sharp white teeth. Without even a tremble in her voice, the little girl said, "Leopard, come here. I want you." The leopard obediently walked over to her. Then she said, "Leopard, take me to the rising sun, that I might throw this white stone into it and make my people free."

"Your wish is my command," said the leopard. He bent down so the little girl could climb on his giant back, and off they raced. But wherever they went, the sun was nowhere to be found. The sky was heavy with clouds, the rivers were all dried up, the birds didn't sing, there weren't any blossoms or fruit. Many times the little girl felt hungry and thirsty, but there was nothing to eat or drink. On and on they went for two days, but still they did not see the sun. Then they came to the bottom of a large, white, nearly vertical cliff. The leopard said, "Little girl, I can go no further, for this is the domain of the king cobra."

The little girl looked around, but she could not see a cobra. So she called out in a firm voice, "Cobra, come here. I want you." At that, almost right in front of her, rose a king cobra with a massive head, a hissing, forked tongue and beady eyes. He was looking right at her, and his scaly body rose and it rose until he was nearly 12 feet high. The little girl looked right at him, and said, "Cobra, take me to the top of this white cliff, that I might throw this stone into the sun and make my people free." There was a long silence, then the king cobra said, "Your wish is my command."

He lowered his huge head, and the little girl climbed on to it. He lifted her high, and started slithering up the cliff. Higher and higher he carried the little girl. The night darkened as they climbed. When they were about half way up, the skies began to clear and the stars came out. Strong winds began to blow and howl around them and nearly knocked the little girl off. But she hung on tight. Then, in the last hour before dawn, when they were almost to the very top, the king cobra stopped. "Little girl," he said, "I can go no further, for this is your domain." He set her down on the slope and the little girl reached up and dug her fingers into the rock. She pulled herself up the cliff, panting, hand over hand, aching with the effort, until at last she grasped the rim of the very top and pulled herself over. She looked off into the distance and saw the first light of sunrise spreading on the horizon. She was overwhelmed by how far away it was, and a feeling of hopelessness overtook her. She lay down, thinking, "I can't do it. It is too far away," and she started to cry.

For the first time in her life, she cried so deeply that even her bones and nerves cried. She cried and cried and cried. Then, inside her, she suddenly had the memory of the radiant man she had seen in the jungle. She felt the love inside her again and she stirred out of her misery. She knew not how but she had to do it. She took that white stone out of her pocket, held it in her right hand, faced the dawning sky, and with total trust she threw that stone as hard as she could.

A great explosion of light from inside her bones flashed through her body: violet, green and gold; colors more beautiful and radiant than anyone had ever seen. And her whole body was filled with celestial music. Instantly, a transformation occurred. Her physical body became healthy, magnificent and radiant. She could stand and walk. She knew who she was and how she had gotten there. She remembered her name. She was the most beautiful princess in all the world. And for the first time, she let out a belly laugh that echoed throughout the jungle. At that, the birds began to sing, the flowers blossomed, fruit appeared on the trees and all of the 12 great rivers flowed once more with sparkling, pure water.

She jumped off the cliff and landed on the floor of the forest. There to greet her was the king cobra, 12 feet tall, and the giant black leopard, seven feet tall, and all three of them danced and played together. Everywhere around them there was celebration. Then she thought about the people in the community, and instantly she found herself, with the leopard and the cobra, standing in the middle of the village. When the evil men saw the radiant warrior girl with the giant leopard and the king cobra, many of them ran away in fear. But others did not want to give up their slaves, so there was a great battle. The cobra and the leopard killed all of the evil men, and the people were finally free.

The people came to her and they did not recognize her, for she was no longer a crippled little girl but a strong, radiant woman. And they said to her, "Who are you, that you are so powerful? What is your name?" "Let me dance for you, " said the princess. As she danced, all of the people were restored instantly to perfect physical health and then they danced with her. Then the princess stopped and said to them, "There is a new, white stone in the secret compartment of the sacred hut. On the bottom of the white stone is your name. And when you know *your* name, you will know who I am."

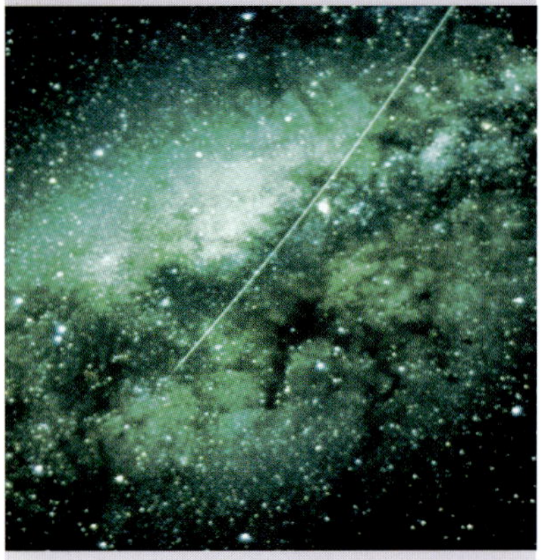

Beyond the Iris

The intermediate goal of Rayid is to help people to understand the deeper patterns that are creating symptoms of distress in their personality or body. This understanding comes gradually but even the act of observing a pattern can begin to alleviate the symptoms associated with it. There are, however, traps for the unwary.

Using a simple allegory, let's say that you keep slipping and falling at a particular place in your house and you don't know why. Then one day you look down and see that there is water on the floor that you haven't noticed before. "Ah," you say, "this is the reason I keep making the same mistake. This is the reason I keep falling down and hurting myself in the same way. Now I see the water on the floor." And you mop it up. In the Rayid Method, this would be equivalent to using therapies that balance the existence of the observed problem (water) and alleviate the symptoms by reducing the number of times that you fall. But you haven't actually done anything about the cause of the problem itself.

So you may return to the same spot a few days, weeks, months or even years later and find that you still slip and fall in the same place. Again you see that there is water there. Again you mop it up. After doing this a few times, you may learn to walk very carefully whenever you have to step on the slippery patch. You fall even less now, meaning that your symptoms are much improved.

If you are the inquisitive type, you may also get curious about where the water is coming from. "What is creating this pattern in my life?" you ask, "Why is this pattern here?" You start to observe the pattern and, looking up for the first time, you realize that the water on the floor is coming from a leak in the ceiling. Investigating further, you find that the leak in the ceiling is coming from the bathroom next to your parents' bedroom upstairs. "Ah," you say, with newfound understanding, "I see where it's coming from. It's coming from my mother and my father. *They* are the cause of this."

By gaining insight into the apparent origins of your emotional trauma, you can begin to feel better about yourself because you now get the idea that your symptoms are not your *fault*. You start to explore your relationship with your parents and discover that your left-brained or right-brained tendencies seem to have a lot to do with your mother's and father's behavior toward you in early childhood. Realizing this, you then start to blame your mother or your father for their leaky toilet, which you are now convinced is the source of your own problem, the pool of water on the floor. So you may spend months or years, even a lifetime, trying to learn more about your mother and father, or your grandparents, or your relationships with siblings, trying to understand the cause of your problems. This kind of analysis can be a seductive trap, a grand illusion. It's very easy to say, "I am this way because my father was a cold, mental type," or "I am this was because my mother was an angry, emotional type." But if you take a really good look at your parents, you will find that they had a similar set of potentially traumatic experiences in their lives. And you can repeat this process of assigning blame back through countless generations. Who are we going to blame as the source of all this pain?

It does no good to look for the light in the dark. While it is true that the family tree has a lot to do with creating the conscious personality, it does no good to overanalyze the unconscious patterns of your mother and father simply to find fault with them. You could spend years patching your ceiling without ever stopping the leak. You could spend years blaming your parents and exploring their plumbing before realizing that the leak is coming from a hole in the roof, not from their toilet.

The source of the leak lies beyond your conscious mind. Your problems come from somewhere that even your subconscious cannot reach. Who knows how the hole in the roof got there? Who really knows the origin of the patterns in your family tree? Who knows where that small meteor came from that put a hole in your roof one dark night, creating the leak that eventually created the pool of water on the floor?

When using the Rayid Method, it is our responsibility to understand that, just as the problem has many levels to it, so does the solution. With any symptom, we need to be aware of all of the levels of causation. Do we just clean up the physical body (the water on the floor) or do we also deal with issues in the conscious mind (the leak in the ceiling)? Do we stop our therapy at the the level of the unconscious mind (the hole in the roof) or do we also try to address some spiritual truth far beyond what we may see or comprehend (the meteor)? The goal of Rayid therapies is to address each one of these levels. In practice, treatment initially emphasizes the physical body and its nutritional needs, moving on to the conscious mind and the unconscious personality, but we should always bear in mind the big picture.

So if you're going to clean up somebody's physical symptoms with vitamins, minerals or bodywork, it is also incumbent on you to begin cleaning up the relationship patterns, the conscious and unconscious mind, and to understand how to use spiritual laws that transcend the hole in the roof, that transcend the laws of cause and effect, so as to free the individual from the damaging effects of meteors that continue to assail the unconscious from places unknown.

You are not your personality. The ultimate aim of Rayid is to help people to free themselves from the limitations of the personality altogether. The first challenge on this journey is to understand the representative (projected) self, which is what most people think of as *the* personality. Then there is the structural or constitutional self, the core personality, which is really a deeper, more pure expression of one's genetic endowment. But ultimate freedom involves going beyond the limitations of the body, mind and emotions. Ultimate freedom is to experience the true self, the presence within, and to be present in all three levels of self simultaneously.

Recognize that the true self in you, who you *really* are, is already complete. The true self already exists inside the physical body and, because it is a spiritual presence, it is already perfect. It always has been. The physical body and the mind can become sensitive to it through the accumulation of knowledge, appropriate therapies and cleansing. But no amount of knowledge will make you free unless you *use* your understanding to unlock the prison door and step out of your limited definition of yourself.

Your personality is a vehicle that you can use to move through life in pursuit of freedom. It is the means by which you travel and it enables you to meet and relate to others who can help you find the way. By studying Rayid you are learning to understand how your vehicle works. The purpose in understanding your vehicle is so that you can become a better driver. If you simply get lost in a fascination with the way in which all the parts fit together, and what makes the vehicle go, you have missed the point.

While you are learning to be proficient at driving your car, to be adept at reading the instruments, using the accelerator, brake and clutch, while you are learning to use the entire vehicle of your personality, remember that you are not the vehicle, you are not your personality. It is better that you never learn to use Rayid than that you use it to limit yourself. You are not the car, you are the driver. And the car has a destination.

Most personalities have forgotten that they are not their car. When Jewels speak of themselves, they say, "I am a thinking, mental type." But they are not, they are more. That is merely the vehicle through which they communicate. Most people are in bondage to their personality and to the ego mechanism that is constructed by their genealogy. Rayid can change that.

The iris is a map of the personality. It can show you how to find your true self but that is all. It does not define you. Reach beyond the iris to your true self. Go beyond the limitations of your personality. And remember that the part of you that knows who you *really* are will never need any training, any information and never did.

Be free.

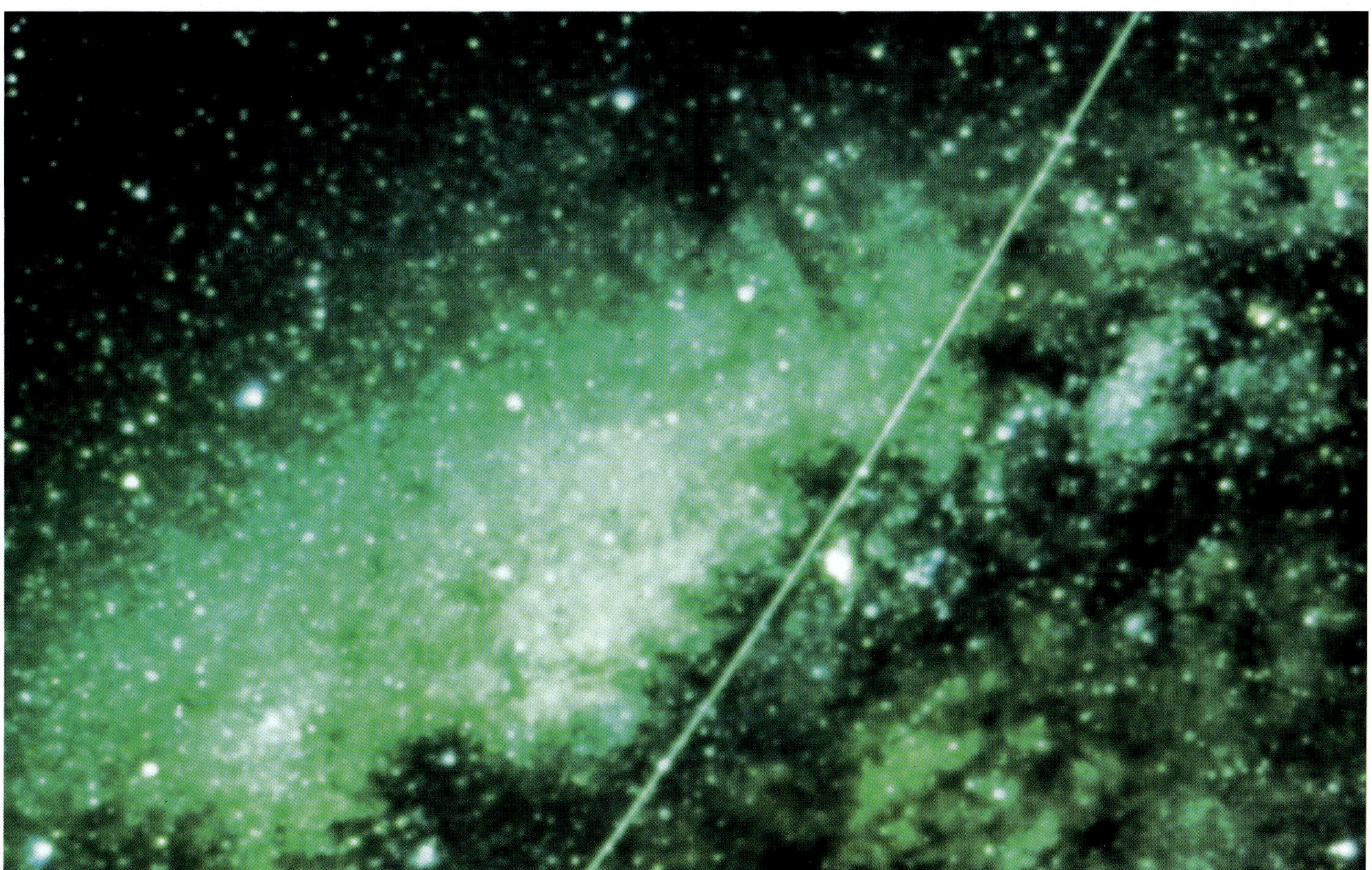

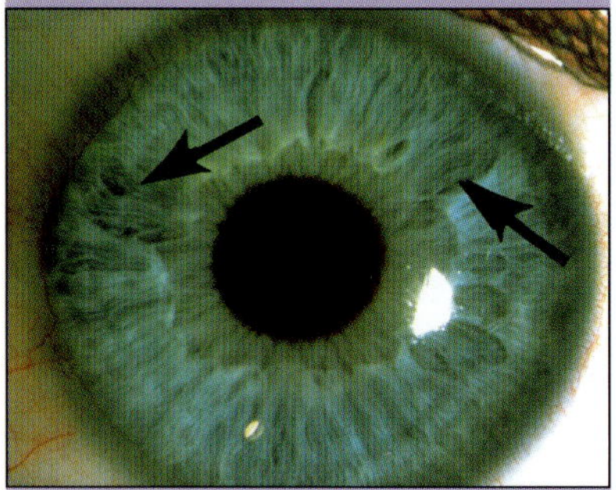
Stream-Flower

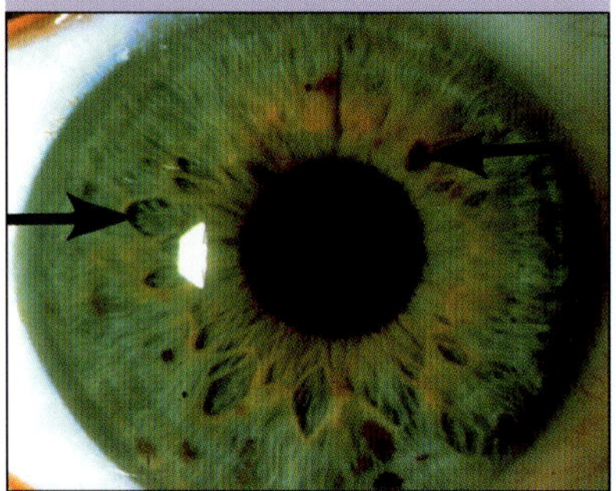
Shaker-Jewel

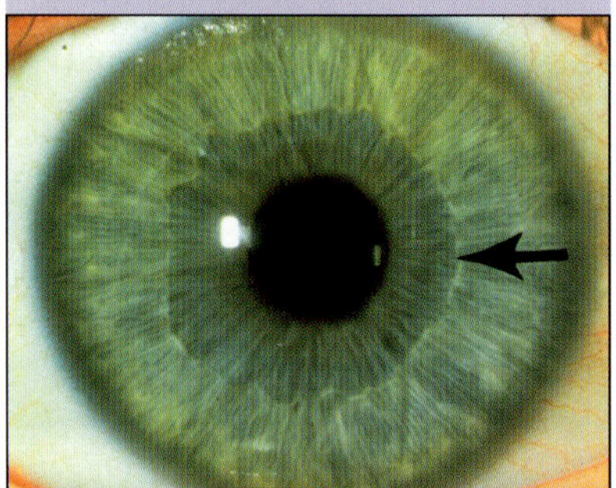
Extrovert Stream

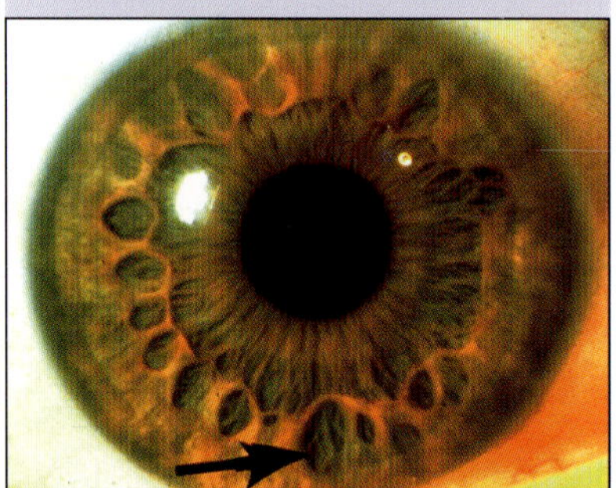
Flower (emotional type)

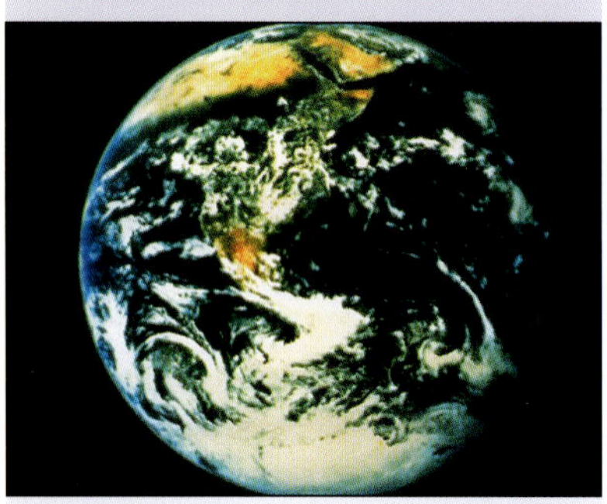

Glossary

Words in italics are cross-references to other glossary entries.

Characteristic Used interchangeably with the word *trait*.

Combination structure Any iris structure that is a combination of the four *primary structures*, such as Stream-Flower, Shaker-Jewel, etc. See also *Constitutional structure* and *Secondary structure*.

Constitutional structure The classification of the underlying iris *pattern*, derived from an impression of the overall appearance of the iris rather than individual *traits*. See *Structure*. In the Rayid Method, there are a total of 12 structural classifications: four *primary structures*, four main *combination structures* and four additional structural combinations that are not covered in this book because they are not essential to the successful application of Rayid and because it usually requires considerable experience in order to correctly identify them. These complex combinations are: Shaker-Stream, Shaker-Stream-Jewel, Shaker-Stream-Flower and Triple Processor.

This term is also used to refer to the individual's physiological and psychological makeup, since the Rayid Method asserts that there is a direct correlation between iris structure, personality and physical characteristics.

Driver The descriptive, nonjargon term used to describe the *Shaker* personality.

Emotional type The descriptive, nonjargon term used to describe a person with a *Flower* personality.

Extremist type Another term used to describe a person with a *Shaker* personality.

Extrovert An outwardly-directed person with a need for social interaction and external gratification.

Eye gender An expression meaning, if the trait is found in the left eye it reflects or affects the relationship with the mother or women and, if it is found in the right eye, it is associated with the individual's experience of the father or men.

Eye sex Another term for *eye gender*.

Father eye See *Right eye*.

Feminine eye See *Left eye*.

Fiber Collectively, the light streaks or lines radiating out from the pupil to the periphery of the *iris*. These fibers are actually strands of muscle tissue. If there is an "absence of fiber" in an area of the iris, it means that there is a lower concentration of muscle fibers close to the surface of the eye in that area, i.e. they are deeply submerged in the iris. Sometimes the individual fibers are not distinguishable because they are so densely packed ("density of fiber"), because they are a similar color to the rest of the iris in that area or because of heavy deposits of pigment overlaying the fibers.

Flower An emotional, feeling-oriented person. One of the four primary structural types in the Rayid system.

flower Rounded openings in the fibers of the iris. Appears in the text with a lower-case 'F' to distinguish it from the personality type.

Hemispheric dominance The human brain is divided vertically into two halves, or hemispheres, that are joined by a corridor of nerve fibers called the corpus callosum. Most people tend to use one half of their brain more than the other and so are said to be left-brained or right-brained. Each hemisphere has an essentially different way of processing information. Because of this, certain differences in personality between people can be attributed to the fact that they are left- or right-brain dominant.

Introvert An inwardly directed person with the need for a quiet environment and inner gratification.

Iris The round, colored portion of the eyeball that surrounds the pupil. It has muscles that adjust the size of the pupil to regulate the amount of light entering the eye. These muscle fibers are often discernible as individual light streaks or lines (occasionally referred to as *streams*) radiating out from the pupil to the periphery of the iris.

Jewel A thinking, intellectual person. One of the four primary structural types in the Rayid system. Also referred to as the mental type.

jewel Dot-like concentrations of pigment in the iris, ranging in color from light gold to black. Appears in the text with a lower-case 'J' to distinguish it from the personality type.

Kinesthetic type Another term used to describe a person with a *Stream* personality. The word "kinesthetic" is used as it is in classical psychology, to describe a person with a sensory, tactile orientation.

Left eye When interpreting the eyes, remember that the left eye is actually on the right as you look at a person, and that this eye relates to the right hemisphere of the brain, since most of the left side of the body is connected to the right hemisphere. The left eye is sometimes referred to as the "mother eye" or the "feminine eye" because it reveals traits associated with the individual's relationship to his mother or to women in general.

Left-brained A person whose abilities and traits indicate a tendency primarily to use the left hemisphere of the brain. See *Hemispheric dominance*.

Masculine eye See *Right eye*.

Mental type Another term used to describe a person with a *Jewel* personality.

Mother eye See *Left eye*.

Pattern A catch-all phrase that encompasses iris *traits* and *structures* and is also used when referring to personality characteristics and relationship attractions.

Primary structure The four main iris types, which represent the main building blocks of personality in the Rayid system: *Jewel, Flower, Shaker* and *Stream*.

Positions Individual iris *traits* that give detailed information about the personality.

Rayid Model The theoretical framework underpinning the *Rayid Method*. Its core tenet is that the iris of the eye provides a guide to an individual's psychological makeup, his behavioral patterns and his physiological strengths and weaknesses. Another key element of the Rayid Model is the notion that all of these characteristics and patterns are transgenerational in nature, that they are inherited from the individual's genetic predecessors.

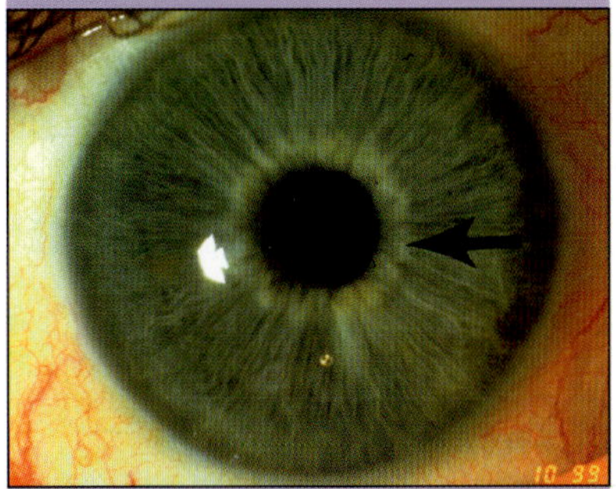

Introvert Stream

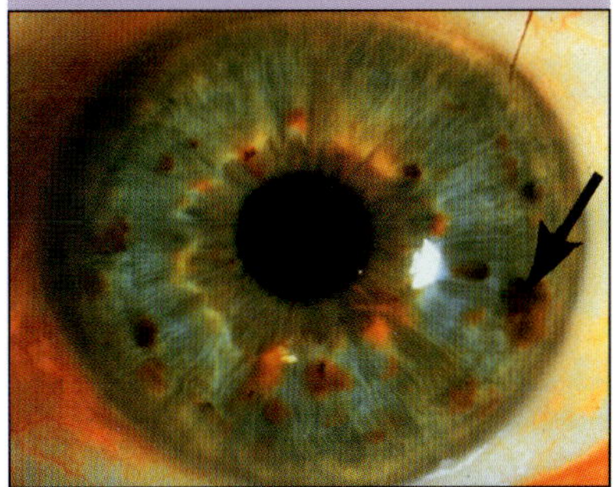

Jewel (mental type)

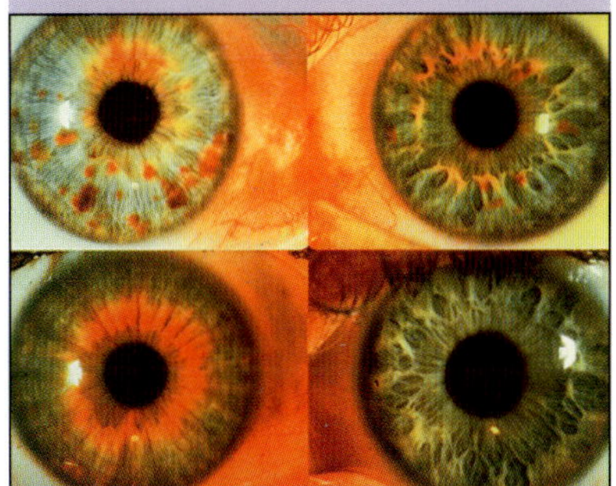

The four primary structures

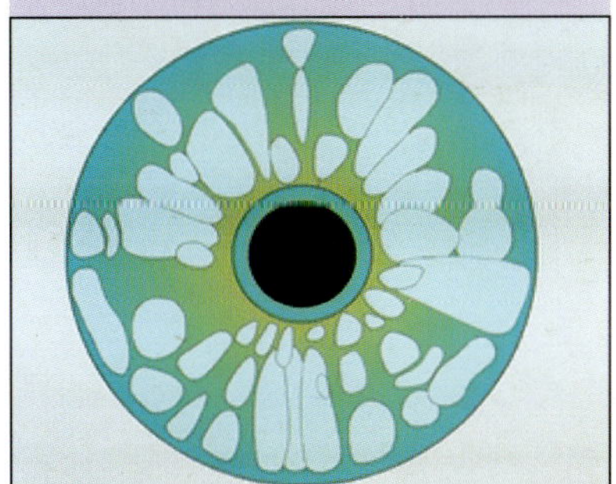

Iris positions, left eye

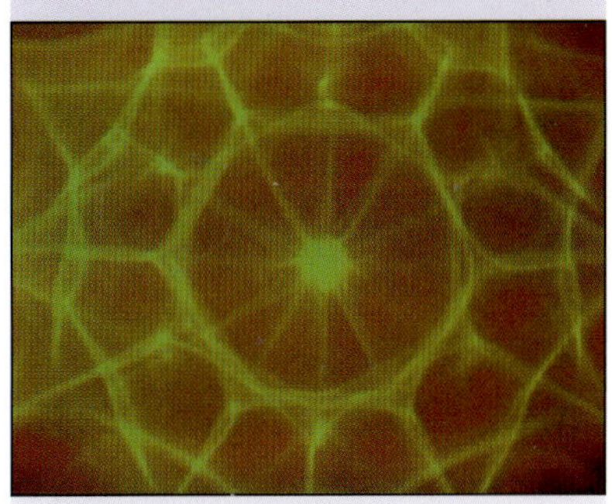

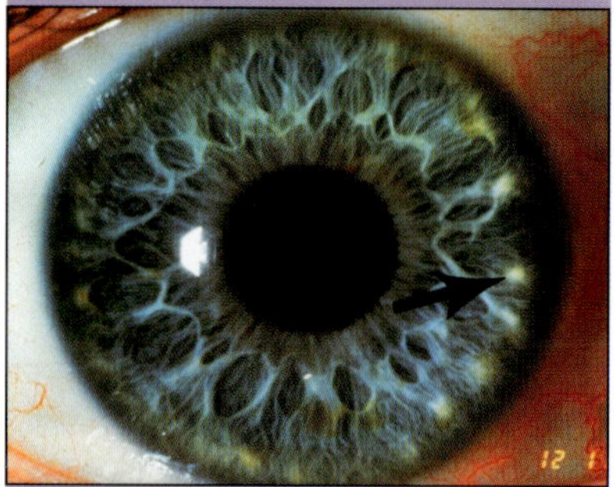

Ring of Harmony

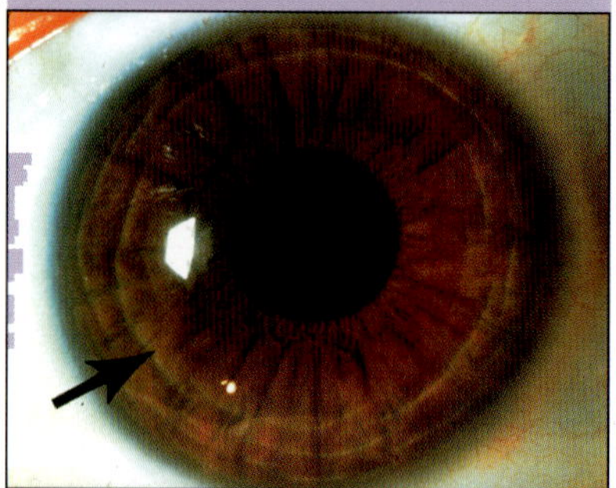

Ring of Freedom

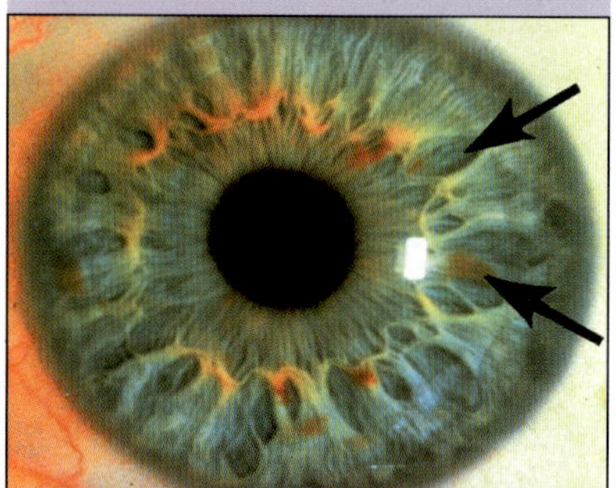

Shaker

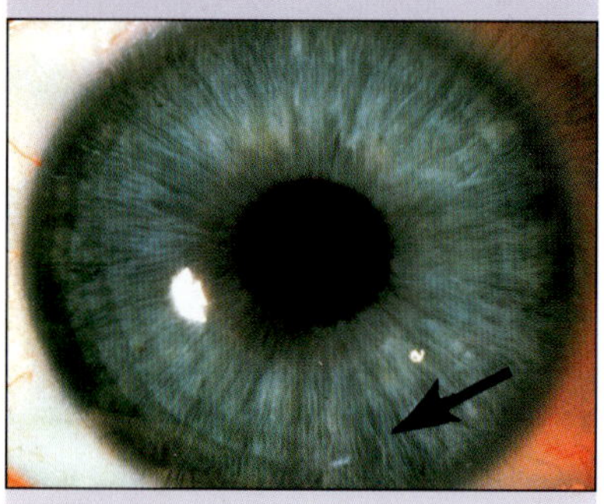

Stream

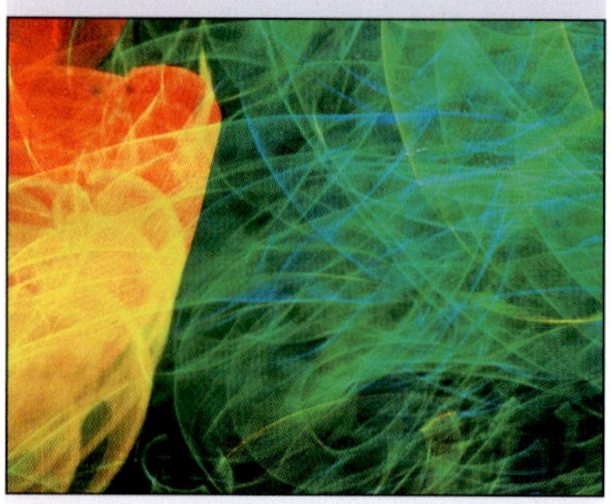

Rayid Method The system of iris interpretation developed independently by Denny Johnson through inspiration and subsequent empirical testing using behavioral research methods. Although it refers primarily to the interpretive procedures used to determine an individual's *constitutional structure*, the Rayid Method also encompasses the therapeutic recommendations made to mobilize the person's innate healing powers. Often simply called "Rayid," this system is not used to diagnose or treat illness; rather, it is used to help the individual to free himself from self-limiting, unconscious attitudes and behaviors that can have physiological and psychological symptoms. Proof of the Rayid Method's accuracy and effectiveness is to be found in the considerable body of supporting case studies from practitioners all over the world.

Right eye When interpreting the eyes, remember that the right eye is actually on the left as you look at a person, and that this eye relates to the left hemisphere of the brain, since most of the right side of the body is connected to the left hemisphere. The right eye is sometimes referred to as the "father eye" or the "masculine eye" because it reveals traits associated with the individual's relationship to his father or to men in general.

Right-brained A person whose abilities and traits indicate a tendency primarily to use the right hemisphere of the brain. See *Hemispheric dominance*.

Ring A structural configuration in the iris that forms a circular pattern centered on the pupil. Ring patterns are not always a complete circle. Some rings are always found at the periphery of the iris, others can be found closer to the pupil.

Sclera The white portion of the eyeball, which surrounds the *iris*.

Secondary structure When the underlying iris pattern is that of a *Shaker* or *Stream* (two of the *primary structures*) but the person also has some jewels or flowers in the iris, the person is classified as a Shaker-Jewel, Stream-Flower, etc. and the Jewel or Flower element of the classification is then referred to as the secondary structure. See *Combination structure*.

Shaker An action-oriented, progressive person. One of the four primary structural types. Also called a driver or an extremist type.

Stream A physically oriented, intuitive person. One of the four primary structures. Also called a kinesthetic type.

streams A term used by some Rayid practitioners to refer to the light streaks or lines radiating out from the pupil to the periphery of the *iris*. More commonly referred to as "iris fibers," they are actually strands of muscle tissue. See *Fiber*. Appears in the text with a lower-case 'S' to distinguish it from the personality type.

Structure A fundamental characteristic of the iris that affects the overall interpretation of the personality. This term is used when describing the 12 *constitutional structures* (Shaker-Jewel, Flower, Triple Processor, etc.) and the iris *rings*. The terms *characteristic* and *trait* are used when referring to individual jewels, flowers and streams in the iris. The term is sometimes used to mean personality type, since each of the constitutional structures represents a distinct personality. For the sake of brevity, this book describes individuals by their iris structures; for example, using the expression "Harmony pattern" instead of referring to "a person with a Harmony pattern." This does *not* mean that we think of a person as being their eye structure. Far from it ...

Trait Used in two senses: 1. A distinct aspect of personality; 2. A specific element of iris structure (e.g. a flower, jewel or stream). Traits in the iris correlate with specific personality traits.

The Team

Denny Ray Johnson
The originator of the Rayid Method of Iris Interpretation, Denny has established the Rayid Model as one of the most powerful modern tools for understanding the personality. An international lecturer, author and behavioral researcher, he has been developing and teaching Rayid since 1978. An inspiring and captivating presenter who has done over 250 radio and television interviews (between 1978 and 1995), Denny introduced Rayid to a media audience of more than 30 million people in 17 countries.

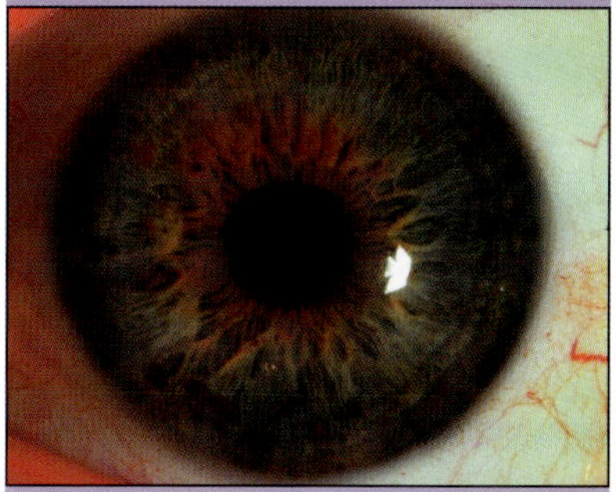

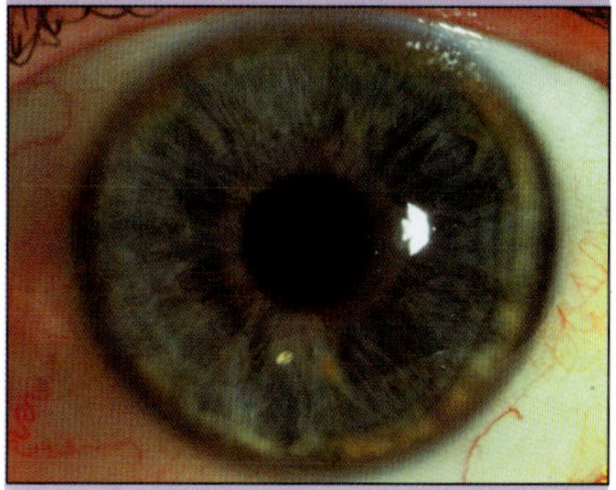

Douglas C. Thompson
Founder of LENA Medical Photo Design Systems in 1984, Douglas designed the LENA AR, the only computerized, automatic and portable iris camera system in the world. He has worked closely with Denny Johnson and the National Iridology Research Association. The LENA AR has owners in 22 countries, and was used to photograph the irises depicted in this book. For more information, write to: 412 N. Coast Highway, B-177, Laguna Beach, CA 92651, USA.

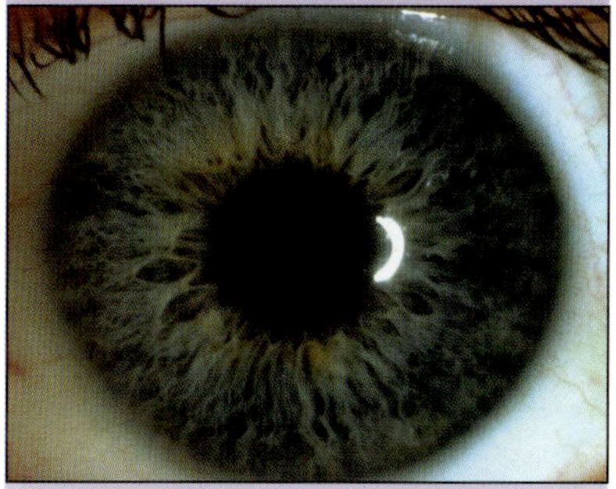

J. Erik Ness
An established writer and editor in the fields of deep ecology, technology and alternative health, Erik has more than ten years of experience in publishing on both sides of the Atlantic. He has been producing educational and promotional materials about the Rayid Method of Iris Interpretation since meeting Denny in January 1991. He was appointed Editor-in-Chief of Rayid Publications in May 1993.

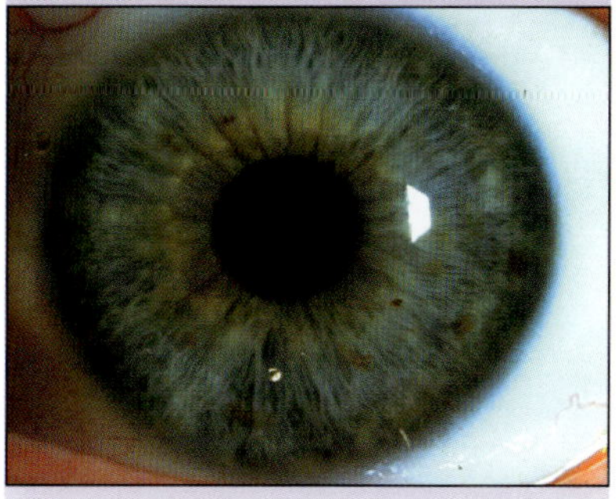

Deborah Alexia Monroe
A long-time supporter of Denny's work who has been involved with the Rayid Method for more than a decade, Alexia spent countless hours sorting through thousands of iris slides, taking notes and focusing Denny's creative energy in preparing the raw material for this book. She edited one of Denny Johnson's earlier works, *Touch Starvation in America*, in 1985.

Acknowledgements

I thank the unseen hand that guides the inspiration that at times seems so compelling; the many individuals who have combined to create one effect; the great wonder and miracle that is the continually unfolding mystery that is life; the many thousands of people who have shared with me the light within their eyes and have acted as my teachers to bring into greater realization the earthly meaning of this profound inspiration; friends and associates who have been so loving and patient with my relentless quest for all-knowing bliss amidst the practicalities of everyday life; my son Nathaniel for his joyful reminders of what is truly important. And I thank those who have helped this book come into fruition: Erik for his diligent and comprehensive editing to piece together endless threads of abstraction; Deborah Alexia for her great attention to detail and the gentleness by which it is realized; Lucinda and Nancy for the heartfelt manner of their day-to-day encouragement and support. The others are too numerous to mention, except that they all exist as one.

Photography and Illustration Credits

All photographs by Douglas Thompson with the LENA AR iris camera except: 4-up of iris structures (Introduction), Rayid International; Illustration of iris fiber types (Chapter 1), Rayid International; Primary and combination structure symbols (Chapter 1), Erik Ness; Schematic diagram of combination structures (Chapter 1), Erik Ness; Introversion and extroversion diagrams (Chapter 2), Rayid International; Diagrams of iris regions (Chapter 4), Erik Ness; Diagrams of iris positions (Chapter 4), Rayid International; Diagram of family tree (Chapter 5), Rayid International; *Vibratory Channels* illustration (Chapter 5), Rayid International; Vibrational pyramid (Chapter 7), Rayid International; *Stages of Healing* chart (Chapter 7), Rayid International; Brain-wave cycles (Chapter 7), Rayid International; *Angel's Wings* sequence (Chapter 7), Erik Ness; Stories for Children illustration (Chapter 7), Dawn Sklener; *Beyond the Iris* photo, NASA.

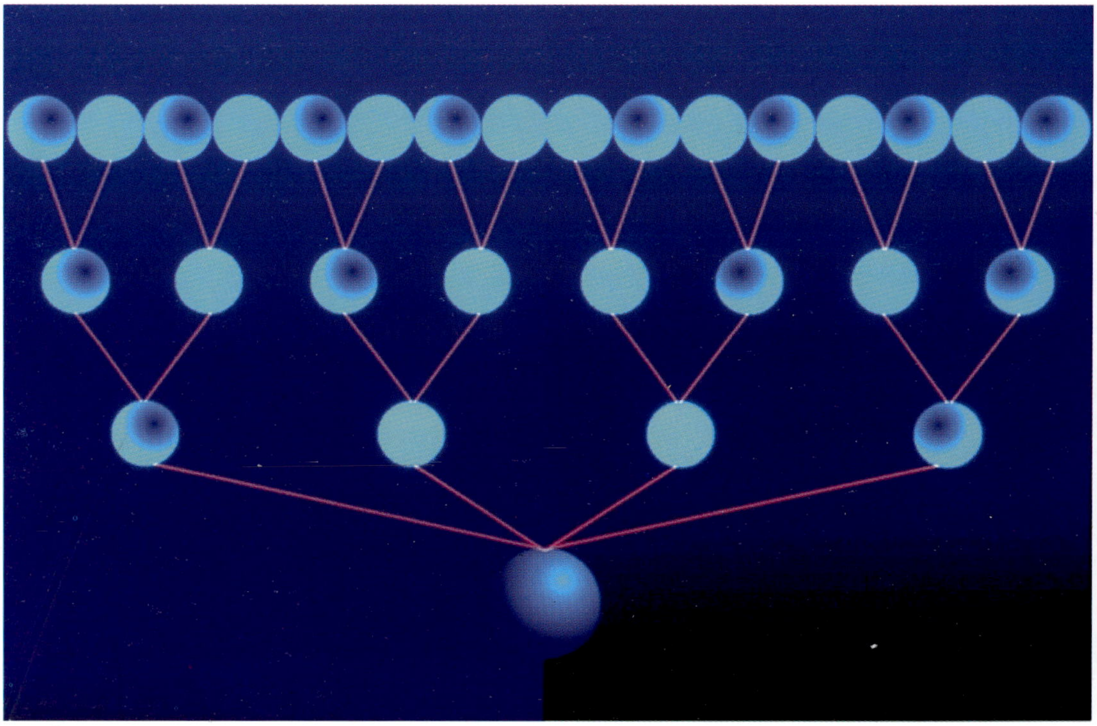

For more information about Rayid, write to
Rayid International • P.O. Box 17367 • Boulder, Co 80308 • USA